Behavioural Medicine
in Cardiovascular Disorders

Behavioural Medicine in Cardiovascular Disorders

Edited by

T Elbert
Psychologisches Institut
Universität Tübingen, FRG

W Langosch
Benedikt-Kreuz Rehabilitation Zentrum, FRG

A Steptoe
Psychology Department
St George's Hospital Medical School
London, UK

D Vaitl
Klinische Psychologie FB 06
Universität Giessen, FRG

A Wiley Medical Publication

JOHN WILEY & SONS
Chichester · New York · Brisbane · Toronto · Singapore

Distributed in the United States of America, Canada and Japan by
Alan R. Liss Inc., 41 East 11th Street, New York, NY 10003, USA.

Library of Congress Cataloging in Publication Data:

Behavioural medicine in cardiovascular disorders.

(A Wiley medical publication)
Includes bibliographies and index.
1. Hypertension — Psychosomatic aspects.
2. Coronary heart disease — Psychosomatic aspects.
3. Arrhythmia — Psychosomatic aspects.   4. Cardiovascular
system — Diseases — Psychosomatic aspects.   I. Elbert,
Thomas. II. Series. [DNLM: 1. Arrhythmia — psychology.
2. Behavior Medicine.   3. Coronary Disease — psychology.
4. Hypertension — psychology.   WG 340 B4193]
RC685.H8B36   1988   616.1′2   87-21068
ISBN 0 471 91770 2

British Library Cataloguing in Publication Data:

Behavioural medicine in cardiovascular disorders.
1. Cardiovascular system — Diseases —
Psychological aspects.   2. Behavior therapy
I. Elbert, T.
616.1′06   RC669
ISBN 0 471 91770 2

Phototypeset by Dobbie Typesetting Service, Plymouth, Devon
Printed in Great Britain at The Bath Press, Avon

Contents

List of Contributors

M. ARICKX, *Limburgs Universitair Centrum, Belgium*

H. D. BASLER, *Institut für Medizinische Psychologie, Universität Marburg, FRG*

J. BECKERS, *Centrum Geestelijke Gezondheidszorg, St Truiden, Belgium*

M. P. F. BERGER, *Department of Education, University of Twente, The Netherlands*

N. BIRBAUMER, *Department of Psychology, Pennsylvania State University, PA, USA*

H. BORCHERDING, *Benedikt Kreutz Rehabilitations Zentrum, Bad Krozingen, FRG*

G. BRODNER, *Benedikt Kreutz Rehabilitations Zentrum, Bad Krozingen, FRG*

L. BUCHHOLZ, *Klinikum, Universität Heidelberg, FRG*

B. DWORKIN, *The Milton S. Hershey Medical Center, Pennsylvania State University, USA*

B. EBERT-HAMPEL, *Medizinische Psychologie, Universität Münster, FRG*

A. EHLERS, *Fachbereich Psychologie, Philipps-University, Marburg, FRG*

TH. ELBERT, *Abt. Klinische und Physiologische Psychologie, Universität Tübingen, FRG*

R. R. ENGEL, *Abt. Klinische Psychologie, Psychiatrische Klinik der Universität München, FRG*

M. ERNST, *Psychiatry Department, Beth Israel Medical Center, New York, USA*

H. R. GOHLKE, *Zentralinst. für Herz-Kreislauf-Regulationsforschung der AdW, Berlin, GDR*

P. GROSSMAN, *N.I.A.S., Wassenaar, The Netherlands (now at Freiburg University, FRG)*

B. HEINRICH, *Zentralinst. für Herz-Kreislauf-Regulationsforschung der AdW, Berlin, GDR*

V. HOMUTH, *Zentralinst. für Herz-Kreislauf-Regulationsforschung der AdW, Berlin, GDR*

M. HONGENAERT, *Limburgs Universitair Centrum, Belgium (now at the Catholic University, Leuven, Belgium)*

K. H. L. JANSSEN, *Department of Psychology, Tilburg University, The Netherlands*

M. KESSLER, *Forschungsstelle für Psychotherapie, Stuttgart, FRG*

W. KUHMANN, *Abt. Klinische Psychologie, Wuppertal, FRG*

U. KNUST, *Zentralinst. für Herz-Kreislauf-Regulationsforschung der AdW, Berlin, GDR*

W. LANGOSCH, *Benedikt Kreutz Rehabilitations Zentrum, Bad Krozingen, FRG*

W. LARBIG, *Abt. Klinische and Physiologische Psychologie, Tübingen, FRG*

W. LUTZENBERGER, *Abt. Klinische and Physiologische Psychologie, Tübingen, FRG*

J. MARGRAF, *Fachbereich Psychologie, Philipps University, Marburg, FRG*

W. MORGENSTERN, *Klinische Sozialmedizin, Universität Heidelberg, FRG*

E. NÜSSEL, *Klinische Sozialmedizin, Universität Heidelberg, FRG*

A. E. PHILIP, *Department of Clinical Psychology, Royal Edinburgh Hospital, Edinburgh, UK*

T. G. PICKERING, *Hypertension Center, New York Hospital, Cornell Medical Center, New York, USA*

R. PIETROWSKY, *Abt. Angew. Physiologie, Universität Ulm, FRG*

E. RICHTER-HEINRICH, *Zentralinst. für Herz- Kreislauf-Regulationsforschung der AdW, Berlin, GDR*

B. ROCKSTROH, *Abt. Klinische und Physiologische Psychologie, Universität Tübingen, FRG*

E. ROSKIES, *Department of Psychology, University of Montreal, Canada*

W. T. ROTH, *Department of Psychiatry and Behavioral Sciences, Stanford University School of Medicine, USA*

E. RÜDDEL, *Medizinische Universitätsklinik, Innere Medizin, Universität Bonn, FRG*

R. SCHEIDT, *Klinische Sozialmedizin, Universität Heidelberg, FRG*

W. SCHEUERMANN, *Klinische Sozialmedizin, Universität Heidelberg, FRG*

K. H. SCHMIDT, *Zentralinst. für Herz-Kreislauf-Regulationsforschung der AdW, Berlin, GDR*

K. SIEGRIST, *Herz-Kreislauf-Klinik, Bad Berleburg, FRG*

J. E. SKINNER, *Baylor College of Medicine, The Methodist Hospital, Department of Neurophysiology, Houston, USA*

A. STEPTOE, *Department of Psychology, St George's Hospital, Medical School, University of London, UK*

C. B. TAYLOR, *Department of Psychiatry and Behavioral Sciences, Stanford University School of Medicine, USA*

D. VAITL, *Klinische Psychologie, Universität Giessen, FRG*

H. VERTOMMEN, *Catholic University, Leuven, Belgium*

J. VINCK, *Limburgs Universitair Centrum, Belgium*

A. VON EIFF, *Medizinische Universitätsklinik, Innere Medizin, Bonn, FRG*

B. WALTER, *Medizinische Universitätsklinik, Innere Medizine, Universität Bonn, FRG*

G. WIEDEMANN, *Städt. Krankenhaus Bogenhausen, Abt. für Psychosomatische Medizin, München, FRG*

R. WIEDEMANN, *Zentralinst. für Herz- Kreislauf-Regulationsforschung der AdW, Berlin, GDR*

K. WYBITUL, *Benedikt Kreutz Rehabilitation Zentrum, Bad Krozingen, FRG*

W. ZANDER, *Gauting, FRG*

Preface

Cardiovascular disorders have become the major cause of death in the industrialized world (see Table 1). Although modern medicine has achieved considerable success with acute infections, the evidence forces us to abandon unidimensional, biological models for cardiovascular disorders. Instead it is necessary to take into account social, behavioural, emotional, and personality factors as well. The first steps towards biopsychosocial models of disease have been taken (e.g. Weiner, 1977; Engel, 1977; Pomerleau and Brady, 1979; Melamed and Siegel, 1980; Pinkerton *et al.*, 1982). The influence of psychological factors on genesis and aetiology is well documented for a number of cardiovascular disorders. In addition, recent research has improved our understanding of the ways in which psychological conditions may interact with physiological regulatory mechanisms, leading to new approaches to treatment and prevention.

The purpose of this book is to outline basic psychophysiological mechanisms in the development of cardiovascular disorders and to discuss recent developments in the behavioural management of these conditions. The two strands

Table 1. Major causes of death (from Vester, DVA Stuttgart, 1976)

	1850	1920	1975
Typhoid	++++	+++	−
Diphtheria	++++	+++	−
Smallpox	++	−	−
Puerperal fever	+++	++	−
Cardiovascular disease	+++	++++++++++	+++++++++++++++++++++++++++++
Cancer	+++	++++++	+++++++++++++
Tuberculosis	++++	++++	(+)
Pneumonia	++++++	+++++	+
Liver and gall	+++	+++	+
Infant mortality	++++	+++	(+)
Infirmity of age	+++++	++++	−
Intermittent fever etc.	++	++	−

of research — on aetiology and intervention — must go hand in hand if genuine gains are to be made in patient care. Current work has reached the point where results are becoming increasingly relevant to the practitioner and there is a need for practical implementation of techniques on a large scale. At the same time, insights into the psychophysiological link between social conditions and medical problems must be at the heart of treatment and provide guidelines for the development of new therapeutic interventions.

Several of the contributors to this volume participated in the 1985 Annual Meeting of the European Association of Behaviour Therapy (EABT) in Munich. There, the suggestion was made to assemble in a single volume recent cardiovascular research relevant to behavioural medicine. Consequently, the book emphasizes European research. The scope of the volume has, however, been expanded considerably to take account of exciting developments in behavioural research on cardiovascular disorders from other parts of the world. The contributions have been divided into four sections reflectings four growth areas, and these are concerned with psychophysiological aspects of essential hypertension, behavioural management of hypertension, prevention and rehabilitation of coronary heart disease, and behavioural aspects of cardiac arrhythmia and related problems. Each section is preceded by an introduction that outlines the issues considered in the chapters. It is our hope that the resulting collection will stimulate further research in the field of behavioural medicine for the benefit of patients suffering from these life-threatening, debilitating disorders.

REFERENCES

Engel, G. L. (1977). The need for a new medical model: A challenge for biomedicine. *Science*, **196**, 129–136.

Melamed, B. G. & Siegel, L. J. (1980). *Behavioral Medicine. Practical Applications in Health Care*, Springer-Verlag, New York.

Pinkerton, S., Hughes, H. and Wenrich, W. W. (1982). *Behavioral Medicine. Clinical Applications*, Wiley, New York.

Pomerleau, O. F. and Brady, J. P. (1979). Behavioral medicine: Theory and practice, Williams and Wilkins, Baltimore.

Weiner, H. (1977). *Psychobiology and Human Disease*, Amsterdam, Elsevier.

Acknowledgement

The editors gratefully acknowledge the advice of Dr Brigitte Rockstroh.

SECTION I

Essential Hypertension: Psychophysiology

INTRODUCTION TO SECTION I

Much of the work in cardiovascular psychophysiology had been restricted to observations of the ways in which psychological processes might affect heart rate, blood pressure, and occasionally more sophisticated measures of cardiovascular control. As for psychosomatic diseases in general, theoretical models, which describe the mechanisms underlying physiological alterations due to psychological processes, are lacking. In his chapter, Dworkin has elaborated a comprehensive hypothesis about the pathophysiology of essential hypertension, suggesting an interaction between elevated blood pressure and pain regulatory mechanisms. Activation of the baroreceptor reflex arc may result in central inhibitory effects (Lacey and Lacey, 1970). Baroreceptor activity is transmitted to the cerebral cortex via several subcortical structures, including the nucleus tractus solitarius, locus coeruleus, and the hypothalamus. Dampening of brainstem arousal and cortical deactivation, resulting from baroreceptor firing, would reduce the aversiveness of noxious stimulation, and hence reinforce blood pressure elevation. Under frequent stressful conditions, hypertension could develop through operant conditioning with the baroreceptors adapting their sensitivity to the ensuing pressor responses.

Dworkin's model is based on a detailed understanding of the role the baroreceptors may play in long-term blood pressure regulation and essential hypertension. This area is reviewed in Chapter 1 by Kessler and Pietrowsky. The available evidence points to a diminished baroreflex sensitivity in subjects with elevated blood pressure.

Another issue which remains unclear is the extent to which elevations of blood pressure can produce reliable reductions of pain sensitivity in human experimental subjects. As reported in Chapter 3, Rockstroh and coauthors have approached this question by employing either mechanical stimulation of the baroreceptors using neck suction or pharmacological manipulation of the blood pressure with a vasoconstrictor. These studies have evaluated the effects of baroreceptor stimulation on electrical brain activity and on pain thresholds. Unlike normotensives, subjects with elevated blood pressure levels tend to tolerate more intense electric stimulation, when the baroreceptors have been activated. A marked reduction of electrical negative brain potentials during baroreceptor firing confirms the view that baroreceptor afferent impulses exert a dampening effect on cortical structures. The distribution of the potential changes across the scalp is related to tonic blood pressure, a finding which may reflect differences in the predisposition for the development of essential hypertension.

Later on, this view is emphasized in Chapter 16 by Skinner, which elaborates the involvement of the brain in the dual autonomic cardiac innervation. An increment in both sympathetic and parasympathetic inputs is favoured by high amplitudes of slow cortical negativity, resulting in cardiac vulnerability. On the

3

other hand, baroreceptor stimulation reduces this negativity indicative of cortical excitability. In other words, brain and cardiovascular activity appear to be linked in a feedback loop, influencing each other.

Another question raised by Dworkin, concerns the responses induced by stress. A laboratory study on autonomic stress responses is presented by Wiedemann, Engel and Zander in Chapter 4. By means of radio plays and an interview, the authors had induced specific emotions prior to stress situations, varying on a passive–active dimension. Whereas group differences between hypertensives and normotensives were rather small, the different test situations produced differential patterning of physiological responses.

Extending blood pressure measurement from the laboratory to clinical practice in the home seems essential for the understanding of factors affecting this variable. The predictive power of theoretical models has to be tested ultimately in everyday life. As Pickering points out in Chapter 5, ambulatory measurement also improves evaluation of both the prognosis and the response to treatment of individual patients. In fact, one-third of the patients are misclassified as being hypertensive if the diagnosis is based only on measurements in unfamiliar settings. It remains a challenge for future psychophysiology to study responses and interactions in the field. Pickering's work presents an important step in that direction.

REFERENCE

Lacey, J. and Lacey, B. (1970). Some autonomic–central nervous system interrelationships. In P. Black (Ed.), *Physiological Correlates of Emotion*, Academic Press, New York.

Behavioural Medicine in Cardiovascular Disorders
Edited by T. Elbert, W. Langosch, A. Steptoe and D. Vaitl
© 1988 John Wiley & Sons Ltd

1

Baroreceptor Sensitivity and Hypertension

Manfred Kessler* and Reinhard Pietrowsky
*Forschungsstelle für Psychotherapie, Stuttgart and
Department of Applied Physiology, University of Ulm, FRG*

INTRODUCTION

This chapter deals with the sensitivity of the baroreceptor reflex in normo-tensives, borderline hypertensives and essential hypertensives. Furthermore the effect of physical exercise or mental stress on baroreflex sensitivity will also be discussed. In this connection the theory of Dworkin et al. (1979), which predicts that essential hypertension can be learned through operant conditioning, is of interest. They suggested that in aversive situations the acute rise of blood pressure can be negatively reinforced via baroreceptor stimulation. If this were true, it would raise the question: does the baroreflex diminish over time and, if so, is hyperalgesia a result of profound essential hypertension? In a study of Randich (1982) spontaneously hypertensive rats (SHR), receiving electric stimulation, exhibited hyperalgetic behavior.

The often reported result, that under tonic high blood pressure baroreceptor activity is not elevated but remains constant or is even diminished (Bristow et al., 1969; Takeshita et al., 1975; Eckberg, 1979), implies a change in the baroreceptor reflex. Two possible mechanisms for diminished baroreflex sensitivity will be discussed. First, a direct loss of baroreflex sensitivity is frequently seen in hyper-tension. Second, a resetting of the baroreceptor sensitivity to a higher blood pressure level, namely an elevated threshold for baroreceptor firing, will also be discussed. The buffer mechanism of the baroreflex then starts its function to lower blood pressure. Thereby it is also likely that these two mechanisms occur together, the result being both a loss of sensitivity and resetting.

Regarding the effects of physical exercise and mental stress, two questions arise: first, to what extent is the baroreflex reduced through sympathetic activity; and, second, do hypertensives differ from normotensives in this respect?

*Permanent address: Forschungsstelle für Psychotherapie, Christian-Belser Str. 79a, 7 Stuttgart 70, FRG.

METHODOLOGY OF BAROREFLEX SENSITIVITY MEASUREMENT

Two different techniques were used to determine baroreflex sensitivity. One was the phenylephrine technique, developed by Smyth *et al.* (1969). This is based on the relation between an actual rise in blood pressure (stimulus side), induced by an injection of phenylephrine, and reflexive heart rate deceleration (reaction side). The resulting regression coefficient (slope) of the regression line shows the prolongation of the R–R interval related to a 1 mmHg rise of the systolic blood pressure. The slope can be used as an index (in ms/mmHg) of baroreflex sensitivity. A steep slope indicates a high baroreflex sensitivity and a shallow one the opposite.

In the second technique, neck suction, a cuff which encloses the neck of the subject is used. With this technique it is possible to stimulate the carotid arterial stretch receptors by applying subatmospheric pressure in the cuff. This procedure increases the transmural pressure around the carotid artery. The baroreceptors cannot distinguish this signal from an internal rise in blood pressure and, hence, they will fire. Evoked changes in heart rate and blood pressure are then used to estimate baroreflex sensitivity. The success of this technique in stimulating the arterial baroreceptors was demonstrated in several studies (e.g. Eckberg *et al.*, 1975; Forsman and Lindblad, 1983; Mancia *et al.*, 1979; Toon *et al.*, 1984). About 60 per cent of the reduction in pressure to subatmospheric levels was transferred to the baroreceptors in the carotid sinus.

There are important differences between these two techniques. First, the baroreceptor stimulation by injection of vasoactive substances such as phenylephrine is characterized by a gradually increasing but transient rise of blood pressure. In contrast, the direct method by neck suction causes a quick and lasting change of baroreceptor activity. These differences in latency and duration of baroreceptor stimulation may lead to different physiological processes. Another difference between the two techniques lies in their measurable dependent variables. In the phenylephrine technique only heart rate alterations are measurable after injection of vasoactive substances. Using the neck suction device variations in blood pressure itself or peripheral blood flow, which are not directly influenced, can also be measured. Therefore neck suction is the favored technique where more than one limb of the baroreflex is to be investigated or if the whole cardiovascular reaction pattern is of interest.

Karemaker and Borst (1980) and Karemaker (1985) criticized the assumption of a linear relation between blood pressure and heart period (R–R interval) in determining baroreflex sensitivity. They found that the resulting curves had an upward concavity. A second point of criticism concerned the established custom of correlating systolic pressure with the duration of the next heart period. This implies that the baroreflex takes more than one heart period to counteract a pressure change by way of a change in heart period. Karemaker (1985) pointed out that the best correlations between changes in blood pressure and heart period were to be found when systolic pressure was correlated with the duration of the same heart period in which they occurred, provided that heart period was not shorter than about 800 ms. When the heart period was shorter, systolic pressure was observed to correlate best with the duration of the next heart period.

From these results, Karemaker formulated a computational time domain model to estimate baroreflex sensitivity. The formula:

$$I_n = \alpha_0 S_n + \alpha_1 S_{n-1} + c$$

(I_n = interbeat interval, S_{n-1} = systolic pressure, c = constant) describes the fast, vagally mediated, baroreflex effect on the nth systolic pressure on the duration of the nth interval. If resting heart period is shorter than about 800 ms, $\alpha_0 = 0$ and α_1 is in operation; at longer heart periods α_0 can offer a sufficient description and $\alpha_1 = 0$. To incorporate the slowly varying sympathetic effects to heart period, the formula had to be extended to:

$$I_n = \alpha_0 S_n + \alpha_1 S_{n-1} + \alpha_2 \ (S_{n-3} + S_{n-4} + S_{n-5}) + c.$$

Wesseling and Settels (1985) describe a model that allows for the estimation of baroreflex sensitivity with the aid of frequency domain techniques (e.g. spectral analysis). For a comparison and discussion of the adequacy of the two models to estimate baroreflex sensitivity, see Mulder (1985).

BAROREFLEX SENSITIVITY IN HYPERTENSION

Two studies (Bristow et al., 1969; Takeshita et al., 1975), in which phenylephrine was used to elevate blood pressure, demonstrated that baroreflex sensitivity was diminished in patients with established hypertension. The slope of the regression line was markedly shallower compared with that of normotensive subjects. Takeshita et al. (1975), who also investigated subjects with borderline hypertension, showed that the slopes of these subjects were located between those of normotensives and hypertensives. A negative correlation between blood pressure level prior to phenylephrine injection and the regression coefficient for each subject was reported. This result indicates that with increasing tonic blood pressure level baroreflex sensitivity decreases linearly.

The authors of these two studies suggest that the shallower slopes in patients with borderline hypertension, and especially in those with established hypertension, are a sign of a direct loss of baroreflex sensitivity. A resetting of baroreceptor sensitivity would be characterized by the same slopes and differs only with respect to the blood pressure level of the subjects. A closer inspection of the results in the study from Bristow et al. (1969), however, shows that in hypertensives the slope, as well as the offset point of the regression line of blood pressure, is changed. This indicates that in these patients a change of sensitivity of the baroreflex (resetting) as well as a change of the sensitivity of the baroreceptors may have occurred.

Eckberg (1979) employed neck suction in two groups of borderline hypertensives — one with high systolic blood pressure, the other with low systolic blood pressure — to investigate baroreflex sensitivity. The results were identical to those of the studies reported above. Borderline hypertensives have a diminished baroreflex sensitivity compared with normotensives.

There is agreement between the reported studies, that in hypertension a change of the baroreceptor reflex is established in the direction of reduced efficiency of the reflex.

Mancia *et al.* (1978, 1979, 1980) also showed that an acute blood pressure change via neck suction is followed by different reflexive changes of the blood pressure in normotensives and established hypertensives. However, they concluded that the reason for these results is not a change in baroreflex sensitivity, but a resetting of the sensitivity of baroreceptors in hypertensives. In hypertensives the baroreflex was more sensitive to a rise in blood pressure. Under this condition the baroreflex can develop its maximum discharge. In normotensives the inverse reaction was observed. This implies that in subjects with normal tonic blood pressure, baroreceptors are near their maximum rate of discharge. In hypertensives, on the other hand, there is little activity in the baroreceptors under tonic blood pressure levels. Indeed, there is a greater allowance for an elevation of baroreceptor discharge in response to a rise in blood pressure. As the authors suggested, a smaller dilatability of the arterial walls in established hypertension could be responsible for this effect.

Now a discussion of the two measures (heart rate and blood pressure) used to determine baroreflex sensitivity will be undertaken. Because of the different reaction courses of heart rate and blood pressure in response to baroreceptor stimulation, the question arises as to which of these two measures would be better for the determination of the sensitivity of the reflex arc.

Changes in heart rate are directly controlled through the baroreceptor reflex, so this is an appropriate measure to determine the sensitivity of the baroreflex. Blood pressure is in fact also regulated through reflex reactions following stimulation of the baroreceptors (e.g. change of peripheral resistance and cardiac output). But we have to consider the possibility that different reflex mechanisms come into force, perhaps with different latencies. In this sense changes of blood pressure seem to be a critical measure for the determination of baroreflex sensitivity. If the question to be answered is whether or not in hypertension an alteration of regulation of blood pressure occurs through the baroreceptors, then those changes of blood pressure might be the appropriate measure, in which changes in heart rate are included.

It is possible that the different results obtained are partly due to the choice of dependent variable. In the studies where baroreflex sensitivity was validated on heart rate (Smyth *et al.*, 1969; Takeshita *et al.*, 1975; Eckberg, 1979) the authors found diminished baroreflex sensitivity in subjects with hypertension. However, when blood pressure was the dependent variable used to determine baroreflex sensitivity (Mancia *et al.*, 1978, 1979), no differences in baroreflex sensitivity between normotensives and hypertensives were found. Taking these conflicting findings together, it can be assumed that in subjects with hypertension there is indeed a diminished baroreflex sensitivity relative to the reflexive heart rate response. The overall regulation of blood pressure would not yet be affected, since this deficiency could be compensated for by other mechanisms.

Simon *et al.* (1977) investigated the influence of parasympathetic and sympathetic activity on baroreflex sensitivity. After determining the basal baroreflex sensitivity of normotensives and hypertensives they first injected propranolol to reduce sympathetic activity and then atropine to block parasympathetic influences. After each injection they determined baroreflex sensitivity. The dose of atropine at which the regression between blood pressure and heart rate was zero, was taken as an index of parasympathetic activity. The dose of atropine required in order to block parasympathetic activity was negatively correlated with tonic diastolic blood pressure in normotensives, but not in hypertensives. That is, normotensives displayed less parasympathetic activity under conditions of higher average diastolic blood pressure. Since this could not be found in hypertensives, the finding indicates that in subjects with established hypertension there is a disturbance of parasympathetic regulation. It can therefore be assumed that a neurogenic factor underlying essential hypertension might be a disturbance of the balance between sympathetic and parasympathetic activity.

Finally the relationship between baroreflex sensitivity and age should be discussed. Gribbin *et al.* (1971) showed that baroreflex sensitivity, calculated by the phenylephrine technique, declines progressively with age in both hypertensives and normotensives. In hypertensives compared with normotensives, in general, baroreflex sensitivity was diminished. Randall *et al.* (1978) investigated the possibility that a loss of dilatability of the arterial walls might be responsible for the diminished baroreflex sensitivity seen in older people and/or hypertensives. They also showed that baroreflex sensitivity is negatively correlated with age and tonic blood pressure, although each variable worked independently with regard to baroreflex sensitivity. Interestingly, there was no influence of arterial dilatability on the correlation between age and baroreflex sensitivity, but there was such an influence on the correlation between blood pressure and baroreflex sensitivity. Furthermore, baroreflex sensitivity was significantly correlated with the dilatability of the arterial walls. Therefore, it may be assumed that a loss of arterial dilatability has an important mediating function between tonic blood pressure and baroreflex sensitivity. The decline of baroreflex sensitivity with age might be due to a possible degenerative change in the nerve endings of the baroreceptor reflex arc, as assumed by the authors.

Similar results were obtained by Conway *et al.* (1983), who demonstrated an inverse relationship between age and baroreflex sensitivity in borderline hypertensives.

EFFECTS OF PHYSICAL EXERCISE AND MENTAL STRESS ON BAROREFLEX SENSITIVITY

The background to these studies is to be found in the hypothesis that the baroreflex is also active during exercise (Heymans and Neil, 1958), that is the tachycardia accompanying exercise is influenced by the baroreflex. Two studies (Bevegard and Shepherd, 1966; Robinson *et al.*, 1966) provide evidence for this hypothesis. Under conditions of baroreceptor stimulation, the reduction in blood pressure and heart rate during supine exercise (bicycle ergometer) was the same as when at rest. The degree of changes of heart rate and blood pressure brought about by an injection of nitroglycerine also did not differ compared at rest (Robinson *et al.*, 1966). Therefore it seems that the sensitivity of the baroreceptor system does not alter during exercise. Indeed, a large number of studies have shown that baroreflex sensitivity is reduced during physical exercise. McRitchie *et al.* (1976) demonstrated that the arterial baroreflex is turned off during rigorous exercise and that it does not modify significantly the cardiovascular response to such exercise (running). Dogs with total arterial baroreceptor denervation displayed the same magnitude of cardiovascular changes (e.g. increase in cardiac output, and heart rate, reduction of total peripheral resistance) as intact dogs. These results indicate that the normal tachycardia seen in rigorous exercise may occur even in the absence of an intact arterial baroreflex. Furthermore, the results suggest that the tachycardia was mediated either by central mechanisms or, since the vagi were intact, by inputs from lung receptors in the chest wall, somatic afferents, low pressure receptors or some combination of these. The studies of Pickering *et al.* (1971), Eckberg *et al.* (1976) and Bristow *et al.* (1971) indicate that physical exercise is associated with a reduction of baroreflex sensitivity. The decrease of the reflex is proportional to the tachycardia caused by physical exercise until a heart rate of $150\,\mathrm{min}^{-1}$ is reached. At higher heart rates no more reflex cardiac slowing was observed in response to a provoked rise in blood pressure (Bristow *et al.*, 1971). They also showed that the relation between pulse interval and arterial pressure during exercise takes the form of a loss of baroreflex sensitivity (shallower slope) as well as a resetting of the reflex (the points representing the values before phenylephrine injection of pulse interval and systolic blood pressure during exercise did not lie on the line for rest). An increase in heart rate brought about by a change of posture (from lying to a standing position) was also associated with a fall in baroreflex sensitivity (Pickering *et al.* 1971). However, Eckberg *et al.* (1976) using neck suction were not able to observe a difference in baroreflex sensitivity between lying and standing positions. Indeed, injection of propranolol increased significantly baroreflex sensitivity in the standing position. Eckberg *et al.* (1976) concluded that baroreflex sensitivity increases with orthostatic change. Under normal circumstances this effect is masked by beta-adrenergic stimulation, which was eliminated in this study by propranolol.

Therefore it seems that the role of the arterial baroreflex in the regulation of cardiovascular changes during exercise is much smaller and more complicated than formerly assumed. In the study of Pickering *et al.* (1972) the possible mechanisms underlying the decline of baroreflex sensitivity during exercise were examined. They investigated the baroreflex bradycardia in man during rest and exercise before and after autonomic blockade of the heart. The parasympathetic efferents to the heart were blocked by atropine and the sympathetic influences on the heart by propranolol. Atropine abolished baroreflex sensitivity both in rest and during exercise. Propranolol augmented it slightly at rest, but had no effect on it during exercise. Therefore it can be assumed that the reflex is mediated via parasympathetic nerves, and that the response declines during exercise as the parasympathetic tone is withdrawn. Given the effects of propranolol during exercise it might be suggested that the peripheral sympathetic–parasympathetic balance cannot account solely for changes in baroreflex sensitivity. Central nervous control, predominantly during exercise, can also account for baroreflex sensitivity.

On the other hand, there is evidence that peripheral parasympathetic–sympathetic interaction is important for the sensitivity of the reflex. In this study isoprenaline (which induces a tachycardia by acting on cardiac $beta_1$ and $beta_2$ adrenergic receptors) was also given to subjects. If the cardiac reflex response were indeed unaffected by the sympathetic–parasympathetic balance, only a shift of the reflex regression line in the direction of tachycardia without altering their slope would be caused by isoprenaline. However, isoprenaline diminished the slopes. Therefore the parasympathetic–sympathetic influence at the sinoatrial node seems to be important for baroreflex sensitivity too.

To summarize, the results of Pickering *et al.* (1972) suggest that changes of baroreflex sensitivity can occur not only at the baroreceptors itself but also at the sinoatrial node or by central mediation of the reflex. There is evidence from animal work that central modulation of the baroreflex control of heart rate can occur. Hilton (1962) showed that stimulation of the defense area in the anterior hypothalamus reduced the baroreflex effect on heart rate.

Sleight *et al.* (1978) tested the effect of mental arithmetic on baroreflex sensitivity in one hypertensive, three borderline hypertensive and three normotensive subjects. The result was that baroreflex sensitivity decreased significantly during mental arithmetic tasks in all subjects. In the subject with the essential hypertension baroreflex sensitivity was low during a control session (no mental arithmetic). During mental arithmetic no significant slowing of the heart rate occurred in response to the phenylephrine injection. Sleight *et al.* (1978) concluded that this finding suggests that the defence of alerting conditions (mental stress) depresses baroreflex control and thus contributes to a rise in blood pressure seen at this time. The reduction of baroreflex sensitivity during mental stress may have parallels to the observation that patients with essential hypertension showed a rise in pressure when they were confronted with a doctor. Littler et al. (1975), in Sleight et al. (1978) observed that these patients display the highest pressures while in hospital; away from hospital the pressure may be much lower or normal.

The results of this study suggest that mental stress might be a risk factor in hypertension because it brings about a reduction in baroreflex sensitivity. In other words: it may be possible that under mental stress the baroreceptor reflex cannot maintain its control of blood pressure by means of heart rate deceleration.

An interesting comparison to this study can be made with that of Forsman and Lindblad (1983). Mental stress was induced by a color/word conflict task and baroreflex sensitivity was determined by the neck suction technique. Mean levels of heart rate and blood pressure during the color/word task indicated that this kind of stress induction was successful. Decreases in heart rate and systolic blood pressure consequent upon neck suction were not different between mental stress and control conditions. Therefore non-specific mental stress did not influence the ability of carotid sinus baroreceptors to decrease heart rate or blood pressure in response to sustained changes in baroreceptor input. This is opposite to the conclusion of Sleight et al. (1978) that mental stress decreases baroreceptor sensitivity. In their discussion Forsman and Lindblad (1983) pointed out that differences in stimulation of the baroreceptors (and therefore in physiological processes) could be responsible for the differing results (see methodology). The different kinds of induced stress may also have contributed to these results.

A study by Conway et al. (1983) points to the importance of central nervous influences on the baroreflex mechanism. Baroreflex sensitivity was highest during sleep with decreased blood pressure and this sensitivity decreased with graded mental arousal (reading, mental arithmetic) introduced upon waking. Mental arithmetic was necessary in order to decrease baroreflex sensitivity to a level lower than the baseline awake value. These results lend further support to the hypothesis that inputs from higher centers, by way of the medulla (e.g. nucleus tractus solitarii), are responsible for differing baroreflex sensitivity between wakefulness and sleep. It seems that during the day the baroreflex is partly inhibited by these central inputs. At night this inhibition is released and the baroreflex becomes more sensitive. This may be due to a reduction in blood pressure and also to its smaller variability during sleep. Therefore it seems possible that baroreflex sensitivity determines the level of blood pressure and heart rate rather than vice versa. That a restoration of blood pressure during sleep to the daytime level did not affect the sensitivity of the reflex (Smyth et al., 1969), supported this view. The earlier discussion of Pickering et al.'s (1972) work regarding central nervous influences (examined by autonomic blockade of heart rate), is also relevant in this view. Finally these results suggest that baroreflex activity is also involved in the medium-term regulation of blood pressure during day and night, in addition to its well-known role in buffering acute changes in blood pressure. Mancia *et al.* (1986) investigated the relationships between baroreflexes, blood pressure and heart rate variations in hypertensive subjects. Baroreflex sensitivity was determined by the phenylephrine as well as the neck suction technique. Several indices of blood pressure and heart rate variability (in the form of standard deviations) were estimated over a 24-hour period. Calculations were drawn from within half hours (short-term variations), between half hours (long-term variations) and for 2-hour periods during the day and also separately during the night.

With either technique baroreflex sensitivity was significantly inversely related to measurements of blood pressure variability, supporting the results of Conway *et al.* (1984). These authors report an inverse relationship between baroreflex sensitivity in the response to vasopressor drugs (e.g. epinephrine), the fall in blood pressure with sleep and the spontaneous variability in systolic blood pressure and heart rate during night. In the study of Mancia *et al.* (1986), heart rate variability was always positively correlated with baroreflex sensitivity. Therefore, stimulation of baroreceptors exerted opposite effects to blood pressure and heart rate. This enhancement of heart rate may represent, as the authors suggested, a means by which baroreflexes alter cardiac output to achieve blood pressure stabilization.

These findings support the role of the baroreflex in buffering blood pressure variations. The fact that this mechanism operated independently of the duration and occurrence during a 24-hour period (i.e. including sleep) is interesting, and agrees with the conclusion of Conway *et al.* (1983, see above) that inputs from higher centers are involved in the regulation of blood pressure via the baroreflex mechanism. Additionally the description by Mancia *et al.* (1986) of consistently low correlation coefficients (< 0.5) between baroreflex sensitivity and different measures of blood pressure variation supported this view. In their discussion Mancia *et al.* (1986) concluded that central factors may cause parallel blood pressure and heart rate changes. Baroreflexes are likely to be involved in both changes. In the former case this might involve a reduction in the size of central influences in blood pressure oscillations, while the latter baroreflexes might induce a series of short-term changes in heart rate in a direction opposite to that of blood pressure changes. The activity of the baroreflexes in increasing heart rate variability takes place without modifying the centrally dependent tendency of heart rate to run in parallel to blood pressure changes throughout the 24-hour cycle. This parallelism would be characterized by smaller blood pressure and larger heart rate oscillations when baroreflexes are effective and by larger blood pressure and smaller heart rate oscillations when they are ineffective.

This is in agreement with Conway *et al.* (1984), who demonstrated that subjects with the most sensitive reflexes showed marked variation in heart rate

(R–R interval) during the day and tended to have a lower level of blood pressure. Conversely, a smaller variation in heart rate and a wider range in systolic blood pressure was observed in subjects with insensitive reflexes.

SUMMARY

The effects of arterial baroreceptor stimulation on normotensives and borderline hypertensives or essential hypertensives were discussed. The question considered was: does elevated blood pressure reduce baroreflex sensitivity?

Two means of determining baroreflex sensitivity have been applied. The first involves the injection of vasoactive substances (e.g. phenylephrine) to produce a rise in blood pressure while the second involves mechanical arterial baroreceptor stimulation via neck suction. The differences between these two methods were discussed.

The overall result from such studies was that in subjects with elevated blood pressure baroreflex sensitivity is diminished. Nevertheless, explanations of diminished baroreflex sensitivity have differed. Sometimes it has been interpreted as a direct loss of baroreflex sensitivity (e.g. Bristow et al., 1969; Takeshita et al., 1975) while other authors have suggested a resetting of baroreflex sensitivity to a higher threshold (e.g. Mancia et al., 1978, 1979, 1980).

Most studies investigating the effects of physical and mental exercise on baroreflex sensitivity indicate that under these conditions baroreflex sensitivity is diminished.

With regard to the theory of Dworkin et al. (1979) the possibility that the negative reinforcing effect of baroreceptor stimulation decreases with sustained high blood pressure can not be excluded.

Baroreflex regulation may be modulated in more than one way: by the balance between sympathetic and parasympathetic activity (Pickering et al., 1972) and, more importantly, through influences from the central nervous system (Conway et al., 1983; Mancia et al., 1986). Finally it seems that the baroreflex is also involved in the long-term regulation of blood pressure, in addition to its well-known short-term regulation role. In this case inputs from higher centers are also important.

REFERENCES

Bevegard, B. S. and Shepherd, J. T. (1966). Circulatory effects of stimulating the carotid arterial stretch receptors in man at rest and during exercise. *Journal of Clinical Investigation*, 45(1), 132–142.

Bristow, J. D., Honour, A. J., Pickering, G. W., Sleight, P. and Smyth, H. S. (1969). Diminished baroreflex sensitivity in high blood pressure. *Circulation*, 39, 48–54.

Bristow, J. D., Brown, E. B., Cunningham, D. J. C., Howson, M. G., Strange Petersen, E., Pickering, T. G. and Sleight, P. (1971). Effect of bicycling on the baroreflex regulation of pulse interval. *Circulation Research*, 28, 582–592.

Conway, J., Boon, N., Vann Jones, J. and Sleight, P. (1983). Involvement of the baroreceptor reflexes in the changes in blood pressure with sleep and mental arousal. *Hypertension*, **5**(5), 746–748.

Conway, J., Boon, N., Davies, C., Vann Jones, J. and Sleight, P. (1984). Neural and humoral mechanisms involved in blood pressure variability. *Journal of Hypertension*, **2**(2), 203–208.

Dworkin, B. R., Filewich, R. J., Miller, N. E., Craigmyle, N. and Pickering, T. G. (1979). Baroreceptor activation reduces reactivity to noxious stimulation: implications for hypertension. *Science*, **205**, 1299–1301.

Eckberg, D. L. (1979). Carotid baroreflex function in young men with borderline blood pressure elevation. *Circulation*, **59**(4), 632–636.

Eckberg, D. L., Cavanaugh, M. S., Mark, A. L. and Abboud, F. M. (1975). A simplified neck suction device for activation of carotid baroreceptors. *Journal of Laboratory and Clinical Medicine*, **85**, 167–173.

Eckberg, D. L., Abboud, F. M. and Mark, A. L. (1976). Modulation of carotid baroreflex responsiveness in man: effects of posture and propranolol. *Journal of Applied Physiology*, **41**(3), 383–387.

Forsman, L. and Lindblad, L. E. (1983). Effect of mental stress on baroreceptor-mediated changes in blood pressure and heart rate and on plasma catecholamines and subjective responses in healthy men and women. *Psychosomatic Medicine*, **45**(5), 435–445.

Gribbin, B., Pickering, T. G., Sleight, P. and Peto, R. (1971). Effect of age and high blood pressure on baroreflex sensitivity in man. *Circulation Research*, **29**, 424–431.

Heymans, C. and Neil, E. (1958). *Reflexogenic Areas Cardiovascular System*. Little, Boston.

Hilton, S. M. (1962). Inhibition of baroreceptor reflexes on hypothalamic stimulation. *Journal of Physiology*, **164**(9), 56 p–57 p.

Karemaker, J. M. (1985). Short-term regulation of blood pressure and the baroreceptor reflex. In Orlebeke, J. F., Mulder, G. and van Dooren, L. J. P. (Eds), *Psychophysiology of Cardiovascular Control*, Plenum Press, New York, pp. 55–68.

Karemaker, J. M. and Borst, C. (1980). Measurement of baroreflex sensitivity in hypertension research. In Sleight, P. (Ed.), *Arterial Baroreceptors and Hypertension*, Oxford University Press, Oxford, pp. 455–461.

Mancia, G., Ludbrook, J., Ferrari, A., Gregorini, L. and Zanchetti, A. (1978). Baroreceptor reflexes in human hypertension. *Circulation Research*, **43**(2), 170–177.

Mancia, G., Ferrari, A., Gregorini, L., Parati, G., Ferrari, M. C., Pomidossi, G. and Zanchetti, A. (1979). Control of blood pressure by carotid sinus baroreceptors in human beings. *The American Journal of Cardiology*, **44**, 895–902.

Mancia, G., Ferrari, A., Ludbrook, J. and Zanchetti, A. (1980) Carotid baroreceptor influences on blood pressure in normotensive and hypertensive subjects. In Sleight, P. (Ed.), *Arterial Baroreceptors and Hypertension*, Oxford University Press, Oxford, pp. 484–491.

Mancia, G., Parati, G., Pomidossi, G., Casadel, R., Di Rienzo, M. and Zanchetti, A. (1986). Arterial baroreflexes and blood pressure and heart rate variability in humans. *Hypertension*, **8**(2), 147–153.

McRitchie, R. J., Vatner, S. F., Boettcher, D., Heyndrickx, G. R., Patrick, T. A. and Braunwald, E. (1976). Role of arterial baroreceptors in mediating cardiovascular response to exercise. *American Journal of Physiology*, **230**(1), 85–89.

Mulder, L. J. M. (1985). Model based measures of cardiovascular variability in the time and the frequency domain. In Orlebeke, J. F., Mulder, G. and van Dooren, L. J. P. (Eds), *Psychophysiology of Cardiovascular Control*, Plenum Press, New York, pp. 333–352.

Pickering, T. G., Gribbin, B., Strange Petersen, E., Cunningham, D. J. C. and Sleight, P. (1971). Comparison of the effects of exercise and posture on baroreflex in man. *Cardiovascular Research*, **5**, 582–586.

Pickering, T. G., Gribbin, B., Strange Petersen, E., Cunningham, D. J. C. and Sleight, P. (1972). Effects of autonomic blockade on the baroreflex in man at rest and during exercise. *Circulation Research*, **30**, 177–185.

Randall, O., Esler, M., Culp, B., Julius, S. and Zweifler, A. (1978). Determinants of baroreflex sensitivity in man. *Journal of Laboratory and Clinical Medicine*, **91**(3), 514–519.

Randich, A. (1982). Sinoaortic baroreceptor reflex arc modulation of nociception in spontaneously hypertensive and normotensive rats. *Physiological Psychology*, **10**(2), 267–272.

Robinson, B. F., Epstein, S. E., Beiser, G. D. and Braunwald, E. (1966). Control of heart rate by the autonomic nervous system. *Circulation Research*, **19**, 400–411.

Simon, A. Ch., Safar, M. E., Weiss, Y. A., London, G. M. and Milliez, P. L. (1977). Baroreflex sensitivity and cardiopulmonary blood volume in normotensive and hypertensive patients. *British Heart Journal*, **39**, 799–805.

Sleight, P., Fox, P., Lopez, R. and Brooks, D. E. (1978). The effect of mental arithmetic on blood pressure variability and baroreflex sensitivity in man. *Clinical Science and Molecular Medicine*, **55**, 381s–382s.

Smyth, H. S., Sleight, P. and Pickering, G. W. (1969). Reflex regulation of arterial pressure during sleep in man: a quantitative method of assessing baroreflex sensitivity. *Circulation Research*, **24**, 109–121.

Takeshita, A., Tanaka, S., Kuroiwa, A. and Nakamura, M. (1975). Reduced baroreceptor sensitivity in borderline hypertension. *Circulation*, **51**, 738–742.

Toon, P. D., Bergel, D. H. and Johnston, D. W. (1984). The effect of modification of baroreceptor activity on reaction time. *Psychophysiology*, **21**(5), 487–493.

Wesseling, K. H. and Settels, J. J. (1985). Baromodulation explains short-term blood pressure variability. In Orlebeke, J. F., Mulder, G. and van Doornen, L. J. P. (Eds), *Psychophysiology of Cardiovascular Control*, Plenum Press, New York, pp. 69–97.

Behavioural Medicine in Cardiovascular Disorders
Edited by T. Elbert, W. Langosch, A. Steptoe and D. Vaitl
©1988 John Wiley & Sons Ltd

2

Hypertension as a Learned Response: The Baroreceptor Reinforcement Hypothesis

Barry Dworkin
The Pennsylvania State University College of Medicine, Hershey, PA 17033, USA

In a study of workers at the Volvo factory in Sweden, Jonsson and Hansson (1977) found a reliable positive correlation between hearing loss and blood pressure. They reasoned that individuals with a history of chronic exposure to noise would have suffered hearing loss in proportion to the amount of exposure; thus, by studying the relationship between auditory threshold and blood pressure it was possible to infer the quantitative effect of chronic noise exposure on hypertension. In their conclusions they proffered a tentative hypothesis about the mechanism of noise-induced chronic hypertension. They said, '. . . the most reasonable explanation to the presented findings is that prolonged exposure to a stressful stimulus may have caused repeated rises in blood pressure leading to circulatory adaptations and a permanent rise in blood pressure.' (p. 87).

This chapter offers an hypothesis and supporting data about the pathophysiology of essential hypertension. The hypothesis differs in several important ways from the one reflected in the conclusions of the Volvo study. Figure 1 shows the general structure of the two models. Each begins with certain noxious environmental events; these may be simple stimuli such as noise or somatic pain, or more complex psychological events with meaning only in a relatively specific social context. In either case the direct consequence of this centripetal process is a central state of discomfort or aversiveness. In the conventional scheme (Figure 1, top) there is an hypothesized centrifugal pathway, which transduces central aversiveness into a peripheral physiological response or symptom. For hypertension this is usually thought to be some combination of humoral and neural mechanisms, which eventually effect an elevation of blood pressure. The linear causal sequence terminates in the familiar multiple tissue pathology of hypertension.

In Figure 1 bottom the initial and final processes are the same as in Figure 1 (top): noxious environmental stimuli produce aversiveness, and chronically

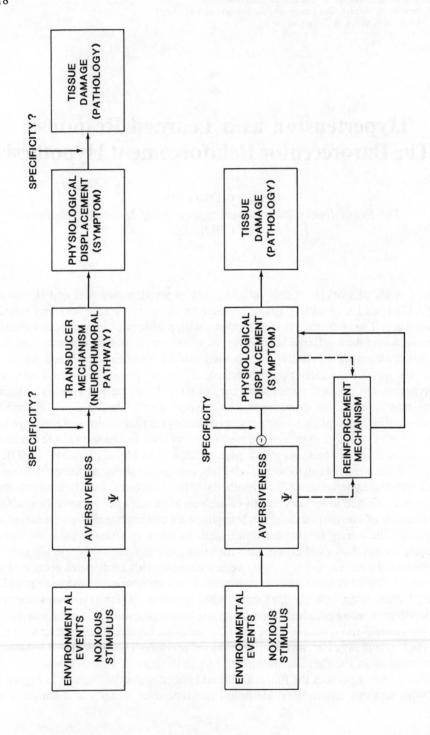

19

Figure 1. Diagrams delineating the pathogenesis of psychosomatic disease. The top panel depicts the conventional scheme and the bottom the baroreceptor reinforcement theory. The first two blocks are identical: a disturbing environmental event produces a central state of aversiveness. The event could be either a simple sensory stimulus or a more complex pattern of events. The state of aversiveness is a hypothetical construct which functionally resembles the physiological drive state of S–R learning theory.

In the conventional model (top) the drive state acts through an innate pathway to produce a symptom. For example, electric shock induced pain, through adrenal medullary mechanisms, releases epinephrine into the circulation, causing vasoconstriction, augmented cardiac output and the symptom of elevated blood pressure. The model can also be conceptualized as a sequence of unidirectional monotonic transfer functions, so that an increment in any block in the chain will produce a proportional increment in subsequent blocks, but have no effect on prior blocks. For example, a beta-blocker would be expected to reduce the blood pressure elevation, but not the perceived aversiveness of a shock.

In the feedback or instrumental learning model (bottom) the drive state need not have a direct effect on the symptom, but the symptom must have an effect on the drive state; specifically, the symptom must reduce the level of aversiveness. The reduction in aversiveness is a reinforcing stimulus, which rewards and strengthens the symptom. In this model partial pharmacological block of the pathways leading to expression of the symptom may have only a temporary effect on the magnitude of the symptom, because reduced symptom strength will cause increased aversiveness and consequently increased motivation to learn use remaining pathways to increase symptom strength and achieve relief.

20

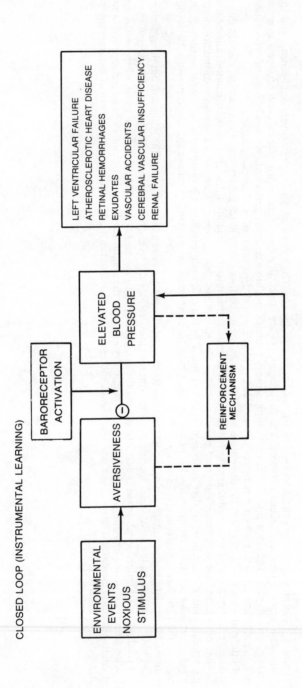

CLOSED LOOP (INSTRUMENTAL LEARNING)

ENVIRONMENTAL EVENTS NOXIOUS STIMULUS

AVERSIVENESS

BARORECEPTOR ACTIVATION

ELEVATED BLOOD PRESSURE

REINFORCEMENT MECHANISM

LEFT VENTRICULAR FAILURE
ATHEROSCLEROTIC HEART DISEASE
RETINAL HEMORRHAGES
EXUDATES
VASCULAR ACCIDENTS
CEREBRAL VASCULAR INSUFFICIENCY
RENAL FAILURE

Figure 2. A schematic of the baroreceptor reinforcement theory of essential hypertension. The same scheme as the bottom of Figure 1 with the hypothesized physiological reinforcement mechanism for hypertension specified. (See text for evidence that blood pressure elevation can be learned and that activation of the baroreceptors reduces the aversiveness of noxious stimuli.)

elevated blood pressure eventually causes widespread vascular damage; however, in place of the hypothetical neuro-humoral transduction process connecting aversiveness and elevated blood pressure there is a different mechanism which depends upon instrumental learning of blood pressure and an intrinsic baroreceptor mediated reinforcement mechanism.

Both models are consistent with the gross features of clinical and experimental hypertension. There is an experimental study which parallels the Volvo study (Peterson *et al.*, 1981) showing that chronic exposure to realistic patterns of noise causes elevated blood pressure in rhesus monkeys; that the blood pressure varies in the expected manner with noise intensity, and that the hypertension persists beyond the termination of the noise.

Figure 2 delineates the baroreceptor reinforcement theory of essential hypertension in more detail. Aversiveness is understood to be a motivational stimulus; thus, a learnable response which consistently reduces aversiveness will be reinforced and strengthened by instrumental learning. If increased blood pressure is a learnable response, and if a mechanism of reinforcement exists which can reward increased blood pressure by reducing aversiveness, then some forms of essential hypertension could involve learning of high blood pressure. Later in this chapter data are presented to indicate that the baroreceptor system has the necessary pain/anxiety reducing function to close the loop and reinforce blood pressure elevations more or less automatically. This is the second of two critical requirements of the baroreceptor reinforcement hypothesis.

The first requirement of the theory is that elevation of blood pressure is a learnable response. Figure 3 shows data from one of a group of paraplegic

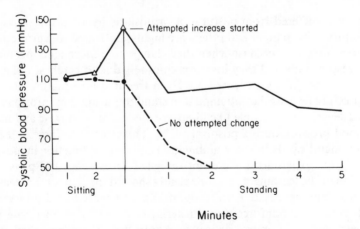

Figure 3. Data from an experiment in which a paraplegic patient was trained with an instrumental learning technique to raise his blood pressure in order to avoid orthostatic hypotension. These trials were typical of data collected after several weeks of training. At the marker he assumes an erect posture using crutches for support; during the trial plotted with a solid line he attempts to keep his blood pressure elevated.

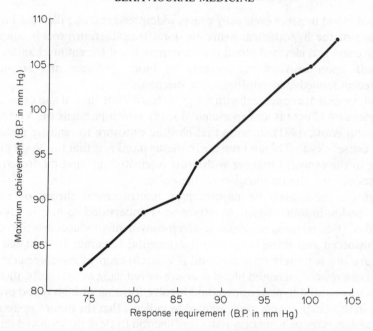

Figure 4. The criterion blood pressure required for a monkey to obtain reinforcement plotted against the blood pressure which was actually achieved during the session (from Plumlee, 1969). The close relationship suggests that the response magnitude is being regulated by a negative feedback mechanism such as instrumental learning.

patients who suffered from postural or orthostatic hypotension secondary to spinal injury. This patient and others are highly motivated to learn to increase their blood pressure, because when they change to a more erect posture their blood pressure falls and they lose consciousness due to cerebral ischemia. In this study spinal injury patients were given frequent information about their blood pressure level as they attempted to stand up; using that information this man and several other people like him were able to learn to raise and maintain their blood pressure during postural shifts. The effect was large and reliable enough to significantly improve ambulation and general function in most cases, and while the experiments were not designed to evaluate the physiological mechanism of the learning, the results clearly showed that humans, at least those with spinal injuries, could learn to significantly increase blood pressure given accurate contingent reinforcement (Pickering *et al.*, 1977). Similar observations have been made in more rigorously controlled blood pressure learning experiments using infrahuman primates: Plumlee (1969) and Benson *et al.* (1969) trained monkeys, and Harris *et al.* (1973), baboons.

Plumlee's study (1969) employed an escape/avoidance procedure in which a tone was triggered by a drop in blood pressure. If the monkey successfully

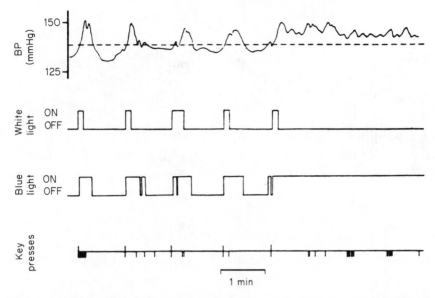

Figure 5. The learning of blood pressure control by squirrel monkeys (from Benson *et al.*, 1969). The white light warns the animal that it is below criterion and will be shocked; the blue light indicates that it has met the blood pressure criterion. In the first cycle of the session the animal terminates the white light by pressing 30 times on a key; in subsequent cycles elevation of blood pressure above 139 mmHg automatically terminates the white light and activates the blue light. By the end of the session blood pressure is consistently above the criterion, and the white light and shock remain off. Similar increases in blood pressure were achieved by three different animals.

increased its pressure within 10 seconds the tone terminated immediately without shock; if it failed, the tone terminated at the end of 10 seconds, but with a shock. All four subjects in the study learned to elevate blood pressure as much as 60 mmHg in response to the warning tone, and showed no change to a second non-shock control stimulus. As further proof that the blood pressure elevation was due to instrumental learning a yoked-control monkey received the same pattern of conditioned stimuli and shock, independent of blood pressure. This monkey did not show blood pressure increases to the warning tone. Another interesting aspect of Plumlee's results is shown in Figure 4. The criterion blood pressure required to obtain reinforcement is plotted against the blood pressure actually achieved during the session; the close relationship is further evidence that the blood pressure elevation was a result of instrumental learning.

Figure 5 shows data from an experiment (Benson *et al.*, 1969) demonstrating the learning of blood pressure control by three squirrel monkeys. A white light was used as a danger stimulus which predicted shock, and a blue light as a safety signal. Each subject was required to make a blood pressure increase to turn off the danger signal and turn on the safety signal. The record shows that each

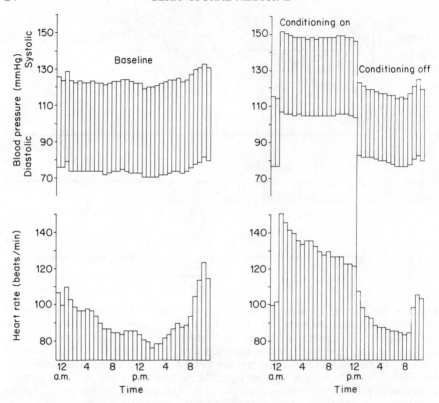

Figure 6. Instrumental learning of large magnitude blood pressure elevation by baboons (from Harris *et al.*, 1973). The animals avoided shock and received food by raising blood pressure during the 'conditioning on' period. Feedback lights similar to those in Benson *et al.* indicated whether pressure was above or below criterion. The criterion was progressively incremented to gradually 'shape' the response.

time the white light was turned on the monkey responded with a blood pressure elevation that extinguished it and temporarily eliminated the danger of shock. As the training session proceeded the baseline blood pressure increased until the blue 'safety' signal was on continuously. When the contingency was reversed, so the monkey was required to lower its blood pressure to extinguish the danger signal — even though the frequency of shock was kept the same, the blood pressure fell toward the pre-experimental control level. The authors found that using instrumental learning, mean arterial pressure could be maintained at 150 mmHg (30 mmHg above control levels) and that the blood pressure level was influenced by the specific shock–blood pressure contingency, rather than the shock density.

Harris *et al.* (1973) studied instrumental learning of blood pressure elevation in baboons and their results are illustrated in Figure 6. The baboons were trained on a 12-hour on/12-hour off schedule. During the 'conditioning on' period they were required to maintain a minimum criterion blood pressure to obtain food and avoid electric shock. The graph shows that the animals were able to learn relatively large magnitude—again 30 mmHg or more—elevations in blood pressure, which were sustained throughout the 12-hour training session, but returned to normal during the 'conditioning off' interval. Harris *et al.* were not successful in their attempts to train other baboons to lower their blood pressure; however, as with the Benson *et al.* study, animals rewarded for lowering pressure did not raise it even though they had the same amount and pattern of shocks and food as the animals specifically reinforced for blood pressure elevation.

These experiments show that neurologically intact primates can learn to substantially elevate blood pressure when a specific reinforcement contingency is in effect; when these results are combined with the data on human spinal cord injury patients, the conclusion that normal humans can learn to elevate blood pressure given appropriate reinforcement seems at least quite plausible.

Assuming that increased blood pressure can be learned with an appropriate schedule of reinforcement, to convincingly argue that blood pressure learning contributes to the pathophysiology of hypertension we must also identify a reinforcement mechanism and explain how it would be activated by elevated blood pressure in a hypertensive patient.

Figure 7 shows the baroreceptors of the carotid sinus; it is well known that they are an important part of the afferent limb of the blood pressure buffer reflexes; that stimulation by distension of the wall results in a reduction in heart rate via the motor neurons in the nucleus ambiguous and vagus nerve, and in general vasodilatation through inhibition of the sympathetic outflow. These effects are illustrated in the lower half of Figure 8. The net action of the reflex is to reduce blood pressure; however, because of their relatively rapid rate of adaptation or resetting, this pressure regulating function of the baroreflexes is probably not important for long-term blood pressure regulation or the pathophysiology of hypertension.

A less well-known aspect of baroreceptor function is their corticofugal inhibitory influence via the ascending reticular activating system. These effects of baroreceptor stimulation, diagrammed in the upper half of Figure 8, resemble those of barbiturate administration: physiological levels of baroreceptor stimulation can reduce the aversiveness of electric shock, attenuate anxiety and even produce sleep.

The first observations of the behavioral effects of baroreceptor stimulation were in 1932 by the Swiss physiologist E. B. Koch. Figure 9 is a sequence of photographs from his 1937 treatise (Koch, 1937) on the irradiation of the autonomic reflexes. The dog had a balloon surgically implanted in a carotid sinus cul-de-sac; as Koch rhythmically inflated the balloon, he observed that the dog became drowsy and, eventually, after several minutes began to sleep. This observation was subsequently verified in the first systematic study of the

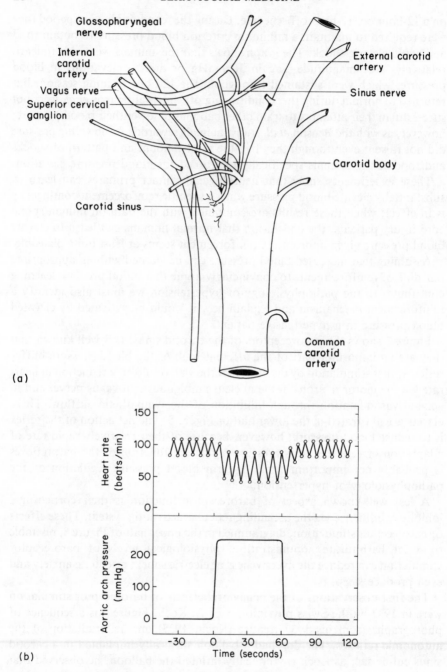

(a)

(b)

Figure 7 (a) and (b) (*see legend on facing page*).

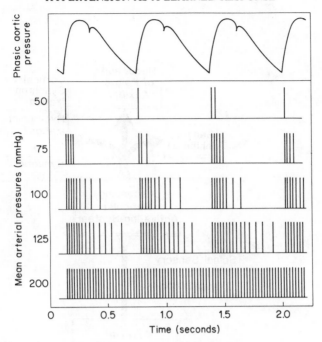

(c)

Figure 7. (a) shows the baroreceptors of the human carotid sinus. (b) shows the usual effect of artificial elevation of blood pressure on heart rate. (c) illustrates the firing pattern of the sinus nerve as a function of baseline blood pressure and pulsatile variations at each level. At very high pressures the baroreceptors fire constantly, but eventually adapt and again begin to reflect the cyclical variations.

supramedullary neurophysiology of the baroreceptors by Bonvallet *et al.* (1953). From their experiments in cats they concluded:

> The main result of these observations is that the afferents from the carotid baroreceptors are capable of producing considerable decreases in electro-cortical activity, and that this effect is independent of any variations in blood pressure or the level of circulating adrenalin. The role of these afferents, then, goes very much beyond that of regulators of vasomotor tone and the activity of the adrenalin-secreting bulbar centers. (Page 1168, our translation.)

Further evidence for the barbiturate-like effect of baroreceptor stimulation is illustrated by the Balinese Islander in Figure 10 who is using mechanical stimulation of the baroreceptors to treat insomnia (Schlager and Meier, 1947).

The sequence of photographs shown in Figure 11 was taken in our laboratory. We prepared rats with venous and arterial cannulas for injecting the alpha-sympathomimetic agent phenylepherine and recording aortic blood pressure.

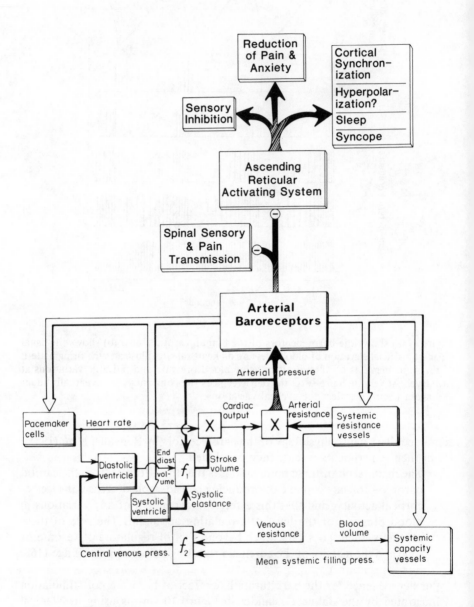

Figure 8. The various components of the peripheral pressure regulating function of the baroreceptors (bottom) and the corticofugal inhibitory influence of the baroreceptors via the ascending reticular activating system (top). Examples of the various responses are given in Figure 7 and in the text.

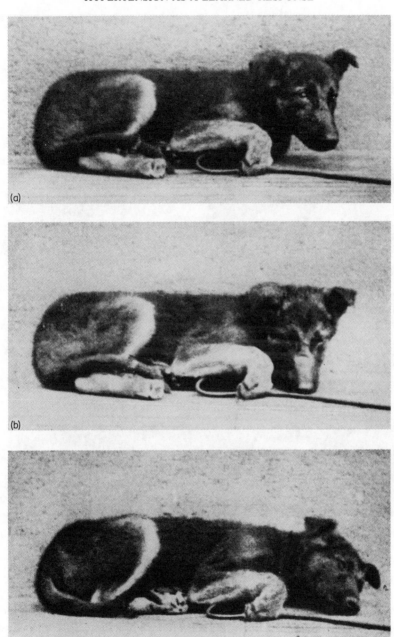

Figure 9. Dog with surgically implanted balloon in a carotid sinus cul-de-sac. Top panel is before the balloon is inflated, middle and bottom panels are during rhythmic balloon inflation: the dog became drowsy, and in the bottom panel began to sleep (from Koch, 1937).

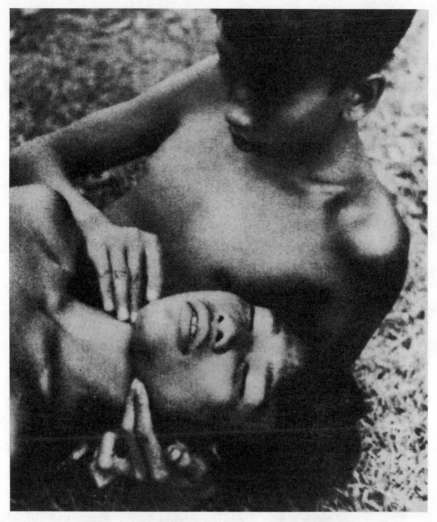

Figure 10. Balinese Islander performing a traditional carotid sinus massage to induce sleep (from Schlager and Meier, 1947).

The rat in the upper series had intact baroreceptors; the rat in the bottom series had a complete surgical denervation of the carotid sinus and aortic arch. The denervation was verified by analysis of the peripheral baroreceptor reflex as shown in Figure 12: the intact rat's heart rate fell when its blood pressure was elevated with phenylepherine but the denervated rat showed no change or possibly a slight increase in heart rate. When these two rats were infused with the same dose of phenylepherine their behavioral responses were very different as illustrated by the photographs in Figure 11. The intact one became very quiet and appeared

TEN MINUTES AFTER INFUSION, INTACT RATS SHOWED SLEEP-LIKE BEHAVIOR:

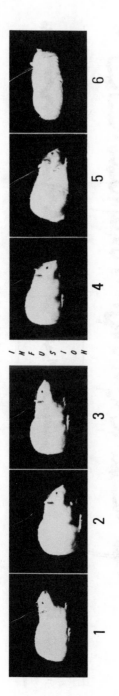

BUT RATS WITH BARORECEPTOR AREAS DENERVATED, DID NOT SHOW SLEEP-LIKE BEHAVIOR:

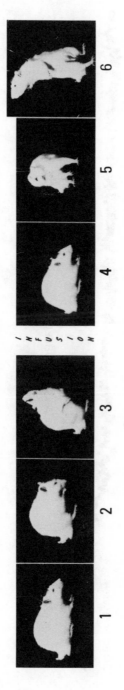

Figure 11. Rat in top series with intact baroreceptors. Rat in bottom series with complete surgical denervation of the carotid sinus and aortic arch. Following injection of phenylepherine, a sympathomimetic which raises blood pressure, the intact animal begins to sleep, as did the dog in Figure 9, but the denervated rat actually became more active.

32

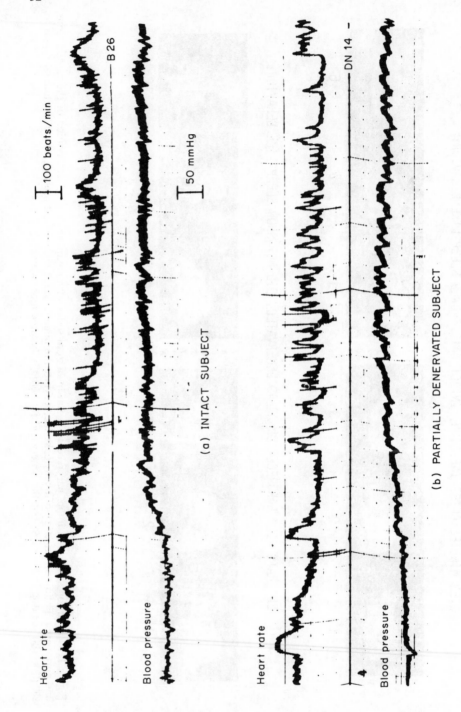

(a) INTACT SUBJECT

(b) PARTIALLY DENERVATED SUBJECT

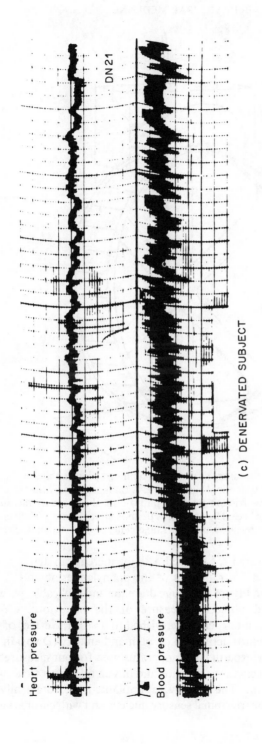

Heart pressure

DN 21

Blood pressure

(c) DENERVATED SUBJECT

Figure 12. Polygraph record of heart rate and blood pressure in intact rat (top panel), partially denervated rat (middle panel), and fully denervated rat (bottom panel). This shows the effect of the surgical denervation procedure on the peripheral baroreceptor mediated bradycardia. Classification of animals as successfully denervated was based on records of this kind.

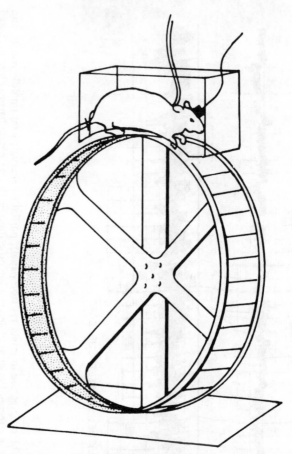

Figure 13. Treadwheel used to measure instrumental running by intact and denervated rats attempting to avoid noxious trigeminal stimulation. A rat is secured by the tail and as it runs the wheel turns on a low-friction pivot. A photo-optical transducer measures the angular displacement of the wheel. The apparatus permits attachment to relatively freely moving animals without complicated swivel arrangements of catheters and electrodes.

to sleep, while the denervated rat showed a slight increase in activity, which is probably due to a direct central effect of the phenylepherine on the brain.

While the effect shown in Figure 11 is quite dramatic and replicable, we wanted a more quantitative and objective measure of the behavioral effect of baroreceptor stimulation; in particular we wished to assess the effect of blood pressure-induced baroreceptor activation on pain and anxiety (Dworkin *et al.*, 1979). Figure 13 shows the experimental apparatus used for our measurements. The large wheel rotates freely as the rat runs and has an odometer to accurately measure the distance run. The rats were implanted stereotaxically with stimulation electrodes in the trigeminal sensory nucleus and with chronic vascular

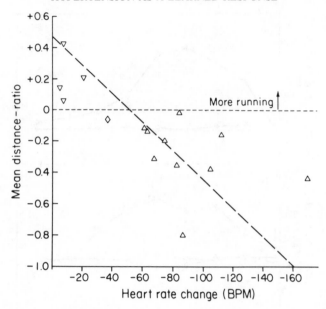

Figure 14. Data showing the relationship between the hypertension-induced change in heart rate and the distance-ratio averaged across all trials for intact (△), denervated (▽), and partially denervated (◇) rats (Dworkin et al., 1979). This correlational analysis supplemented a non-parametric test which revealed reliable differences in the effect of phenylepherine between the denervated and normal animals. The change in heart rate is assumed to be a more direct measure of baroreceptor activation than elevation in blood pressure. Because the peripheral baroreceptor reflex has been eliminated along with the corticofugal connections, the denervated animals are clustered at the left. This experiment did not incorporate controls to exclude the possibility that the behavioral effect was mediated by the heart rate change, because that issue, while important to theories of avoidance behavior, was not particularly relevant to the baroreceptor reinforcement hypothesis. Subsequent experiments (Randich and Maixner, 1984) have shown that the behavioral effect of blood pressure elevation is essentially unchanged when the peripheral reflex bradycardia is blocked by prior administration of methyl atropine.

cannulas; half of the animals were surgically denervated and the other half subjected to a sham operation. The trigeminal electrode was used to administer very accurate and reproducible levels of noxious stimulation, and in an initial phase of the experiment the rats were trained to avoid or escape from the trigeminal stimulation by running or walking 10 cm on the wheel. After daily training both groups were given infusions on the wheel in a counterbalanced sequence of phenylepherine to raise blood pressure, or saline as a control. We found that on days when blood pressure was elevated 50 mmHg by phenylepherine the intact rats showed a significantly reduced tendency to escape from the trigeminal stimulation; in contrast, those denervated showed no effect of blood pressure elevation or a somewhat increased tendency to escape.

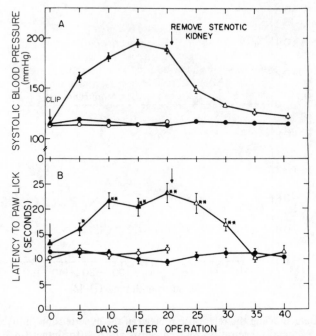

Figure 15. Data showing the relationship between hotplate-induced paw-lick latency and blood pressure in rats subjected to Goldblatt type hypertension (from Zamir and Segal, 1979). This procedure results in a reversible chronic hypertension without drug administration (**$p < 0.001$). Note that the time course of the hypertension and pain sensitivity are similar, but that recovery of pain sensitivity lags the fall in pressure after removal of the stenotic kidney. In another experiment reported in this article a non-thermal pain measure, the Randall-Selitto test, showed the same effect.

The authors found that the paw-lick pain sensitivity could be partially returned to normal by Naloxone; however, this effect has not been consistently observed by other investigators in blood pressure/pain experiments, and at this point the neuropharmacology of the baroreceptor effect remains undefined.

Analysis of the extinction data suggested that baroreceptor stimulation attenuated the anxiety level as well as pain sensitivity. An additional correlational analysis revealed that the tendency to escape or avoid the stimulation was closely related to the degree of baroreceptor activation, as measured by phenylepherine-induced heart rate slowing. These data are presented in Figure 14.

At approximately the same time that we published this experiment (Dworkin et al., 1979) Zamir and Segal (1979) reported similar observations using the Goldblatt renal ischemia method for producing hypertension. Their data (Figure 15) showed a highly reliable relationship between the standard hot plate induced paw-lick latency and blood pressure. Most recently, Randich and Maixner (1984) have described an extensive series of experiments in rats using the thermal tail-flick analgesiometric technique, and several different stimulation

Table 1. Data showing correlation between blood pressure and electrical tooth pulp pain sensitivity in humans (Zamir and Shuber, 1980). None of the subjects were receiving anti-hypertensive medication or showed clinical signs of secondary hypertensive disease. While both sensory threshold and pain threshold changed, this result may be an artifact of the homogeneous and restricted receptor population activated by electrical stimulation of the tooth-pulp (Dworkin et al., 1977; Lee et al., 1985).

Group	Sensory threshold (volts)	Pain threshold (volts)
A		
Systolic	0.708*	0.632*
Diastolic	0.584*	0.539*
B		
Systolic	0.787*	0.782*
Diastolic	0.708*	0.715*

*$p < 0.001$.

methods: they concluded that baroreceptor activation reduced pain sensitivity, and by using atropine in conjunction with phenylepherine, they further showed that the reflex bradycardia was not necessary to the antinociceptive baroreceptor effect.

There are a number of other relevant studies: George Adam's group (Adam et al., 1963a,b) has shown that denervation reduces behavioral inhibition as indicated by decreased latency to response to stimuli, and increased neurotic behavior in conflict situations. Zanchetti's laboratory (Bartorelli et al., 1960) reported that reducing baroreceptor stimulation in decerebrate cats elicits sham

Table 2. Data showing the actual mean pain thresholds of hypertensives and normals (from Zamir and Shuber, 1980). The differences are large and highly significant, whereas the average age and weight are almost the same.

Group	Age (years)	Weight (kg)	Systolic blood pressure (mmHg)	Diastolic blood pressure (mmHg)	Sensory threshold (volts)	Pain threshold (volts)
Normotensive	32.3 ± 1.8 (34)	73.3 ± 1.9 (34)	118.7 ± 1.7 (34)	76.8 ± 1.0 (34)	33.0 ± 3.3 (34)	50.1 ± 4.0 (34)
Hypertensive	33.6 ± 2.8 (21)	76.7 ± 2.4 (21)	151.7 ± 2.2** (21)	95.5 ± 1.6** (21)	76.4 ± 5.9** (21)	97.1 ± 6.4** (21)

Different from normotensive controls at *$p < 0.05$.
Different from normotensive controls at **$p < 0.001$ (Student's t-test).

rage, whereas increasing such stimulation inhibits it. And Garsik *et al.* (1983) found that evoked potentials in the medial lemniscus, the classical subthalamic sensory pathway, were reduced by both phenylepherine-induced acute blood pressure elevations and by Goldblatt-type chronic renal hypertension. Finally, several different students in my laboratory (see Dworkin *et al.*, 1979: footnote no. 10) have shown that denervating rats makes them more sensitive to both electric foot shock and the bitter taste of quinine-adulterated water.

Thus, experimental studies using a variety of stimulation and ablation methods and a range of behavioral measures, appear to confirm that baroreceptor activation reduces both the aversiveness of noxious stimuli and the level of anxiety in experimental animals. The interpretation of these experiments is relatively unambiguous, because by employing either direct electrical or mechanical stimulation of the baroreceptors, or surgically denervated control groups they eliminate most confounding variables. Such stringent controls are not possible in human studies; nevertheless, certain non-invasive baroreceptor stimulation techniques such as cervical suction and lower body positive pressure, may prove to be useful in human experiments (see next chapter).

While not a substitute for a randomized experiment, Zamir and Shuber (1980) have made some interesting observations of the relationship between blood pressure and tooth pulp pain sensitivity in humans. Their data (Table 1) show a correlation between blood pressure and pain threshold of greater than 0.70, and, specifically, in Table 2 that hypertensives have pain thresholds nearly twice those of normotensives.

In summary, a substantial body of work has accumulated, indicating that baroreceptor stimulation has many of the properties commonly associated with certain behavioral reinforcers; in particular, its action resembles that of addictive drugs, such as barbiturate: the effect of baroreceptor stimulation is to ameliorate anxiety or reduce the aversiveness of ambient noxious stimuli. Miller *et al.* (1968) showed that rats will learn a response, such as bar-pressing, to obtain intravenous infusions of barbiturate, but only in the presence of an aversive stimulus such as mild electric shock. Similarly, rats trained to run to avoid shock, will run less when their baroreceptors are stimulated by elevated blood pressure.

Assuming, now, that baroreceptor stimulation is an effective reinforcer, and blood pressure elevation a learnable response: since the inevitable consequence of blood pressure elevation is stimulation of the baroreceptors, elevation of blood pressure could be expected to more or less automatically trigger the baroreceptor reinforcement mechanism. In the presence of noxious stimuli or anxiety a patient may learn to elevate blood pressure as a way of self-stimulating his baroreceptors and, consequently, reducing the aversiveness of the situation.

It is in the nature of instrumental learning that under these circumstances, if the blood pressure response is comparatively more effective than other responses or symptoms, it will eventually become the principal way of dealing with aversiveness. Correlatively, once a particular response or symptom is

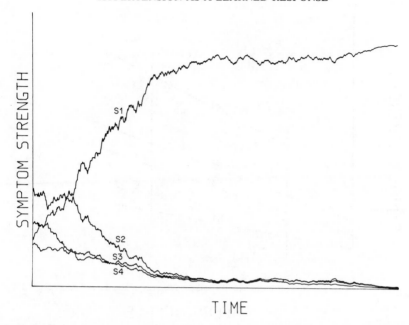

TIME

Figure 16. Monte Carlo computer simulation of a multiple symptom model in which one symptom (S1) has a somewhat higher probability of reducing aversiveness than the other three (S2, S3, or S4). Each response was assigned an initial probability of occurrence, or symptom strength, (S2 > S3 > S1 > S4), and a fixed reinforcement probability (S1 > S4 > S2 > S3; $p(S1)-p(S3) = 0.05$). The sum of the symptom strengths was rescaled to 1.00 at after each iteration. Occurrence and reinforcement of a response increased the subsequent probability by a factor of 1.01. Asymptote was achieved in approximately 500 iterations and the final form of the response distributions proved to be very insensitive to all parameters except the rank order reinforcement probabilities. The model helps verify the common intuition that a response with a higher probability of achieving reinforcement will tend to 'crowd out' or dominate the behavioral repertoire.

learned, and the aversiveness of the situation reduced, the motivation for learning additional symptoms is eliminated. For both of these reasons an instrumental learning based hypothesis predicts that a single symptom such as hypertension will emerge and dominate. The graph shown in Figure 16 is from a computer implementation of a multiple symptom model in which one learnable symptom has a somewhat higher probability of reducing aversiveness than the others. The Monte Carlo simulation, which takes into account the decremental effect of the emerging symptoms on motivation, shows that the somewhat more effective symptom (S1) increases in strength over time and that the other symptoms (S2–S4) actually become weaker. This outcome is important because of the documented specificity of psychosomatic symptoms.

When exposed to stress, some patients exhibit elevated blood pressure, others develop gastrointestinal diseases such as duodenal ulcers or irritable bowel

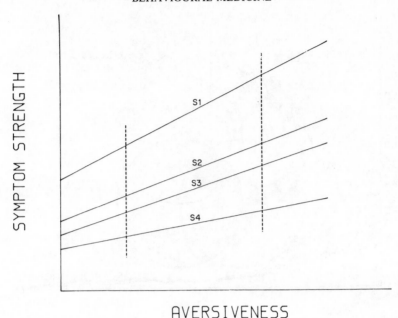

AVERSIVENESS

Figure 17. Hypothetical plot of symptom strength versus aversiveness for a linear or proportional effect model of psychosomatic disease (top panel Figure 1). The curves are based on the assumption that the magnitude of the symptom is proportional to the intensity of aversiveness. Each symptom has a different sensitivity to aversiveness and a different initial strength (due to other sources of variance), but all symptoms increase with aversiveness. If this relationship were accurate for real psychosomatic symptoms, e.g. hypertension, duodenal ulcer, or temporomandibular joint syndrome, the symptoms would tend to be correlated in a given patient population; however, multiple symptom studies have tended to show no effect or a negative correlation, i.e. if a patient has one symptom he is not more likely to have another.

syndrome; others suffer from skeletomuscular disorders such as temporo-mandibular joint syndrome or lower back pain, and still others may develop tumors, asthma, or migraine. But surprisingly few have more than one full-blown psychosomatic symptom (Weiner *et al.*, 1962; Graham *et al.*, 1962a, 1962b; Alexander *et al.*, 1968). Nevertheless, accounting for specificity is a weak point of other psychosomatic models; they either deal with it by invoking an elaborate and complex psychoanalytic doctrine of the symptom specific personality type, or by flatly asserting that for certain individuals one organ system is genetically more sensitive to stressful stimuli than others. While this 'point of least resistance' concept is not superficially illogical (some individuals could undoubtedly have greater vulnerability in certain organs), when examined more critically, it does not, unless organ sensitivity can be all or nothing—a

AT RISK

AVERSIVENESS OF
NOXIOUS STIMULATION

ABILITY TO LEARN TO
RAISE BLOOD PRESSURE

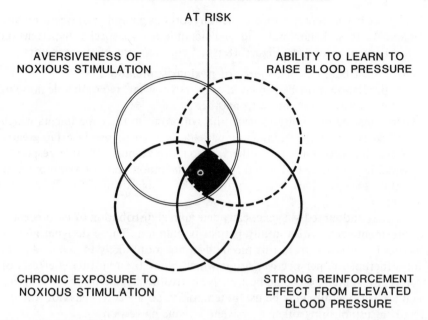

CHRONIC EXPOSURE TO
NOXIOUS STIMULATION

STRONG REINFORCEMENT
EFFECT FROM ELEVATED
BLOOD PRESSURE

Figure 18. Venn diagram showing how an at-risk population for hypertension might develop when the factors of aversiveness, behavior, and genetics intersect. Each factor will have a distribution of strength in a given population. For example, amount of exposure to noxious stimuli may be related to occupation, cultural characteristic such as family structure or urbanization, or the prior learning of non-hypertensive coping strategies. Aversiveness of particular noxious stimuli may depend upon personality or genetic characteristics. The ability to learn to raise blood pressure and the magnitude of the baroreceptor reinforcement effect for a given individual may depend upon specifically inherited anatomical characteristics. The degree to which elevation in blood pressure is learned as a way of reducing discomfort or anxiety will depend upon the way that these factors interact in a particular individual. Thus, although the baroreceptor reinforcement hypothesis is a 'behavioral' theory, it incorporates social and biological variables which have been found to be relevant to the pathogenesis of high blood pressure.

rather unrealistic assumption—explain how an individual can, for example, have a severe case of hypertension without even a trace of gastrointestinal disease or vice versa.

Increased aversiveness would inevitably produce increased symptom strength in all potentially vulnerable organs, even if the effect in one was much larger than in the others. Figure 17, taken from another set of computer generated data incorporating the linear effect model, shows symptom strength plotted against aversiveness. The result of the simulation shows that under the linear model patients with one full-blown symptom would have a statistical increased risk of a second or third psychosomatic symptom; however, the data in the literature indicate the opposite.

Under the baroreceptor reinforcement hypothesis a number of operationally definable factors, behavioral and genetic, interact to specify hypertension as the emergent symptom. Figure 18 is a Venn diagram of these factors.

1. There must be a chronic source of noxious stimulation.
2. The stimulation must be perceived as aversive: what is abominable noise to one person can be great music to another.
3. There must be an ability to learn the symptom: in the experiments which I described some of the animals or patients learned to produce far greater increases in blood pressure than others. Also if other, more effective, responses are available, they may be learned first, and the blood pressure symptom may never fully emerge. This latter point may have significance for therapeutic intervention.
4. There is undoubtedly a genetically determined distribution of baroreceptor reinforcement sensitivities in any patient population. Those deriving greater behavioral advantage from this mechanism are more likely to use it. Again, from a therapeutic perspective, drugs which block the reinforcing effects of baroreceptor stimulation could be effective in treating hypertension; even agents which act peripherally may be useful temporary adjuncts to behavior therapy directed at establishing other aversiveness reducing responses.

In conclusion it should be noted that while there is extensive data supporting the relationship between elevation in blood pressure and those CNS and behavioral phenomena which we ordinarily consider to be associated with reinforcing stimuli, several issues remain to be resolved by future research.

1. Can acute elevations of blood pressure produce reliable reductions of pain and anxiety in human experimental subjects?
2. If so, are these reductions sufficient to reinforce the learning of an instrumental response, and in particular can they reinforce blood pressure elevations?
3. Can stress-induced hypertension be shown to depend upon intact baroreceptor innervation in experimental animals? Peterson's rhesus monkeys that develop hypertension when chronically exposed to realistic patterns of noise would be an excellent preparation for studying the baroreceptor reinforcement hypothesis. Replication of the Peterson experiment with the addition of a group of baroreceptor denervated animals would come close to a critical test of the theory.

REFERENCES

Adam, G., Markel, E., Donath, O., Kovacs, A. and Nagy, A. (1963a). Carotid afferentation and higher nervous activity: activation of higher nervous centres by carotid afferentation. *Acta Physiologica Academiae Scientarium Hungarica*, **23**, 143–153.
Adam, G., Bela, A., Koo, E. and Szekely, J. I. (1963b). Conditioned reflexes of rats deprived of their carotid innervation. *Acta Physiologica Academiae Scientarium Hungarica*, **23**, 339–353.

Alexander, F., French, T. M. and Pollock, G. H. (1968). *Psychosomatic Specificity.* University of Chicago Press, Chicago.

Bartorelli, C., Bizzi, E., Libretti, A. and Zanchetti, A. (1960). Inhibitory control of sinocarotid pressoceptive afferents on hypothalamic autonomic activity and sham rage behavior. *Archives of Italian Biology*, **98**, 308–326.

Bonvallet, M., Dell, P. and Hiebel, G. (1953). Sinus carotidien et activite electrique cerebrale. *C. R. Society of Biology*, **147**, 1166–1169.

Benson, H., Herd, J. A., Morse, W. H. and Kelleher, R. T. (1969). Behavioral induction of arterial hypertension and its reversal. *American Journal of Physiology*, **217**, 30–34.

Dworkin, B. R., Lee, M. H. M., Zaretsky, H. H. and Berkeley, H. A. (1977). A precision toothpulp stimulation technique for the assessment of pain threshold. *Behavioral Research Methods Instrumentation*, **9**, 463–465.

Dworkin, B. R., Filewich, R. J., Miller, N. E., Craigmyle, N. and Pickering, T. G. (1979). Baroreceptor activation reduces reactivity to noxious stimulation: Implications for hypertension. *Science*, **205**, 1299–1301.

Garsik, J. T., Low, W. C. and Whitehorn, D. (1983). Differences in transmission through the dorsal column nuclei in spontaneously hypertensive and Wistar Kyoto rats. *Brain Research*, **271**, 188–192.

Graham, D. T., Kabler, J. D. and Graham, F. K. (1962a). Physiological responses to the suggestion of attitudes specific for hives and hypertension. *Psychosomatic Medicine*, **24**, 159–169.

Graham, D. T., Lundry, R. M., Benjamin, L. S., Kabler, J. D., Lewis, W. C., Kunish, N. O. and Graham, F. K. (1962b). Specific attitudes in initial interviews with patients have different 'psychosomatic' diseases. *Psychosomatic Medicine*, **24**, 257–266.

Harris, A. H., Gilliam, W. J., Findley, J. D. and Brady, J. V. (1973). Instrumental conditioning of large-magnitude, daily, 12-hour blood pressure elevations in the baboon. *Science*, **182**, 175–177.

Jonsson, A. and Hansson, L. (1977). Prolonged exposure to a stressful stimulus (noise) as a cause of raised blood-pressure in man. *The Lancet*, **I**, 86–87.

Koch, E. B. (1937). Die irradiation der pressoreceptorischen kresilaufrefdlexe. In Schweitzer, A. (Ed.), *Die Irradiation Autonomer Reflex*. Karger, Basel.

Lee, M. H. M., Zarestky, H. H., Ernest, M., Dworkin, B. and Jonas, R. (1985). The analgesic effects of aspirin and placebo on experimentally induced tooth pulp pain. *Journal of Medicine*, **16**, 417–428.

Miller, N. E., Davis, J. D. and Lulenski, G. C. (1968). Comparative studies of barbiturate self-administration. *Journal of the Additions*, **3**, 207–214.

Peterson, E. A., Augenstein, J. S., Tanis, D. C. and Augenstein, D. G. (1981). Noise raises blood pressure without impairing auditory sensitivity. *Science*, **211**, 1450–1452.

Pickering, T. G., Brucker, B., Frankel, H. L., Mathias, C. J., Dworkin, B. R. and Miller, N. E. (1977). Mechanisms of learned voluntary control of blood pressure in patients with generalized bodily paralysis. In Beatty, J. and Legewie, H. (Eds), *Biofeedback and Behavior*. Plenum Press, New York.

Plumlee, L. (1969). Operant conditioning of increases in blood pressure. *Psychophysiology*, **6**, 283–290.

Randich, A. and Maixner, W. (1984). Interactions between cardiovascular and pain regulatory systems. *Neuroscience and Biobehavioral Reviews*, **8**, 342–367.

Schlager, E. and Meier, T. (1947). A strange Balinese method of inducing sleep. *Acta Tropica*, **4**, 127–134.

Weiner, H., Singer, M. T. and Reiser, M. F. (1962). Cardiovascular responses and their psychological correlates: a study in healthy young adults and patients with peptic ulcer and hypertension. *Psychosomatic Medicine*, **24**, 477–497.

Weiss, S. and Baker, J. P. (1933). The carotid sinus reflex in health and disease: its role in the causation of fainting and convulsions. *Medicine*, **12**, 297–354.

Zamir, N. and Segal, M. (1979). Hypertension-induced analgesia: changes in pain sensitivity in experimental hypertensive rats. *Brain Research*, **160**, 170–173.

Zamir, N. and Shuber, E. (1980). Altered pain perception in hypertensive humans. *Brain Research*, **201**, 471–474.

APPENDIX

A new non-invasive method for studying the behavioral effects of baroreceptor stimulation in humans

The baroreceptors appear to have important effects on arousal and pain perception (Dworkin *et al.*, 1979), which could have implications for the etiology and treatment of hypertension, but because of the invasive nature of most techniques for stimulating the baroreceptors, demonstrations of baroreceptor influences on behavior have been largely confined to animal experiments. Clinical observations and correlational studies suggest that similar effects exist in humans, however, experimental studies in patients and normal subjects are needed to estimate the magnitude of the effects and to establish the relationship of ascending baroreceptor influences to hypertension.

Of the several methods for experimental stimulations of the carotid sinus baroreceptors in humans, only the pressure-regulated external neck chamber produces an adequate, reliable physiological effect and is sufficiently non-invasive to permit extensive behavioral studies. The operation of the neck chamber is based upon a simple physical principle: since the baroreceptors are actually stretch receptors in the wall of the carotid sinus and respond to the pressure difference between the inside and outside of the sinus, an extravascular pressure change influences the receptors exactly as does an equal magnitude opposite signed intravascular change. For example, lowering the pressure in the tissue surrounding the sinus by 20 cmH$_2$O will cause the receptors to fire as if the intravascular pressure had been increased by 20 cmH$_2$O. In contrast to this conceptual elegance actual implementation of the neck chamber technique has proved awkward. Most neck chambers are quite large and resemble either a deep-sea diver's helmet perforated by a mouth tube to permit free breathing or relatively large rigid cylinders resting on the shoulders and sealed with a rubber diaphragm above the chin (Thron *et al.*, 1967; Ludbrook *et al.*, 1977; Kober and Arndt, 1970). These cumbersome devices enclose relatively large volumes of air, and transmit pressure changes to the extra-carotid tissue uniformly and quantitatively, but also relatively slowly.

While the neck chamber has been used extensively for human physiology (Mancia and Mark, 1983; Mark and Mancia, 1983), there are few studies in the psychophysiological literature employing the neck chamber to study baroreceptor influences on behavior. This is most likely because neck suction

Neck chamber phase diagram

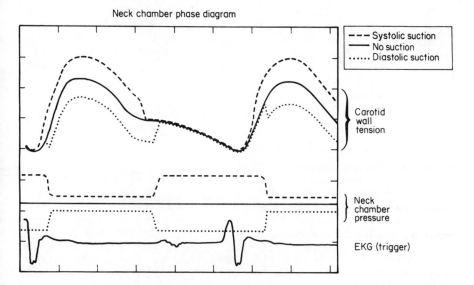

Figure A1. The solid curve is the normal pulse pressure wave as reflected in carotid sinus wall tension. When the QRS complex directly triggers a brief application of suction (dashed curves), the negative pressure burst in the neck chamber adds to the systolic peak pressure and results in an enhanced pulse amplitude; however, if the suction pulse is delayed until diastole (dotted curves) the suction instead elevates the effective diastolic level and, thus, reduces the systolic–diastolic difference.

is a perspicuous, somewhat annoying stimulus, and it is difficult to arrange a suitably convincing, psychologically equivalent 'placebo' condition. The neck chamber may produce a relatively 'pure' physiological stimulus, but psychologically its effects are complicated; without an appropriate control procedure, it is difficult to be confident that an observed behavioral effect is due only to the pressure differential created across the sinus wall and not simple distraction from the suction associated sensation.

So far the best control devised has been to compare the effects of positive and negative neck pressure. Using this technique, which assumes that pressure in the neck chamber should have similar general sensory effects to suction, but opposite effects on the sinus wall, Rockstroh *et al.* (Chapter 3) have demonstrated reliable effects on slow cortical potentials, and on reactivity to cutaneous electric shock. The results of these experiments are generally concordant with previous animal studies: baroreceptor stimulation (negative neck pressure) both induces cortical positivity and attenuates the reactivity of borderline hypertensive subjects to noxious stimulation as compared to the placebo (positive neck pressure) condition.

A simplified neck chamber developed by Eckberg *et al.* (1975) consists of a malleable hemi-ellipsoidal shell of thin lead sheet, which is placed below the

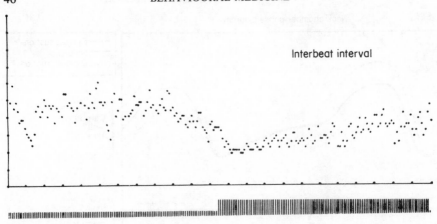

Figure A2. The interbeat interval response to systolic-suction/diastolic-pressure (low marker), and diastolic-suction/systolic-pressure (higher marker) in a 27-year-old male normotensive subject. There were 113 heart beats under each condition, and both the suction and pressure were limited to 20 cmH$_2$O. The mean pressure per cardiac cycle was 0 ± 2 cmH$_2$O.

chin so that the apex spans between the mandibles and the clavicle and the tapering poles wrap toward, but do not reach, the back of the neck. The edges of the metal are covered with high density closed cell rubber foam to improve the subject's comfort and insure a conforming seal against the skin. The edges of the chamber can be manually reformed to accommodate individual variations in surface anatomy. In its simplest application the chamber is connected through a port and hose to the suction inlet of a conventional domestic vacuum cleaner. The arrangement can easily develop a pressure of more than -60 cmH$_2$O, and Eckberg (1976) has shown that considerable lower levels are effective physiological stimuli. The Eckberg chamber has been criticized by some baroreceptor physiologists because it fails to completely encircle the neck and, thus, may produce non-uniform tissue pressure (Mancia and Mark, 1983, p. 755); however, the more compact design also has an advantage: the relatively low included volume facilitates the rapid changes in pressure necessary to dynamically stimulate the sinus at frequencies approximating those of the cardiac cycle.

We have recently developed a neck suction baroreceptor stimulation technique, which we believe will be more practical for behavioral studies. It is based on the original design of the Eckberg *et al.* (1975) chamber and subsequent observations by Eckberg (1976) on the effectiveness of briefly applied pulses of suction delivered during different phases of the cardiac cycle. Because the carotid stretch receptors are at least as sensitive to rate of change as static levels of pressure, it is possible to manipulate receptor firing rate through changes in pulse amplitude. *Application of a brief external suction burst during systole enhances the pulse amplitude by addition with the intravascular pressure peak;*

whereas exactly the same brief external burst applied later, in diastole, reduces the pulse amplitude. Figure A1 illustrates this effect. To the subject, who is unaware of the phase relationship to the cardiac cycle, the two conditions are perceptually indistinguishable, but as the data in Figure A2 show, the cardiovascular consequences are quite different.

Figure A1 does not show the resultant effect of the mean arterial pressure (MAP). In the procedure exactly as described above the virtual MAP, i.e. mean wall tension, in the sinus, would be elevated under both neck pressure–cardiac cycle phase relationships; however, the MAP can be independently determined by using positive as well as negative neck chamber pressures. In fact the data upon which Figure A2 is based were collected using alternating positive and negative neck chamber pressures with the magnitudes adjusted to a resultant zero average pressure over each cardiac cycle. Assuming a reasonably linear relationship between the neck chamber and extra-sinus pressure (Eckberg and Eckberg, 1982; Bronk and Stella, 1932; Kalkoff, 1957; Kober and Arndt, 1970) except for activation of reflex mechanisms, the MAP should not be affected.

References to appendix

Bronk, D. W. and Stella, G. (1932). Afferent impulses in the carotid sinus nerve. *Journal of Cell and Comparative Physiology*, **1**, 113–130.

Dworkin, B. R., Filewich, R. J., Miller, N. E., Craigmyle, N. and Pickering, T. G. (1979). Baroreceptor activation reduces reactivity to noxious stimulation: Implications for hypertension. *Science*, **205**, 1299–1301.

Eckberg, D. L. (1976). Temporal response patterns of the human sinus node to brief carotid baroreceptor stimuli. *Journal of Physiology*, **258**, 769–782.

Eckberg, D. L., Cavanaugh, M. S., Mark, A. L. and Abboud, F. M. (1975). A simplified neck suction device for activation of carotid baroreceptors. *Journal of Laboratory Clinical Medicine*, **85**, 167–173.

Eckberg, D. L. and Eckberg, M. J. (1982). Human sinus node responses to repetitive, ramped carotid baroreceptor stimuli. *American Journal of Physiology*, **242**, H638–H644.

Kalkoff, W. V. (1957). Pressorezeptorische Aktionspotentiale und blutdruckregulation. *Verhandlungen der Deutschen Gesellschaft für Kreislaufforschung*, **23**, 397–401.

Kober, G. and Arndt, J. O. (1970). Die cruck-durchmesser-beziehung der A. carotis communis des wachen menschen. *Pflugers Archiv*, **314**, 27–39.

Ludbrook, J., Mancia, G., Ferrari, A. and Zanchetti, A. (1977). The variable-pressure neck-chamber method for studying the carotid baroreflex in man. *Clinical Sciences and Molecular Medicine*, **53**, 165–171.

Mancia, G. and Mark, A. L. (1983). Arterial baroreflexes in humans. In Shepherd, J. T. and Abboud, F. M. (Eds), *The Handbook of Physiology: The Cardiovascular System*. Williams and Wilkins, Baltimore, pp. 755–793.

Mark, A. L. and Mancia, G. (1983). Cardiopulmonary baroreflexes in humans. In Shepherd, J. T. and Abboud, F. M. (Eds), *The Handbook of Physiology: The Cardiovascular System*. Williams and Wilkins, Baltimore, pp. 795–813.

Thron, H. L., Brechmann, W., Wagner, J. and Keller, K. (1967). Quantitative untersuchungen uber die bedeutung der gefassdehnungsreceptoren im rahmen der kreislaufhomoiostase beim wach menchen. *Pflugers Archiv*, **293**, 68–99.

Behavioural Medicine in Cardiovascular Disorders
Edited by T. Elbert, W. Langosch, A. Steptoe and D. Vaitl
©1988 John Wiley & Sons Ltd

3

The Influence of Baroreceptor Activity on Pain Perception

Brigitte Rockstroh*, Barry Dworkin[†],
Werner Lutzenberger*, Wolfgang Larbig*, Monique Ernst[‡],
Thomas Elbert*, and Niels Birbaumer[§]

*Department of Clinical and Physiological Psychology,
University of Tübingen, FRG
[†]Hershey Medical Center, Hershey, PA, USA
[‡]Psychiatry Department, Beth Israel Medical Center, New York, NY
[§]Department of Clinical Psychology, Pennsylvania State University,
University Park, PA, USA

Activation of the baroreceptor reflex arc is likely to result in central inhibitory effects (Lacey and Lacey, 1970; Bonvallet et al., 1953). On the basis of behavioral, as well as pharmacological data suggesting a relationship between elevated blood pressure (BP) and pain regulatory mechanisms, Dworkin (Dworkin et al., 1979; see also Randich and Maixner, 1984) concluded that the baroreceptor induced reduction in pain sensitivity may serve as a reward (negative reinforcement) in learning to elevate blood pressure. The reinforcing effects may be due to cortical deactivation, or dampening of brain-stem arousal (Puizillout et al., 1984) with baroreceptor firing. As a consequence hypertension would be favoured through operant conditioning, in chronic pain or under frequent stressful conditions.

While experimental evidence from deafferentation studies supports the view that the sinoaortic baroreceptor reflex arc is related to antinociception (Dworkin et al., 1979), this covariation has to be further validated for humans. As a measure for the influence of baroreceptor stimulation on brain activation, slow brain potentials (SPs) can be recorded from the intact human brain. SPs (the contingent negative variation, CNV) are influenced by afferent arousal pathways originating in the reticular formation. Negative SPs result from depolarization of apical dendrites in the upper cortical layers (Caspers et al., 1984), whereas cortical positivity may indicate inhibition spreading in the upper cortical layers.

In an earlier study (see Larbig *et al.*, 1985) we investigated pain tolerance to an intense electric shock, as well as slow brain potentials (SPs) under the influence of an alpha-sympathomimeticum (Norfenefrin, Novadral). Pain tolerance was evaluated by response latency to terminate the shock and by subjective ratings. In a within-subject cross-over design effects of 5 to 15 mg Norfenefrin were compared with the effects of a saline placebo. In contrast to subjects with low blood pressure borderline hypertensives (with systolic BP above 130 mmHg and diastolic BP above 90 mmHg) showed higher BP elevation, larger heart rate decrease, and increased pain tolerance in response to Norfenefrin as compared to the placebo condition; the terminal CNV (negative slow potential shift) was reduced in amplitude under Norfenefrin, especially in borderline hypertensives. This result strengthens the idea of an antinociceptive influence of baroreceptor activity only for borderline hypertensives. Normotensives showed decreased pain tolerance with drug induced BP elevation. This raises the question, whether the observed differences would covary in all subjects equally well with tonic BP or whether the regulatory loops would be different in normotensives and borderline hypertensives (or also in essential hypertensives).

The present study I investigated this hypothesis by measuring electro-cortical responses (EEG synchronization, slow event related potentials) and pain sensitivity during mechanical stimulation of the pressoreceptors in the area of the carotid sinus.

STUDY I

Method

Twenty male volunteers (mean age 23 years) were selected with either normal ($n = 10$, systolic below 120 mmHg, diastolic below 90 mmHg) or elevated blood pressure ($n = 10$, systolic values between 130 and 160 mmHg, diastolic values above 90 mmHg). The sample was selected from a population of healthy university students, who were totally naive with respect to their BP. For each subject, blood pressure was measured under resting conditions in a sitting position on 2 days different from the day of the experimental session at the same time of the day. Subjects were assigned to the normotensive group, if all systolic values were below 120 mmHg and all diastolic values were below 90 mmHg, or to the group of borderline hypertensives, if all systolic values were above 130 mmHg and diastolic values were above 90 mmHg. (These subjects are labeled borderline hypertensives here, although this would not fit precisely with the WHO definition of hypertension and borderline hypertension.) The group average for the normotensives turned out to be 115.8 ± 0.6 mmHg (range 113–118 mmHg), for borderliners 138.3 ± 1.7 mmHg (range 134–152 mmHg); a t-value of $t(18) = 12.5$ characterizes the separation within the independent variable. The respective values for diastolic BP are 76.3 ± 3.6 mmHg for the normotensives and 82.5 ± 4.5 mmHg for borderline hypertensives.

Every subject participated in one experimental session; subjects were asked neither to consume any caffeine containing nutrition nor to smoke prior to the experimental session.

Baroreceptor activity was manipulated by varying carotid sinus transmural pressure. This was realized by changing the external cervical pressure within a cuff around the neck for periods of 6 s. A negative external cervical pressure (suction) would be expected to produce a stretching of the carotid sinus, and hence an increase in baroreceptor activity (Eckberg *et al.*, 1975; Eckberg *et al.*, 1976; Toon *et al.*, 1984). Thirty-two trials with reduced atmospheric pressure in the cuff (baroreceptor stimulation) were interspersed pseudo-randomly with 32 trials with slight excess pressure (control). The two different conditions were associated with two signal tones. For half of the subjects, a high-pitched tone was presented for 6 s during pressure reduction and a low-pitched tone during the control trials. This relationship was reversed for the other half of the sample.

The ECG was recorded from the lower rib cage (V1–V5). *Heart rate* (HR), converted from R–R intervals, was averaged for each subject and condition (suction, control) across trials. *Pulse volume amplitude* (PVA) was scored during each R–R interval as the maximal change (peak to peak) in photo-plethysmographic finger pulse. *Pulse transit time* (PTT) was calculated from the upstroke of the R-wave to the point in time when the pulse wave reached its maximum. Statistical significance of differences was evaluated by analyses of variance (ANOVA) with the between-subjects factor *groups* and the within-subjects factor *condition* (suction–blow control).

For the evaluation of *event-related potentials*, a DC record of the EEG was obtained from frontal (F_z), central (C_z, C_3, C_4), and parietal (P_z) leads referred to shunted earlobes. In order to control for eye-movement artifacts in the EEG, the changes in the ocular dipole field (vertical, lateral, and radial) were monitored according to Elbert *et al.* (1985). A digital band pass (8 to 12 Hz), based on the algorithm of complex demodulation (Lutzenberger *et al.*, 1985) served to obtain a continuous record of the alpha-power of each 100 ms point.

Pain sensitivity was evaluated by applying an electrical stimulus to the left ventral forearm; electric stimulation started 4 s after the beginning of each pressure change and increased in intensity; subjects were asked to interrupt the stimulus by pressing a button whenever it would become uncomfortable (i.e., annoying and at pain threshold). Subjects were informed that an electric shock would be used during the experiment, and that they would set its maximal intensity themselves. The shock was administered via concentric Tursky electrodes. Shock intensity ranged from 0.2 mA at the beginning of the shock work-up procedure to a maximum of 3.0 mA, the highest value administered to any subject. During each trial shock

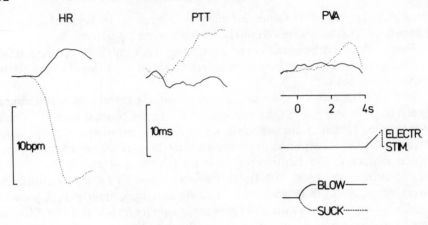

Figure 1. Time course of the cardiovascular responses heart rate (HR), pulse transit time (PTT), and pulse volume amplitude (PVA) during 1 s pre-stimulus baseline and 4 s pressure change interval averaged across Ss and trials.

intensity increased linearly so that its maximal intensity would be reached after 2 s. Thus, a reaction time of 1 s means that the subject interrupted shock application at 50% of its maximal possible intensity.

Results

Figure 1 illustrates the cardiovascular effects of the stimulation; these results are similar to those reported by Toon *et al.* (1984), confirming that the stimulation method had indeed the desired effects on the baroreflex. As compared to the blow control, a baroreflex during suction was indicated by a significant HR deceleration ($F(1,18) = 123.7$, $p < 0.001$), increased pulse volume amplitude (PVA), i.e., vasodilation ($F(1,18) = 5.1$, $p < 0.05$), and a prolonged pulse transit time (PTT, $F(1,18) = 8.3$, $p < 0.01$). Cardiovascular measures did not discriminate between the groups.

Overall, borderline hypertensives (B) tolerated the electrical stimulus longer than normotensives (N) (Figure 2). Mean reaction time (RT) was 1.083 ± 0.069 s for N and 1.371 ± 0.047 s for B (groups: $F(1,18) = 11.9$, $p < 0.01$). Furthermore, borderline hypertensives delayed their button press under baroreceptor stimulation, while normotensives demonstrated the reversed relationship. Mean RT difference (suction-control) for N was -33 ± 12 ms, $t(9) = 2.77$, $p < 0.05$; for B $+34 \pm 11$ ms, $t(9) = 3.12$, $p < 0.05$. The interaction between groups and condition reaches $F(1,18) = 17.2$ ($p < 0.01$).

Event-related desynchronization of the EEG (Figure 3) was generally more pronounced in B than in N, reaching a maximal reduction of 22% in B but only 16% in N (groups: $F(1,18) = 6.2$, $p < 0.05$). Four seconds after pressure

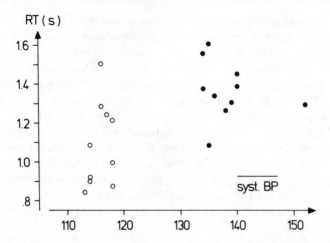

Figure 2. Reaction times (RT in seconds) averaged across all trials for every subject. Circles represent normotensives (N), dots borderline hypertensive (B) subjects.

change onset, i.e., the second prior to the onset of the electrical stimulation, alpha power values had returned to baseline in N, while the alpha block was still persistent (by 8%) in B ($F(1,18) = 12.1, p < 0.05$). Pre-trial absolute alpha-power did not differ between groups. EEG desynchronization proved not to be sensitive for pressure manipulation.

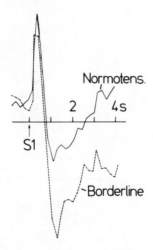

Figure 3. Event-related desynchronization of the precentral (mean of C_3 and C_4) EEG as indicated by the change in mean alpha power during the 4 s suction/control interval, calculated separately for N and B.

Pressure change onset signalled the onset of electrical stimulation 4 s later. During such anticipatory intervals a slow surface-negative potential, a contingent negative variation (CNV), is commonly observed (Walter, 1964; Rockstroh *et al.*, 1982; Rohrbaugh and Gaillard, 1983). As illustrated by Figure 4, a CNV typical in morphology and scalp distribution developed under control conditions. Baroreceptor stimulation markedly reduced the terminal CNV at all recording sites $(F_z - C_z - P_z$: $F(1,18) = 16.6$, $p < 0.01$; $C_3 - C_z - C_4$: $F(1,18) = 14.5$, $p < 0.01)$. This reduction, however, differed in scalp distribution between groups (see Figure 5): N but not B showed a significant *parietal* CNV reduction $(t(9) = 2.3$, $p < 0.05)$. Furthermore, N but not B exhibited *lateral asymmetry* during baroreceptor stimulation. In normotensives, positivity was prominent at C_3 but not at C_4, the difference being $9.8 \pm 2.9 \mu V$ $(t(9) = 3.35$, $p < 0.01)$ (for the group difference under suction $t(18) = 3.02$, $p < 0.01)$.

Discussion

These results add further evidence for a reduced pain sensitivity under baroreceptor firing, but *only in borderline hypertensives*. This group exhibits the predicted behavior of reduced pain sensitivity under baroreceptor stimulation. The same mechanism could have been responsible for the overall prolonged

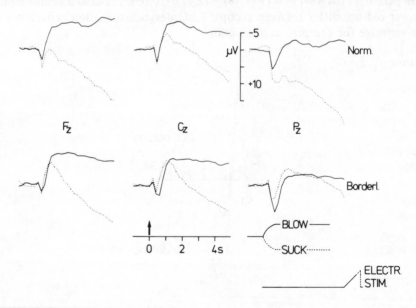

Figure 4. Event-related slow potentials averaged across trials separately for conditions (baroreceptor stimulation: suck, and control: blow) groups (normotensives and borderline hypertensives), and electrode locations along the mid-sagittal line: frontal: F_z, precentral: C_z, parietal: P_z (from Elbert *et al.*, 1988).

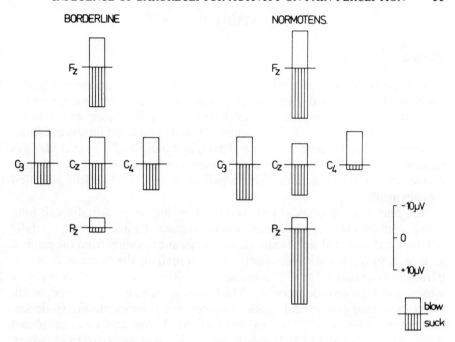

Figure 5. Magnitude of the terminal CNV (in μV) measured as the average voltage during the fourth second (the second prior to the onset of electrical stimulation) separately for the groups (borderline hypertensives, normotensives), conditions (white bars: suck, i.e., baroreceptor stimulation; hatched bars: blow, i.e., control condition), and electrode locations: F_z (mid-frontal), C_z (vertex), P_z (mid-parietal), C_3 (left precentral), C_4 (right precentral).

response latency in B as compared to N. But why is it that N increase their pain sensitivity under baroreceptor stimulation as compared to control conditions? No differences in cardiovascular responsivity could be detected indicating similar effects of baroreceptor afferentation on brain stem and the cardiovascular system. Only central nervous differences may provide an explanatory background for the differential responding to pain stimulation of N and B. Although both groups showed a reduction in negativity under baroreceptor stimulation indicating cortical inhibition, N but not B showed a differential pattern between hemispheres: N's inhibition of the projection areas for the pain afferents (C_4) under baroreceptor stimulation is less pronounced than that in B, but rather more intense at the other recording sites, the effects being significant for P_z, C_3 and (as a tendency) F_z (see Figure 5).

This raised the question, whether N and B have 'different brains' or whether a tonic change in BP by itself would alter the brain's processing of pain stimulation. This question was approached by pharmacological manipulation of tonic BP in normotensives.

STUDY II

Method

In a single-blind, within-subjects, cross-over design, 10 male normotensive volunteers (mean BP 120/79 mmHg) participated in two sessions each, received an alpha-sympathomimeticum (phenylephrine) in one session and a saline placebo in the other session. Phenylephrine was administered intravenously by an infusion at an amount which was determined individually so that HR was reduced by 15% of its baseline value. Saline was infused during the placebo control session. Injection started after a baseline period with four pain sensation measurements.

Pain sensation thresholds were evaluated by means of dental tooth pulp stimulation: Stimulation was delivered to the surface of a dental filling carefully selected on the basis of size, location, resistance, and isolation from the gingival surface. A snugly fitted silicone rubber mold containing the platinum electrode (Grass Instruments E22) was constructed for each subject and provided a moisture-proof electrode assembly. The filling was used as the cathode, which insured identical geometrical relationship between the stimulus electrode and the sensory receptive field over repeated sessions. A solid gold electrode placed in the buccal pouch served as the anode. Electrodes were connected to a constant current stimulus of special design. Stimulation was delivered every 10 s as a train of 200 ms duration consisting of monopolar square 1 ms pulses at 100 Hz. The resistance of the preparation was controlled with an ohmmeter prior to and following the experimental period. Stimulus intensities ranged between 0 and 1000 μA, with an average between 100 and 300 μA. Two perceptual levels were determined by means of the method of ascending limits using uniform current increments of 5 μA. The detection thresholds corresponded to the first level of intensity at which the subject signaled its perception three times in a row. For this determination the subject was instructed to press the button each time he felt anything. The discomfort level corresponded to the drug request threshold. The subject was instructed to press the button when the sensation reaches a level of discomfort, that if persisting, would prompt him to take aspirin. As a measure for the change in subjective discomfort threshold the mean difference in current intensities between drug condition and baseline period was subtracted from the mean difference in current intensities under placebo condition referred to baseline.

The EEG was recorded as reported for study I. EEG desynchronization was evaluated as described above. Furthermore, evoked potentials to tooth pulp stimulation were recorded by applying a series of 50 stimuli between the second and the third threshold determination. Twenty-five stimuli set at a level above the discomfort value and 25 stimuli below discomfort value according to the preceding threshold determination were administered in pseudorandom order.

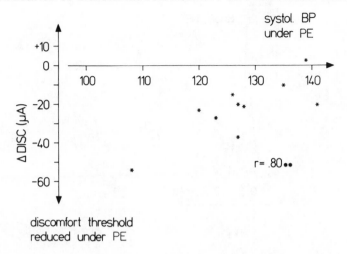

Figure 6. Change in discomfort threshold between phenylephrine and placebo treatment (ordinate) plotted against the baseline systolic BP for every S. Product-moment correlation $r = 0.80$ explains 63% of the variance ($p < 0.01$).

For every measure, the difference in change between placebo and drug conditions, calculated as the difference between baseline and placebo minus the difference between baseline and drug is reported.

Results

Relative to placebo conditions phenylephrine treatment resulted in an average *heart rate* (HR) decrease compared to the baseline mean of 67 bpm by 9.4 ± 2.0 bpm ($F(1,9) = 21.2$, $p < 0.01$), in an average increase of the *systolic BP* by 7 mmHg ($F(1,9) = 6.3$, $p < 0.01$) and of the *diastolic BP* by 10 mmHg ($F(1,9) = 20.3$, $p < 0.01$).

Figure 6 illustrates that 9 out of 10 Ss reduced their *discomfort threshold* to dental tooth pulp stimulation during baroreceptor stimulation by a mean of $22.4 \pm 8 \mu A$ ($t(9) = 4.64$, $p < 0.01$). This reduction correlated with the pre-experimental systolic BP ($r = 0.78$, $p < 0.01$), as well as with systolic BP under phenylephrine ($r = 0.80$, $p < 0.01$), while the relationship to the experimentally induced HR deceleration via baroreceptor stimulation was less pronounced (absolute HR decrease $r = 0.55$, $p < 0.1$; relative HR decrease: $r = 0.63$, $p < 0.05$). The *detection* threshold was neither significantly correlated with the cardiovascular parameters nor significantly affected by the experimental manipulations.

No treatment effect on the EEG synchronization measure could be found (see Figure 7).

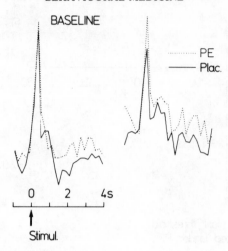

Figure 7. Event-related EEG desynchronization in response to the tooth pulp stimulation. Traces are averaged across Ss, the electrode locations and the two levels of stimulus intensity, separately for the two sessions with either drug (dotted) or placebo (solid) treatment. Left graph: superimposed traces for the baseline period (prior to injection), right graph: superimposed traces for the period after drug or placebo injection. Upward direction indicates increase in alpha power. Except for a general increase in synchronization across each session, no systematic difference would be observed.

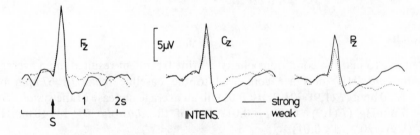

Figure 8. Event-related slow brain potentials in response to tooth pulp stimuli above (solid) and below (dotted) discomfort threshold averaged separately for electrode locations across Ss and trials (negativity up).

A parietocentral ($F(2,18) = 5.0$, $p < 0.05$) slow positive wave in the slow *event related potential* to pain stimuli with an intensity above and below discomfort threshold, which peaks after 0.7 s, was sensitive to stimulus intensity ($F(1,9) = 11,6$, $p < 0.01$). This suggests that this positive slow wave should be considered a cortical indicator of pain perception. The more, since (across subjects) the slow wave amplitude correlated with the subjective change in discomfort threshold. This is true for slow waves elicited by weak (below discomfort threshold) stimuli ($r = 0.57$, $p < 0.1$), as well as for slow waves in response to strong stimuli ($r = 0.66$, $p < 0.05$; see Figure 8). The slow wave amplitudes elicited by the two different stimulus intensities correlated with $r = 0.73$, $p < 0.05$ across subjects. Similarly to the discomfort threshold, the pre-experimental systolic BP correlated with the positive slow wave in response to the weak ($r = 0.69$, $p < 0.05$), as well as for the strong stimulus ($r = 0.57$, $p < 0.1$).

Discussion

Similarly to the normotensives' behavior in the first study, subjects in the second study demonstrated decreased pain sensation threshold under baroreceptor stimulation induced by pharmacological means. The experimentally induced tonic increase in BP did not reverse the relationship between pain sensation and baroreceptor activity. Furthermore, there is a discriminative effect of baro-receptor stimulation on pain sensitivity related to the pain sensory level: no effect is proven on low pain level (pain detection) but an inhibitory effect is obvious on higher pain level (discomfort). The differences in EEG measures between N and B in the first study cannot be attributed to a transient change in tonic BP, since no similarity with the B patterns was induced under phenylephrine. Instead, the high correlation between pre-experimental BP values and change in discomfort threshold points again at a constitutional difference between normotensives and borderline hypertensives. Assume that humans differ with respect to their psychophysiological circuits. In subjects in whom a BP increase, and hence an increase in baroreceptor firing, reduces the aversiveness of noxious stimulation, the BP increase can serve as a reward. If those subjects are exposed to painful or stressful conditions they would be frequently reinforced for blood pressure elevations. Higher BP would be the consequence of visceral learning depending upon environmental conditions (Dworkin, Chapter 2). If this mechanism is influential and if a sample of subjects is selected from a uniform population exposed to the same environmental conditions, then BP increase should reduce the aversiveness of noxious stimulation in those subjects with elevated BP much more than in normotensives. This assumption is supported by the present study. Dworkin's model would also predict that the same subjects with elevated BP should have a higher ability to learn to raise BP. This has to be proven by further studies.

Acknowledgements

Research was supported by the Deutsche Forschungsgemeinschaft and the W. and H. Mazer Foundation.

REFERENCES

Bonvallet, A., Dell, P. and Hiebel, G. (1953). Sinus carotidian et activité électrique cérébrale. *Compte rendu des séances de la Société de biologie*, **147**, 1166.

Caspers, H., Speckmann, E.-J. and Lehmenkühler, A. (1984). Electrogenesis of slow potentials of the brain. In Elbert, T., Rockstroh, B., Lutzenberger, W., Birbaumer, N. (Eds), *Self-Regulation of the Brain and Behavior*. Springer, Heidelberg, pp. 26–41.

Dworkin, B., Filewich, R., Miller, N., Craigmyle, N., Pickering, T. (1979). Baroreceptor activation reduces reactivity to noxious stimulation: Implications for hypertension. *Science*, **205**, 1299–1301.

Eckberg, D., Cavanaugh, M., Mark, A. and Abboud, F. (1975). A simplified neck suction device for activation of carotid baroreceptors. *Journal of Laboratory and Clinical Medicine*, **85**, 167–173.

Eckberg, D., Abboud, A. and Mark, A. (1976). Modulation of carotid baroreflex responsiveness in man: Effects of posture and propanolol. *Journal of Applied Physiology*, **41**, 383–387.

Elbert, T., Lutzenberger, W., Rockstroh, B. and Birbaumer, N. (1985). Removal of ocular artifacts from the EEG—A biophysical approach to the EOG. *Journal of Electroencephalography and Clinical Neurophysiology*, **60**, 455–463.

Elbert, T., Rockstroh, B., Lutzenberger, W., Kessler, M., Pietrowsky, R. and Birbaumer, N. (1988). Baroreceptor stimulation alters pain sensation depending on tonic blood pressure. *Psychophysiology*, **25**, 25–29.

Lacey, J. and Lacey, B. (1970). Some autonomic-central nervous system interrelationships. In Black, P. (Ed.), *Physiological Correlates of Emotion*. Academic Press, New York, pp. 205–277.

Larbig, W., Elbert, T., Rockstroh, B., Lutzenberger, W. and Birbaumer, N. (1985). Elevated blood pressure and reduction of pain sensitivity. In Orlebeke, J., Mulder, G. and van Doornen, L. (Eds), *Psychophysiology of Cardiovascular Control*. New York, Plenum, pp. 113–122.

Lutzenberger, W., Elbert, T., Rockstroh, B. and Birbaumer, N. (1985). *Das EEG*. Springer, Berlin.

Puizillout, J., Gaudin-Chazal, G. and Bras, H. (1984). Vagal mechanisms in sleep regulation. In Borbely, A. and Valatx, A. (Eds), *Sleep Mechanisms*. Springer, Berlin, pp. 19–38.

Randich, A. and Maixner, W. (1984). Interactions between cardiovascular and pain regulatory systems. *Neuroscience and Biobehaviour Review*, **8**, 343–367.

Rockstroh, B., Elbert, T., Birbaumer, N. and Lutzenberger, W. (1982). Slow Brain Potentials and Behavior. Urban & Schwarzenberg, Baltimore.

Rohrbaugh, J. and Gaillard, A. (1983). Sensory and motor aspects of the contingent negative variation. In Gaillard, A., Ritter, W. and Kok, A. (Eds), *Tutorials in Event Related Potential Research: Endogenous Components*. Elsevier, Amsterdam, pp. 269–310.

Toon, P. D., Bergel, D. H. and Johnston, D. W. (1984). The effect of modification of baroreceptor activity on reaction time. *Psychophysiology*, **21**, 487–493.

Walter, W. G. (1964). The contingent negative variation. An electrical sign of significance of association in the human brain. *Science*, **146**, 434.

Behavioural Medicine in Cardiovascular Disorders
Edited by T. Elbert, W. Langosch, A. Steptoe and D. Vaitl
©1988 John Wiley & Sons Ltd

4

Autonomic Stress Response in Patients with Essential Hypertension

Georg Wiedemann*, Rolf R. Engel[†] and Wolfgang Zander[‡]

Psychiatric Hospital, University of Munich

INTRODUCTION

The concept of a uniform, physiologically and likewise biochemically non-specific reaction to various stress situations in the sense of Selye is becoming more and more doubtful (Mason, 1975). This 'general adaption syndrome' according to Selye is often seen as contrasting with the theory of the biological specificity of emotional events (Lacey, 1967).

In earlier investigations we were able to show that physiological and biochemical reaction patterns differed clearly between healthy subjects and psychiatric patients, depending on whether the stress situation required activity (for instance mental arithmetics) or whether it was to be received passively (example: noise; Engel, 1986). Nonetheless, each stress situation was experienced subjectively as equally unpleasant and stressful by the subjects.

In the study presented here, it was decided to induce specific emotions which go beyond the dimensions of activity/passivity. In order to achieve this goal, short scenes from radio plays were used. In addition, a semi-standardized interview concerning the special conflicts and emotions of individual subjects was conducted.

Apart from the problem of the situational specificity of physiological reactions, the present study also addressed the question of the specific symptoms and physiological reactions of patients suffering from hypertension. This symptom specificity might appear in interaction with the experimental situations, or be independent of them.

*Städtisches Krankenhaus Bogenhausen, Abteilung für Psychosomatische Medizin, Englschalkinger Str. 77, D-8000 München 81, FRG.
[†]Psychiatrische Klinik der Universität München, Abteilung für Experimentelle und Klinische Psychologie, Nußbaumstr. 7, 8000 München 2, FRG.
[‡]Hildegardstr. 30 1/2 D-8035 Gauting, FRG.

METHOD

The sample for the present investigation was composed of 12 healthy subjects and 12 patients with essential hypertension. General selection criteria for all subjects and patients were an age between 20 and 45 and no more than 20% overweight.

All investigations were carried out in an electrically and acoustically shielded room. The session lasted approximately 2 hours. Each experiment consisted of the following experimental situations, which were separated by at least 2 minutes of rest.

Radio Play 1   A man leaves his girlfriend when she tells him she is pregnant: induction of pity (2 minutes duration).

Radio Play 2   The employment of a clerk's son as apprentice is refused by the director of the company: this play induced feelings of anger and rage (4 minutes duration).

Radio Play 3   Scene in which a couple caresses: dimensions of tenderness, security, and happiness are involved (3 minutes).

Passive stress situation   Noise of approximately 95 dB, composed partly of recordings of 'real' noise, for instance traffic noise, aeroplanes, people screaming in a football arena, and partly of the hooting of a sound generator.

Radio Play 4   A mother fears that something terrible has happened to her son: induction of fear (4 minutes duration).

Active stress situation   Mental arithmetic: serial subtraction of 7 from 500, in which the subject had to begin again in case of error (3 minutes duration).

Radio Play 5   An employee tells his wife about his own failure and the success of a colleague in the same company: feelings of inferiority and jealousy (6 minutes duration).

Subsequently a semi-standardized interview was held consisting of 10 areas of interest, in which we attempted to probe problem areas in an individually relevant manner.

All subjects assessed their subjective feelings during the experimental situations retrospectively with the aid of self-rating scales.

During the experiment the following physiological functions were continuously recorded:

1. Parameters of the cardiovascular systems: heart rate and pulse wave velocity, the latter serving as indirect indicator of blood pressure. These measurements were made using an analog computer. For every heart beat, the distance from heart to wrist was divided by the time between the R-wave in the ECG and the arrival of each pulse wave at the wrist.
2. Electrodermal reactions: palmar skin conductance level and the integrated area of the skin conductance responses recorded from the right hand.

3. Components of peripheral skin blood flow: finger pulse amplitude and the finger temperature of the left hand.
4. Electromyogram from the volar surface of the right forearm and from the forehead.
5. Electrogastrogram.
6. Respiratory volume.
7. Forehead temperature.

RESULTS

Physiological data were averaged within the experimental test situations and the rest phases and then subjected to an analysis of variance with one group factor (hypertensive patients/healthy subjects) and one trial factor, involving all nine situations. In order to clarify the possible effects of the radio plays more exactly, an additional analysis of variance was conducted with the trial factor consisting only of the five radio plays.

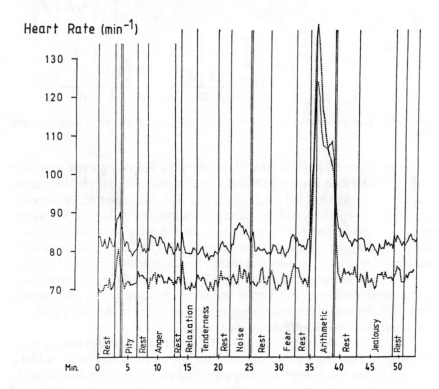

Figure 1. Mean of heart rate in hypertensive patients ($n = 12$, solid line) and controls ($n = 12$, broken line).

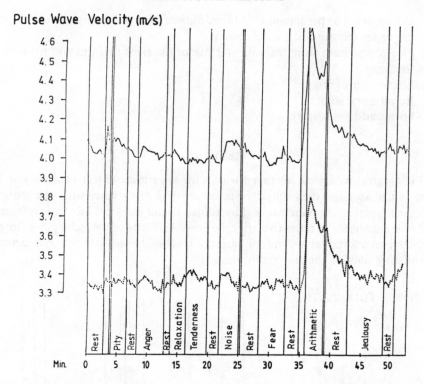

Figure 2. Mean of pulse wave velocity in hypertensive patients ($n = 12$, solid line) and controls ($n = 10$, broken line).

Average values of physiological parameters for the two groups were very similar. A significant main effect could be demonstrated only in the case of pulse wave velocity ($F(1,20) = 9.53$, $p < 0.01$). This was expected, because the hypertensive patients have a higher pulse wave velocity by definition. Situational specific differences between the normo- and hypertensive subjects were demonstrated by the respiratory volume responses ($F(1,22) = 6.64$, $p < 0.025$): An increased respiratory activity was manifest in hypertensive patients subjected to stress (mental arithmetic and noise), while there was little or no such reaction in normotensive subjects. In all other recordings, baseline values and response to standardized test conditions were similar: there were no further significant main effects and no significant interactions.

In contrast to the small group differences, marked differences were demonstrated between the various test situations: mental arithmetic caused a highly significant rise of heart rate (Figure 1) and pulse wave velocity (Figure 2). This was to be expected in the light of our earlier findings. Both of these cardiovascular parameters were distinctly uniform in all other test situations.

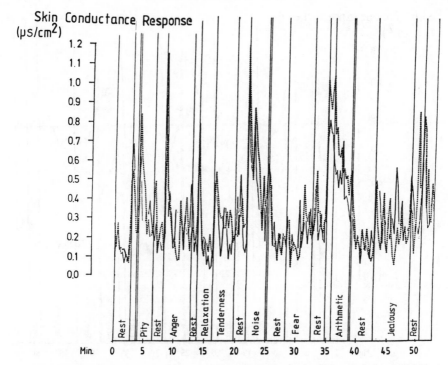

Figure 3. Mean of skin conductance level in hypertensive patients ($n = 11$, solid line) and controls ($n = 12$, broken line).

The very different pattern in the two electrodermal parameters is demonstrated in Figure 3 (skin conductance level) and Figure 4 (skin conductance response). In particular, a phasic increase in skin conductance response appears with every new stimulus, independent of its quality or the activity–passivity dimension. Peripheral blood flow showed a similar response to that seen in the electrodermal parameters, and was consistent with a general orienting response (Sokolov, 1963). The finger temperature, due to its more pronounced inertia, was much slower to respond than the finger pulse amplitude.

The electromyographic variables showed markedly different interactions with the test situations: like the cardiovascular system, the muscle tone on the lower arm (Figure 5) differentiated mainly along an activity–passivity dimension ($F(1,22) = 7.16$, $p < 0.025$) while the muscles of the forehead (Figure 6) covaried significantly with the nature of the radio plays' contents ($F(1,22) = 7.48$, $p < 0.025$). Those with unpleasant, anxiety-provoking contents (radio plays 2, 4, and 5 = aggression, fear, rivalry) caused more forehead muscle tension than the other two radio plays (pity and tenderness).

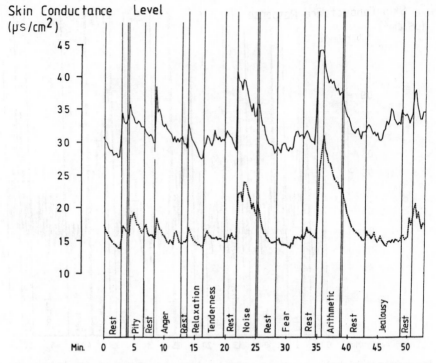

Figure 4. Mean of skin conductance response in hypertensive patients ($n = 12$, solid line) and controls ($n = 12$, broken line).

DISCUSSION

In the experiment presented here, the following two questions were considered in a combined design.

1. Are there specific physiological response patterns demonstrable for certain dimensions of experience (situational specificity)?
2. Are there group specific reaction patterns (symptom specificity) in patients with essential hypertension compared with healthy controls.

In accordance with hypotheses formulated by Lacey and Lacey (Lacey, 1967; Lacey and Lacey, 1974a,b) and later agreed upon by others (e.g. Obrist *et al.*, 1978), cardiovascular parameters differed markedly between situations demanding activity from the subjects and those which had to be endured passively. The activity-demanding situation of mental arithmetic was not felt to be any more unpleasant than the passive noise situation. Engel *et al.* (1980) were able to differentiate the purely motor from the psychological elements of reactions within the cardiovascular system. Since the motor components of mental arithmetic were only responsible for a smaller proportion of the

Forehead - EMG (µV)

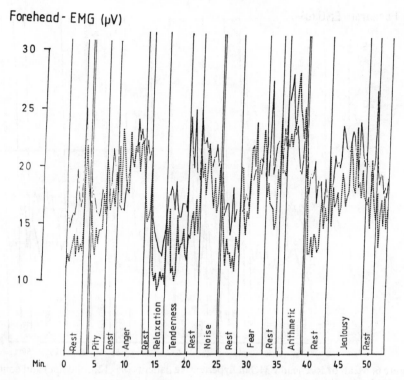

Figure 5. Mean of forearm EMG in hypertensive patients ($n = 12$, solid line) and controls ($n = 12$, broken line).

cardiovascular reaction, the reaction of these parameters is largely induced by cognitive and emotional components. Emotional factors, such as the fear of failure in a publicly performed task (like mental arithmetic) seems to play the most important part in these reactions.

In contrast to this pattern the electrodermal parameters changed in the manner of a non-specific orienting reaction to every new stimulus, depending on its novelty and challenging character. The other qualities of the situation seemed to be insignificant. The parameters of skin blood flow reacted qualitatively in a similar fashion (Engel and King, 1982). The two electromyographic variables reacted as elements of two different systems: that of limb muscles, which (just as the cardiovascular system does) covary with the activity component of a task, and the mimetic muscles, which alone among the physiological functions that were recorded, covaried significantly with the mood contents of the radio plays. In the muscular system, the limb muscles have a mainly preparatory function, while the mimetic muscles have more of an expressive function (Uexküll, 1967).

External factors in the test situation could not be held responsible for this result, since: (1) all test subjects rated the radio plays according to the emotion

Forearm- EMG (µV)

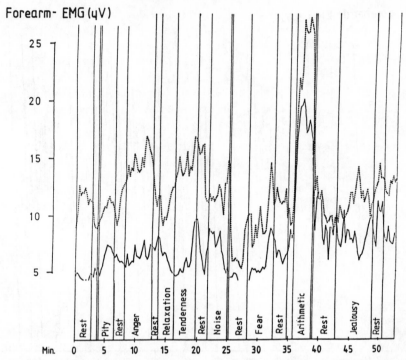

Figure 6. Mean of forehead EMG in hypertensive patients ($n = 12$, solid line) and controls ($n = 12$, broken line).

content that had been intended; (2) the standard situations could be differentiated from each other by different physiological variables in conformity with earlier experiments.

It must be generally concluded that listening to emotional events in a radio play induces certain feelings which are demonstrated in expressive behavior, but does not induce significant variations in autonomic parameters. In future investigations it will be important to place special emphasis on the fact that the experimental situations are experienced by the individual in an immediate and vitally important manner (Stemmler et al., 1983).

The increased respiratory activity of the hypertensive patients in comparison with normotensive subjects during stress (mental arithmetic and noise) can be explained as a preparatory function of the respiratory system. The cardiovascular parameters indicate that hypertensive patients have an increased tonus in the sympathetic nervous system. The hearts of hypertensives must perform more work during rest periods than those of normotensive individuals (raised blood pressure and heart rate); more pronounced sympathetic reactions in circulatory parameters could, however, only be demonstrated for pulse wave velocity.

Otherwise, contrary to the distinct effects produced by the laboratory situations, hardly any group differences were established in this investigation. This may be attributed to the fact that the diagnostic entity of essential hypertension probably consists of several subgroups whose physiological reactions to psychic stress situations are possibly very different. It could be that a separation between hypertension due to increased cardiac output and hypertension due to increased peripheral resistance could open new pathways for research in this area.

Acknowledgement

This study was supported by the Sandoz Foundation for Therapeutic Research.

REFERENCES

Engel, R. R. (1986). Aktivierung und Emotion. Psychophysiologische Experimente zur Struktur physiologischer Reaktionsmuster unter psychischer Belastung. Minerva, München.

Engel, R. R. and King, U. G. (1982). Periphere vaskuläre Reaktionen von Migränepatienten auf psychische und thermale Reize. In Huber, H. P. (Ed.), *Migräne*. München: Urban & Schwarzenberg, 1982, pp. 111–120.

Engel, R. R., Müller, F., Münch, U. and Ackenheil, M. M. (1980). Plasma catecholamine response and autonomic functions during shorttime psychological stress. In Udsin, E., Kvetnansky, R. and Kopin, J. J. (Eds), *Catecholamines and Stress: Recent Advances*. Elsevier, New York, pp. 461–466.

Lacey, J. I. (1967). Somatic response patterning and stress: Some revisions of activation theory. In Appley, M. H. and Trumbull, R. (Eds), *Psychological Stress*. Appleton-Century-Crofts, New York, pp. 14–37.

Lacey, J. I. and Lacey, B. C. (1974a). On heart rate responses and behavior: A reply to Elliott. *Journal of Personality and Social Psychology*, **30**, 1–18.

Lacey, J. I. and Lacey, B. C. (1974b). Studies of heart rate and other bodily processes in sensorimotor behavior. In Obrist, P., Black, A., Breuer, J. and DiCara, L. (Eds), *Cardiovascular Psychophysiology*. Aldine, Chicago, 1974.

Mason, J. W. (1975). A historical view of the stress field. *Journal of Human Stress*, **1**, 6–12 and 22–36.

Obrist, P. A., Gaebelin, C. J., Teller, E. S., Langer, A. W., Grignolo, A., Light, K. C. and Cubbin, J. A. (1978). The relationship among heart rate, carotid dP/dt, and blood pressure in humans as a function of the type of stress. *Psychophysiology*, **15**, 102–115.

Sokolov, E. N. (1963). *Perception and the Conditioned Reflex*. Macmillan, New York.

Stemmler, G., Bruhn, K. and Koch, U. (1983). Eine psychophysiologische Validierungsstudie zum Gottschalk-Gleser-Verfahren: Einführung. In Koch, U. (Ed.), *Sprachinhaltsanalyse in der psychosomatischen und psychiatrischen Forschung*. Beltz, Weinheim, chapter 1.

Uexküll, Th. (1967). *Grundfragen der Psychosomatischen Medizin*. Rowohlt, Hamburg.

Behavioural Medicine in Cardiovascular Disorders
Edited by T. Elbert, W. Langosch, A. Steptoe and D. Vaitl
©1988 John Wiley & Sons Ltd

5

The Study of Blood Pressure in Everyday Life

Thomas G. Pickering

The Cardiovascular Center, New York Hospital-Cornell Medical Center, New York, New York 10021

High blood pressure is now generally regarded as being the result of a number of factors which may be present in different combinations in different subjects. The traditional viewpoint of physicians is that these factors are largely physiological or biochemical, while consideration of the role of behavioral factors has largely been left to psychologists. Recognition of the role of behavioral factors has been limited for a number of reasons. One is the absence of a good animal behavioral model of hypertension, and another is the difficulty in quantifying such factors. It is relatively easy to measure an individual subject's level of sodium intake, but it is very difficult to measure his level of 'stress'. This problem is confounded by the fact that stress is an interactive phenomenon which depends not only on an environmental stimulus, but also on the way this is perceived by the individual.

Most studies on the influence of behavioral factors on hypertension have been carried out in the laboratory, using standardized adversive stimuli, and measuring the respone of blood pressure and other related variables. These studies have led to the unproven assumption that individuals with high levels of cardiovascular reactivity may be predisposed to develop hypertension (Hines and Brown, 1936), and also suffer from the limitation that the stressors that have been used often bear little resemblance to the types of stress that are experienced in real life.

Another traditional view that is rapidly being eroded is that hypertension is a fixed entity. The Joint National Committee (1984) recently attempted to classify individuals according to rigidly defined levels of blood pressure, and based their recommendations for treatment on these definitions. Despite this, it has been known for many years that blood pressure shows great variations, not only because of the effects of different activities and circumstances on blood pressure, but also because of unpredictable factors resulting in variations of pressure when measured in the same situation on different occasions. Since the decisions to start or change treatment depend on very small differences of blood pressure, the circumstances in which blood pressure is measured are becoming increasingly important.

The ability to record blood pressure outside the clinic or laboratory using non-invasive ambulatory monitoring techniques has provided the opportunity to overcome some of these problems. As long ago as 1940, Ayman and Goldshine observed that pressures taken in the clinic might be 30 or 40 mmHg higher than pressures taken at home, and suggested that extending blood pressure measurements in the home might have at least three advantages: first, a better understanding of factors that might affect the level of blood pressure; second, a better evaluation of prognosis in the individual patient; and, third, a better evaluation of the response to treatment. Now, after an interval of nearly 50 years, it appears that all of these predictions are coming true.

TECHNIQUES FOR MEASURING BLOOD PRESSURE IN NATURAL SETTINGS

There are two types of technique for measuring blood pressure outside the clinic or laboratory, and each has advantages and disadvantages. The first is a conventional sphygmomanometer with which the patient can take his or her blood pressure either at home or at the workplace. These range from the mercury sphygmomanometer to semi-automatic electronic devices.

The former is still generally the most reliable method, but is relatively expensive and cumbersome. A large number of electronic recorders is now commercially available, and they have the advantages of being portable and easier to use, and of eliminating observer bias from the readings. Their accuracy is often questionable, however, and each machine must be calibrated with each patient (Pickering et al., 1986). One of the main advantages of this type of recorder is that the patient can keep it at home (or at work), and obtain serial readings over a long period of time. Such a procedure could be of great value in evaluating the effectiveness of an intervention designed to lower the blood pressure in hypertensive patients, or in observing the effects of environmental stressors on blood pressure over long periods of time. Some authors have found that when hypertensive patients first start to record their home blood pressures the pressure tends to decrease over a period of a few weeks (Laughlin et al., 1979), as has commonly been observed with clinic pressures measured serially over time, although we did not find this to be the case in our study (Kleinert et al., 1984).

Figure 1 shows the daily averages of home blood pressures in a single hypertensive patient, whose pressure remained poorly controlled despite taking medication. It shows that blood pressure is higher in the morning than in the

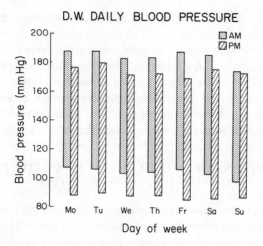

Figure 1. Average values of morning and evening home blood pressures taken by a hypertensive patient over several weeks. Note higher pressures in the morning, except Sunday.

evening, and that the morning pressures tend to be higher on work days (which included Saturday) than on Sunday.

The other, and potentially more useful, method for taking blood pressure in natural settings is with ambulatory blood pressure recorders. Continuous recordings of blood pressure can be obtained using direct intra-arterial pressure recording, but the use of these recorders is limited by their invasiveness and attendant potential hazards. Non-invasive ambulatory recorders have also been developed, and, while they are more convenient and free of any risk, they have the limitations of being less accurate and also of being only able to take readings intermittently. We have found that this last property is not necessarily such a disadvantage because, if the patients are instructed to make a diary entry at the time of each reading, it does permit a precise correlation between blood pressure and changes of physical or mental activity. This has usually not been done with continuous intra-arterial recordings. Another limitation of the inter-mittent recordings is that many of the peaks and troughs of pressure will be missed, so that it is not possible to obtain a true index of blood pressure variability. Mancia's group has shown, however, that if blood pressure recordings are made at least every 30 minutes, a reasonable approximation of the true diurnal variation can be obtained (Di Rienzo et al., 1983).

The non-invasive ambulatory recorders are of two sorts, the semi-automatic and fully automatic. Semi-automatic recorders such as the Remler require the patient to inflate the cuff, and then the machine stores the Korotkoff sounds on tape. From the point of view of behavioral studies, this type is unsatisfactory because the patient has to stop whatever he is doing, and it is often difficult to get readings at preset intervals. In addition, no sleep readings can be obtained.

The recorders that are being most widely used for behavioral studies are the fully automatic recorders. A number of these are now available. The earlier models are somewhat bulky, and do place some limitations on the patients' activities. Second and third generation recorders are now becoming available which are smaller and less obtrusive. It is still true, however, that all such recorders only provide accurate readings when the patient is relatively inactive.

COMPARISONS OF BLOOD PRESSURE IN THE CLINIC AND DURING EVERYDAY LIFE

The fact that blood pressure measured in the clinic is typically higher than pressure measured in the home has considerable theoretical and practical implications. On the theoretical side, it suggests that since the physical activity of the patient is similar in the two situations, the differences are due to psychological factors. On the practical side, it raises the possibility that many patients may be misclassified as being hypertensive. In general, there is a reasonably good correlation between clinic and home blood pressures (with a correlation coefficient of 0.6 to 0.7), but the difference between the two becomes progressively greater with higher overall levels of blood pressure. Thus, for an individual patient, a clinic pressure gives only an approximate estimate of the home blood pressure. The most obvious explanation for this effect, which has been termed 'white coat hypertension', is that it is due to the anxiety associated with a clinic visit. This is probably an oversimplification, however, because the phenomenon may persist after multiple visits, and does not necessarily habituate. It has been suggested that it is of clinical relevance because it reflects an individual's blood pressure response to any type of psychological stress. We have tested this hypothesis, however, and found that it is not necessarily so. We divided 292 patients with borderline hypertension (clinic diastolic pressures between 90 and 104 mmHg) into two groups, according to whether their blood pressure in situations outside the clinic was normal or not (Pickering et al., 1988). There was no difference between the two groups either in the variability of blood pressure or in the difference between work and home pressures, the latter being one possible marker of the blood pressure response to real life stress.

FACTORS INFLUENCING THE DIURNAL VARIATIONS OF BLOOD PRESSURE

It is well known that there is a diurnal pattern of blood pressure variation, with pressures tending to be higher in the morning than in the evening and being lowest at night. There has been some dispute as to whether this represents an intrinsic circadian rhythm, or whether it is determined by changes in activity

(Millar-Craig *et al.*, 1978; Floras *et al.*, 1978). Several lines of evidence support the latter view. First, if the effects of environmental stimuli and changes in physical activity are minimized, the profile of blood pressure during the day becomes relatively flat, with a decrease of about 20% during the hours of sleep. This was shown in a study performed in orthopaedic patients who were immobilized by plaster casts (Athassaniadis *et al.*, 1969). Other studies have shown that the diurnal changes of blood pressure are less pronounced in hospitalized patients than in patients who are in their natural environment (Young *et al.*, 1983). Second, as described below, we have used modelling techniques that suggest that time of day is a less powerful predictor of blood pressure than activity. Finally, a limited amount of evidence indicates that in people who are working night shifts, blood pressure is still lowest during sleep.

Physical activity

So far, there have been relatively few attempts to quantify the relationship between physical and mental activity and ambulatory blood pressure. In a study using intra-arterial blood pressure monitoring in ambulatory subjects, Littler *et al.* (1978) concluded that the highest pressures were generally seen during periods of physical activity, but did not quantify these changes. In a subsequent study, they found that systolic pressure ranged from a peak level of 240 mmHg during intense physical exercise (bicycling) to 120 mmHg during sleep in patients with mild hypertension, whose resting systolic pressure was about 140 mmHg (Watson *et al.*, 1979). Using non-invasive recorders, Dembroski and McDougall (1984) found 'significant' (defined as $p < 0.2$) partial correlations between self-reports of physical activity and blood pressure in 31% of subjects. Schmieder *et al.* (1985) also reported linear correlations between levels of physical activity and systolic pressure.

Another form of exercise, sexual intercourse, may cause very large increases of blood pressure (from 25 to 120 mmHg in systolic, and 24 to 48 in diastolic) and heart rate (Littler *et al.*, 1974a). After orgasm, both pressure and heart rate return to normal within 2 minutes.

During micturition and defecation there are transient swings of pressure, usually a decrease followed by an overshoot, resembling a Valsalva maneuver (Littler *et al.*, 1974b).

Talking is also a potent pressor stimulus, producing increases of both systolic and diastolic pressure of between 10 and 50%. Greater increases are seen in hypertensive than in normotensive individuals (Lynch *et al.*, 1981), and the pressure increase is also a function of the rate of talking (Friedman *et al.*, 1982). The magnitude of the increase is greatly influenced by psychological factors, such as the size of the audience (Thomas *et al.*, 1984), status differences between the speaker and the audience (Long *et al.*, 1982), and the affective content of the speech.

Sleep and wakefulness

During sleep, both systolic and diastolic pressure fall by about 20% (Littler et al., 1975; Pickering, 1980), with the lowest levels occurring during Stage 4 or rapid eye movement (REM) sleep. Thus, pressure tends to be lowest about 2 hours after the onset of sleep and rises immediately on waking (Floras et al., 1978). That the decrease of pressure is due to sleep itself rather than the time of day is shown by the fact that if subjects stay awake all night the pressure falls very little, whereas if they sleep during the day the usual fall is seen. Similar changes are seen in normal and hypertensive subjects.

Ingestion

Eating may have a variable effect on blood pressure. For 3 hours after a meal there may be a reduction of diastolic pressure of about 5 mmHg, but systolic pressure may be unchanged (Fagan et al., 1986). This, together with the fact that heart rate tends to increase, can be attributed to an increased cardiac output. There is a much more pronounced fall of both systolic and diastolic pressure in older subjects (Lipsitz et al., 1983).

Smoking a cigarette has been shown to raise systolic pressure by around 11 mmHg and diastolic by about 5 mmHg both in ambulatory (Cellina et al., 1975) and laboratory studies (Roth et al., 1944). These changes last for about 15 minutes.

Alcohol consumption has been associated with hypertension in a number of epidemiological studies (Larbi et al., 1983). The acute effects of alcohol on blood pressure are variable: in normotensive subjects, some studies have demonstrated a modest increase of blood pressure and heart rate following acute ingestion of alcohol (Orlando et al., 1976), while others have found no change (Gould et al., 1971). Malhotra et al. (1985) studied three groups of subjects both during abstinence and after drinking whiskey before dinner for 5 days. Blood pressure was unaffected in normal subjects; in hypertensives who did not drink regularly, standing blood pressure rose by 13/6 mmHg, while supine pressure was not significantly altered; in hypertensive drinkers, blood pressure was increased in both positions. In another study, conducted in hospital, reintroduction of alcohol to moderate drinkers with hypertension caused a gradual increase of blood pressure over 48 hours (Potter and Beevers, 1984).

Caffeine is another commonly ingested substance that has often been incriminated in cardiovascular disease, including hypertension (Lang et al., 1983), but the evidence for adverse long-term effects is inconclusive (Dawber et al., 1974). In healthy subjects who do not normally take it, caffeine can cause an acute rise of pressure of 14/10 mmHg (Robertson et al., 1978), but in regular caffeine users this increase is smaller (Izzo et al., 1983). Older subjects show a bigger increase of blood pressure. Caffeine may also augment the blood pressure response to acute psychological stress (Lane, 1983). Coffee and cigarettes are often taken together, and a study by Freestone and Ramsay (1982) showed that they may have an additive effect, causing pressure to remain elevated for 2 hours or more.

Mental activity

Both Dembroski and MacDougall (1984) and Schmieder *et al.* (1985) reported some correlations between self-rated mental 'stress' or 'arousal' and blood pressure during non-invasive ambulatory monitoring. We have reported generally higher levels of blood pressure when people are at work than when they are at home, which we have attributed to mental rather than physical factors, because most of our subjects had sedentary jobs (Harshfield *et al.*, 1982; Pickering *et al.*, 1982). Others have reported lesser changes during work (Kennedy *et al.*, 1983) and we are currently testing the hypothesis that subjects in high-strain jobs (characterized by high demands and low control) have higher pressures than those in low-strain jobs.

Driving a car has also been regarded as a potentially stressful activity, but in one study using intra-arterial ambulatory monitoring (Littler *et al.*, 1973), blood pressure remained remarkably stable, except for transient increases during episodes such as overtaking.

In another study of patients with untreated borderline hypertension, we asked patients to record one of four mood states (anxious, angry, happy or sad) on a scale of 1 to 10. Out of a total of around 4000 readings in 90 patients, there were 1152 entries for mood, giving sufficient numbers to analyze the effects of anxiety, anger, and happiness but not sadness. When the mood readings were related to each patient's mean daytime pressure, there was a highly significant effect of mood on blood pressure (Figure 2), which was independent of location and activity (James *et al.*, 1986). Systolic pressure decreased as the intensity

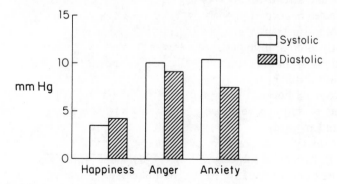

Figure 2. Effects of mood on blood pressure during ambulatory monitoring. The changes are given relative to the subjects' average 24-hour pressure.

of happiness increased, and diastolic pressure increased with the intensity of anxiety. Although anger was associated with increased systolic and diastolic pressure, there was no significant correlation between intensity and pressure, possibly because of the smaller numbers of observations. The effects of mood on blood pressure were most pronounced in subjects with more labile blood pressures.

A QUANTITATIVE ANALYSIS OF FACTORS INFLUENCING DIURNAL BLOOD PRESSURE VARIATIONS

We have attempted a quantitative analysis of factors influencing blood pressure variability in a study of 461 untreated patients with borderline hypertension who wore a monitor for 24 hours during normal daily activities (Clark *et al.*, 1987). They were asked to record their activity and location in a diary at the time of each reading. They were divided into two groups, one of 190 patients who were at home during the entire recording period, and the other of 271 who went to work. Figure 3 shows the observed diurnal profile of blood pressure for the entire group. We first attempted to account for the variability of blood pressure by modeling for time of day, where hour-to-hour differences were compared by a one-way analysis of covariance. This model accounted for 35% of the variation in systolic pressure readings and 30% of diastolic. An alternative procedure was to relate the activity and location of the patients to the changes of pressure. For the group who stayed at home, there were 21 activity–location

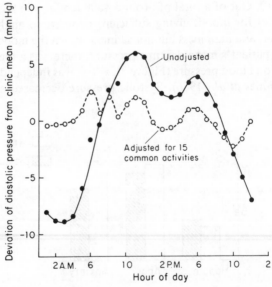

Figure 3. Diurnal variation of diastolic pressure in 461 subjects before and after adjusting for 15 common daily activities including sleep.

combinations which occurred with sufficient frequency (in at least 20 patients) to be included in the analysis. The pressure for each of these was adjusted, using the patient's clinic pressure as a covariate, and the model tested by an analysis of covariance. This model accounted for 41% of systolic and 36% of diastolic variation. The residuals of this model (i.e., the difference between the observed and predicted values) are also plotted in Figure 3, which suggests that the major part of the diurnal variation of blood pressure can be accounted for by the effect of a relatively small number of activities and that, based on this analysis, there is no reason to postulate any circadian rhythm of pressure which is independent of these activities. Combining the models for activity and time of day accounted for only a further 1% of the overall variance of systolic and diastolic pressure. A fourth model was tested in which the effects of a given activity or blood pressure were assumed to be the same regardless of the location. This model used 15 commonly occurring activities, and accounted for 41% of systolic pressure variation and 36% of diastolic. The estimated activity coefficients for this model are shown in Table 1.

When the same modeling procedure was applied to the group who went to work on the day of monitoring, the results were virtually identical. Blood pressure for any given activity was higher than at home by 5/4 mmHg, and readings occurring in other locations (e.g., when travelling) were 10/5 mmHg higher than at home.

Although this modeling procedure can account for a sizeable portion of the overall variation of blood pressure, it is obviously only a first approximation.

Table 1. Average changes of blood pressure associated with 15 commonly occurring activities (Clark et al., 1987).

		Systolic (mmHg)	Diastolic (mmHg)
1.	Meetings	+ 20.2	+ 15.0
2.	Work	+ 16.0	+ 13.0
3.	Transportation	+ 14.0	+ 9.2
4.	Walking	+ 12.0	+ 5.5
5.	Dressing	+ 11.5	+ 9.7
6.	Chores	+ 10.7	+ 6.7
7.	Telephone	+ 9.5	+ 7.2
8.	Eating	+ 8.8	+ 9.6
9.	Talking	+ 6.7	+ 6.7
10.	Desk work	+ 5.9	+ 5.3
11.	Reading	+ 1.9	+ 2.2
12.	Business (at home)	+ 1.6	+ 3.2
13.	Television	+ 0.3	+ 1.1
14.	Relaxing	0	0
15.	Sleeping	− 10.0	− 7.6

Changes are shown relative to blood pressure while relaxing.

Thus, the idea that the effects of each activity can be represented by a single coefficient is an oversimplification, because the intensity of any activity may vary, and individual subjects will have different pressure responses to the same activity, e.g., from differences in baroreflex sensitivity (Conway et al., 1984). In addition, there were many other activities which were not included in the analysis, and no attempt was made to account for changes of mood.

DOES CARDIOVASCULAR REACTIVITY INFLUENCE BLOOD PRESSURE IN EVERYDAY LIFE?

The idea that individuals who demonstrate a high level of cardiovascular reactivity, i.e., an exaggerated pressor response to stressful stimuli, may be at increased risk of future hypertension has become very popular, and it has been suggested that repeated exposure to such stimuli could contribute to the development of sustained hypertension. One requirement of this hypothesis is that it should be possible to demonstrate that individuals who are defined as having a high level of reactivity on the basis of laboratory tests should also demonstrate high reactivity in everyday life. We attempted to do this by comparing the blood pressure response to three commonly used laboratory stimuli—mental arithmetic, playing a video game, and a treadmill exercise test—to ambulatory blood pressure in a group of patients with borderline hypertension (Harshfield et al., 1988). A major problem here is how to define reactivity in real life. If the degree of reactivity is a characteristic of the individual rather than of the nature of the stimuli, there should be some correlation between the reactivity to the laboratory tests and the overall level of variability of blood pressure over 24 hours, since, as we have seen above, we believe that a major part of 24-hour blood pressure variability occurs in response to specific stimuli and activities. In our patients, we found a good correlation between the absolute levels of blood pressure during the laboratory testing and ambulatory monitoring, but no correlations between reactivity (defined as the increase of pressure occurring in response to the laboratory tests) and blood pressure variability over 24 hours. It is not hard to see why such correlations should be weak: first, the intermittent sampling of blood pressure by non-invasive ambulatory recorders means that only a rough estimate of the true blood pressure variability can be obtained; second, differences in ambulatory blood pressure variability may be due to differences in the activities of individual subjects as well as to differences in reactivity. It is also possible that hyper-reactivity may be limited to certain types of stimuli. It is often stated, for example, that subjects with borderline hypertension display an increased reactivity to some stimuli, e.g., mental arithmetic, but not to others, e.g., exercise (Julius et al., 1986). In our series, we also attempted more focal comparisons, for example, relating the increase of pressure during mental arithmetic to the increase of pressure at work relative to the pressure at home. Since most of our subjects had sedentary or clerical types of jobs, there should be a reasonably close resemblance between the two types of activity. Once again, however, we could find no significant correlations. In the study described earlier (Clark *et al.*, 1987), where we examined the effects of activities on ambulatory blood pressure, including a term for individual levels of reactivity did not improve the model. These findings would suggest that it is going to be difficult to demonstrate the role of individual differences in reactivity in influencing the variations of blood pressure in everyday life.

PATHOLOGICAL IMPLICATIONS OF THE EFFECTS OF EVERYDAY ACTIVITY ON BLOOD PRESSURE

The vascular damage caused by hypertension could, in theory, depend on three aspects of blood pressure: the average level over time, the peaks of pressure, or the shape of the arterial waveform. All three measures of pressure could be affected to a greater or lesser extent by the changes of pressure occurring as a result of daily activities.

While it is generally accepted that the average level of pressure is important in this regard, the role of the other two factors has not been adequately tested, either in human or animal studies. Since it is much more certain that behavior can cause acute changes of pressure than chronic changes, the influence of the dynamic aspects of blood pressure on vascular damage is of particular interest to behaviorists. In a cross-sectional study relating ambulatory blood pressure to left ventricular hypertrophy (LVH)—a convenient measure of the long-term impact of blood pressure on the circulation—we found that the correlation between pressure and LVH was closest in subjects who had pressure monitored on a working day (Devereux *et al.*, 1983), suggesting that the intermittent elevation of pressure occurring during work might contribute to the development of LVH, in the same way that the intermittent elevations of pressure in athletes who train for a few hours a day can cause LVH.

The concept of basal blood pressure is an old one, being first introduced by Addis in 1922, and further developed by Smirk (1944), who coined the terms casual and supplemental pressures. The casual pressure, which is the generally prevailing level of blood pressure, is conceived as the sum of the basal pressure and the supplemental pressure, which represents the contributions of daily activity to blood pressure. These concepts still have merit today. Thus, as reviewed above, numerous studies using ambulatory monitoring of blood pressure in free-ranging subjects have shown that the highest levels of blood pressure are usually seen during the morning hours, whereas studies of subjects who are immobile over the 24-hour recording period have shown relatively stable blood pressures during the day, with a fall occurring during sleep, as shown diagrammatically in Figure 1. This daytime pressure is equivalent to the basal pressure. As we have also discussed above, it is our belief that the usual diurnal pattern of blood pressure is to a large extent determined by the superimposition of the

1. Basal BP Changes

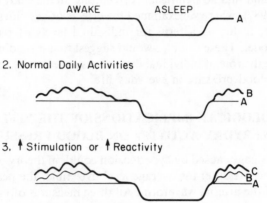

2. Normal Daily Activities

3. ↑ Stimulation or ↑ Reactivity

4. Sustained Elevation

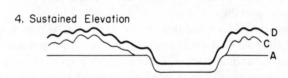

Figure 4. Hypothetical patterns of blood pressure variability. 1: Basal BP changes (A), as observed in subjects immobilized throughout the 24-hour period. 2: Superimposition of normal activities (B) produces the typical diurnal pattern of BP seen in free-living subjects. 3: Increased level of activity (stimulation), or increased BP reactivity to a given stimulus (C) produces enhanced variability of BP over 24 hours. 4: Sustained elevations of BP (D) throughout the 24-hour period, without any increase in reactivity.

effects of everyday activities (the supplemental pressure) on this basal pressure (Figure 2). Higher levels of pressure would occur during the day if there was an increase in either the reactivity of blood pressure to a given activity or in the intensity of activity (Figure 3). In such instances, the blood pressure during sleep would not necessarily be raised. In practice, most studies comparing 24-hour blood pressures in normotensive and hypertensive subjects have shown that while there is some increase in the diurnal variations of pressure, most of the differences can be attributed to differences of basal pressure, with an upward shift of the curve (Figure 4).

REFERENCES

Addis, T. (1922). Blood pressure and pulse rate levels: the levels under basal daytime conditions. *Archives of Internal Medicine*, **29**, 539.

Athassaniadis, D., Drayer, G. J., Honour, A. J. and Cranston, W. I. (1969). Variability of automatic blood pressure measurements over 24 hour period. *Clinical Science*, **36**, 147–156.

Ayman, D. and Goldshine, A. D. (1940). Blood pressure determination by patients with essential hypertension. I. The difference between clinic and home reading before treatment. *American Journal of Medical Science*, **200**, 465–474.

Cellina, G. U., Honour, A. J. and Littler, W. A. (1975). Direct arterial pressure, heart rate, and electrocardiogram during cigarette smoking in unrestricted patients. *American Heart Journal*, **89**, 18–25.

Clark, L. A., Denby, L., Pregibon, D., Harshfield, G. A., Pickering, T. G., Blank, S. and Laragh, J. H. (1987). The effects of activity and time of day on the diurnal variations of blood pressure. *Journal of Chronic Diseases*, **40**, 671–681.

Conway, J., Boon, V., Davies, C., Vann Jones, J. and Sleight, P. (1984). Neural and humoral mechanisms involved in blood pressure variability. *Journal of Hypertension*, **2**, 203–204.

Dawber, T. R., Kannel, W. B. and Gordon, T. (1974). Coffee and cardiovascular disease: Observations from the Framingham study. *New England Journal of Medicine*, **291**, 871–984.

Dembroski, T. M. and MacDougall, J. M. (1984). Validation of the Vita-Stat automated noninvasive ambulatory blood pressure recording device. In Herd, J. A., Gotto, A. M., Kaufmann, P. G. and Weiss, S. M. (Eds), Cardiovascular Instrumentation. NIH Publication No. 84–1654, Bethesda, pp 55–77.

Devereux, R. B., Pickering, T. G., Harshfield, G. A. *et al.* (1983). Left ventricular hypertrophy in patients with hypertension: importance of blood pressure response to regularly recurring stress. *Circulation*, **68**, 470–476.

Di Rienzo, M., Grassi, G., Pedotti, A. and Mancia, G. (1983). Continuous vs. intermittent blood pressure measurement in estimating 24-hour average blood pressure. *Hypertension*, **5**, 264.

Fagan, T. C., Conrad, K. A., Mar, J. H. and Nelson, L. (1986). Effects of meals on hemodynamics: Implications for antihypertensive drug studies. *Clinical Pharmacology and Therapeutics*, **39**, 255–260.

Floras, J. S., Jones, J. V., Johnston, J. A., Brooks, D. E., Hasson, M. O. and Sleight, P. (1978). Arousal and the circadian rhythm of blood pressure. *Clinical Science and Molecular Medicine*, **55**, 39S.

Freestone, S. and Ramsey, L. E. (1982). Effect of coffee and cigarette smoking on the blood pressure of untreated and diuretic-treated hypertensive patients. *American Journal of Medicine*, **73**, 348–353.

Friedman, E., Thomas, S. A., Kulick-Ciuffo, D., Lynch, J. J. and Suginahara M. (1982). The effects of normal and rapid speech on blood pressure. *Psychosomatic Medicine*, **44**, 545–553.

Gould, L., Zahir, M., DeMartino, A. and Gomprecht, R. F. (1971). The cardiac effects of a cocktail. *JAMA*, **218**, 1799–1802.

Harshfield, G. A., Pickering, T. G., Kleinert, H. D., Blank, S. and Laragh, J. H. (1982). Situational variation of blood pressure in ambulatory hypertensive patients. *Psychosomatic Medicine*, **44**, 237–245.

Harshfield, G. A., James, G. D., Schlussel, Y., Yee, L. S., Blank, S. G. and Pickering T. G. (1988). Do Laboratory tests of blood pressure reactivity predict blood pressure variability in real life? *American Journal of Hypertension*, **1**, 168–174.

Hines, E. A. and Brown, G. E. (1936). The cold pressor test for measuring the reactability of the blood pressure: Data concerning 571 normal and hypertensive subjects. *American Heart Journal*, **11**, 1–9.

Izzo, J. L., Ghosal, A., Kwong, T., Freeman, R. B. and Jaenike, J. R. (1983). Age and prior caffeine use alter the cardiovascular and adrenomedullary responses to oral caffeine. *American Journal of Cardiology*, **52**, 769–773.

James, G. D., Yee, L. S., Harshfield, G. A., Blank, S. G. and Pickering, T. G. (1986). The influence of happiness, anger, and anxiety on the blood pressure of borderline hypertensives. *Psychosomatic Medicine*, **48**, 502–508.

The 1984 report of the Joint National Committee on detection, evaluation, and treatment of high blood pressure (1984). *Archives of Internal Medicine*, **144**, 1045–1057.

Julius, S., Weder, A. B. and Hinderliter, A. L. (1986). Does behaviorally-induced blood pressure variability lead to hypertension? In Matthews, K., Weiss, S. M. *et al.* (Eds), *Handbook of Stress, Reactivity and Cardiovascular Disease*. Wiley, New York, pp. 71–82.

Kennedy, H. L., Horan, M. J., Sprague, M. K., Padgett, N. E. and Shriver, K. K. (1983). Ambulatory blood pressure in healthy normotensive males. *American Heart Journal*, **106**, 717–722.

Kleinert, H. D., Harshfield, G. A., Pickering, T. G. *et al.* (1984). What is the value of home blood pressure measurement in patients with mild hypertension? *Hypertension*, **6**, 574–578.

Lane, J. D. (1983). Caffeine and cardiovascular response to stress. *Psychosomatic Medicine*, **45**, 447–451.

Lang, T., Degoulet, P., Aime, F. *et al.* (1983). Relation between coffee drinking and blood pressure: analysis of 6,321 subjects in the Paris region. *American Journal of Cardiology*, **52**, 1238–1242.

Larbi, E. B., Cooper, R. S. and Stamler, J. (1983). Alcohol and hypertension. *Archives of Internal Medicine*, **143**, 28–29.

Laughlin, K. D., Sherrard, D. H. and Fisher, L. (1979). Comparison of clinic and home blood pressure levels in essential hypertension and variables associated with clinic-home differences. *Journal of Chronic Diseases*, **33**, 197.

Lipsitz, L. A., Nyquist, R. P., Wei, J. Y. and Rowe, J. W. (1983). Postprandial reduction in blood pressure in the elderly. *New England Journal of Medicine*, **309**, 81–83.

Littler, W. A., Honour, A. J., and Sleight, P. (1973). Direct arterial pressure and electrocardiogram during motor car driving. *British Medical Journal*, **2**, 273–277.

Littler, W. A., Honour, A. J. and Sleight, P. (1974a). Direct arterial pressure, heart rate, and electrocardiogram during human coitus. *Journal of Reproduction and Fertility*, **40**, 321–331.

Littler, W. A., Honour, A. J. and Sleight, P. (1974b). Direct arterial pressure, pulse rate, and electrocardiogram during micturition and defecation in unrestricted man. *American Heart Journal*, **88**, 205–210.

Littler, W. A., Honour, A. J., Carter, R. D. and Sleight, P. (1975). Sleep and blood pressure. *British Medical Journal*, **3**, 346–348.

Littler, W. A., West, M. J., Honour, A. J. and Sleight, P. (1978). The variability of arterial pressure. *American Heart Journal*, **95**, 180–186.

Long, J. M., Lynch, J. J., Machiran, N. M., Thomas, S. A. and Malinow, K. L. (1982). The effect of status on blood pressure during verbal communication. *Journal of Behavioural Medicine*, **5**, 165–172.

Lynch, J. J., Long, J. M., Thomas, S. A., Malinow, K. L. and Katcher, A. H. (1981). The effects of talking on the blood pressure of hypertensive and normotensive individuals. *Psychosomatic Medicine*, **43**, 25–33.

Malhotra, H., Mehta, S. R., Mathur, D. and Khandelwal, P. D. (1985). Pressor effects of alcohol in normotensive and hypertensive subjects. *Lancet*, **2**, 584–586.

Millar-Craig, M. W., Bishop, C. N. and Raftery, E. B. (1978). Circadian rhythm of blood pressure. *Lancet*, **1**, 795.

Orlando, J., Aronow, W. S., Cassidy, J. and Prakash, R. (1976). Effect of ethanol on angina pectoris. *Annals Internal Medicine*, **84**, 652–655.

Pickering, T. G. (1980). Sleep, circadian rhythms and cardiovascular disease. *Cardiovascular Reviews and Reports*, **1**, 37–47.

Pickering, T. G., Harshfield, G. A., Kleinert, H. D., Blank, S. and Laragh, J. H. (1982). Blood pressure during normal daily activities, sleep, and exercise. Comparison of values in normal and hypertensive subjects. *Journal of the American Medical Association*, **247**, 992–996.

Pickering, T. G., Cvetkowski, B. and James, G. D. (1986). An evaluation of electronic recorders for self monitoring of blood pressure. *Journal of Hypertension*, **4**, 9328–9330.

Pickering, T. G., Boddie, C., James, G. D., Harshfield, G. A., Blank, S. G. and Laragh, J. H. (1988). How common is white coat hypertension? *Journal of the American Medical Association*, **259**, 225–228.

Potter, J. F. and Beevers, D. G. (1984). Pressor effect of alcohol in hypertension. *Lancet*, **1**, 119–122.

Robertson, D., Frolich, J. C., Carr, R. K., Watson, J. T., Hollifield, J. W., Shand, D. G. and Oates, J. A. (1978). Effects of caffeine on plasma renin activity, catecholamines and blood pressure. *New England Journal of Medicine*, **298**, 181–186.

Roth, G. M., McDonald, J. B. and Sheard, C. (1944). The effect of smoking cigarettes, and of intravenous administration of nicotine on the electrocardiogram, basal metabolic rate, cutaneous temperature, blood pressure, and pulse rate of normal persons. *Journal of the American Medical Association*, **125**, 751–767.

Schmieder, R., Rüddel, H., Langewitz, W., Neus, J., Wagner, O. and von Eiff, A. W. (1985). The influence of monotherapy with oxprenolol and nitrendipine on ambulatory blood pressure in hypertensives. *Clinical and Experimental Hypertension*, **A7**, 445–454.

Smirk, F. H. (1944). Casual and basal blood pressures IV, their relationship to the supplemental pressure with a note on statistical implications. *British Heart Journal*, **6**, 176.

Thomas, S. A., Friedman, E., Lottes, L. S., Gresty, S., Miller, C., Lynch, J. J. (1984). Changes in nurses' blood pressure and heart rate while communicating. *Research in Nursing Health*, **7**, 119–126.

Watson, R. D. S., Hamilton, C. A., Reid, J. L. and Littler, W. A. (1979). Changes in plasma norepinephrine, blood pressure and heart rate during physical activity in hypertensive man. *Hypertension*, **1**, 341–346.

Young, M. A., Rowlands, D. B., Stallard, T. H., Watson, R. D. S. and Littler, W. A. (1983). Effect of environment on blood pressure: Home versus hospital. *British Medical Journal*, **286**, 1235–1236.

Essential Hypertension: Implications for Behavioural Management

INTRODUCTION TO SECTION II

The development of behavioural methods for managing essential hypertension has been one of the greatest successes in behavioural medicine. The first uncontrolled studies published nearly 20 years ago were followed by a second generation of research, in which behavioural methods were shown in systematic experiments to be superior to a variety of control conditions (e.g. Patel and North, 1975; Brauer *et al.*, 1979). Contemporary research has moved beyond the stage of simply demonstrating the effects of behavioural interventions, to a new phase. A number of themes are emerging in current investigations, and many of these are illustrated in the five chapters of Section II.

The first general theme is that behavioural intervention is no longer confined to training in relaxation or biofeedback in the clinic. The behavioural approach has expanded to include the use of relaxation as a coping skill, and the modification of other factors known to influence blood pressure, such as body weight, alcohol intake and dietary composition. This is emphasized in the weight control programmes developed by Basler (Chapter 9), and in the incorporation of information concerning exercise, nutrition and lifestyle into the stress management treatments discussed by Walter, Rüddel, and von Eiff (Chapter 7), and Steptoe (Chapter 10). The behavioural management of essential hypertension is becoming multimodal to a much greater extent than hitherto.

The second trend to emerge in these chapters is the concern with mechanism. The notion that stress–management techniques operate through altering autonomic indices of sympathetic activation is proving difficult to confirm. As the experiment described by Vinck and colleagues (Chapter 6) indicates, there are few associations between changes in blood pressure and other autonomic parameters supposedly implicated in the relaxation process. Nor do reactions to standardized stimuli in the laboratory necessarily decline with treatment, as can be seen in the contribution from Richter-Heinrich, Homuth, Heinrich, Knust, Schmidt, Wiedemann and Gohlke (Chapter 8). It is suggested in the chapter by Steptoe that sustained blood pressure reductions may not even depend on regular practice of relaxation exercises. These data all indicate that it may be necessary to look elsewhere in order to understand the therapeutic mechanisms. Some clues emerge from these chapters, where it appears that successful blood pressure reductions are associated with improved coping skills and alterations in the ways in which patients view their social and physical environment. Future research is likely to evaluate cognitive and behavioural change with greater sophistication.

A related theme that can be traced through this section is the concern with individual differences. Although hypertensives do not differ from normotensives in terms of basic psychological dimensions, the studies described here suggest great heterogeneity in the hypertensive population, with a tendency towards differences when more subtle elements of coping are assessed. Thus useful changes may be effected among hypertensives at the psychological as well as physiological levels by behavioural treatment. Another aspect of individual differences is variation in treatment response. This factor has been comparatively neglected in behavioural medicine, yet it is clearly important to be able to identify those people who are most likely to benefit from any particular approach. An interesting comparison is described by Richter-Heinrich *et al.* between responders and non-responders to a behavioural programme, suggesting that certain psychological characteristics might be important in predicting outcome.

The final trend illustrated in these chapters concerns the implementation of research data on a general clinical level. Studies described here indicate that, potentially, behavioural interventions have a very wide scope. Basler and Steptoe indicate that behavioural treatments may be used on a wide range of hypertensives, and not only on subjects with a special interest in self-help or alternative therapy. It is also apparent that behavioural therapies can be administered by trained personnel without medical or psychological qualifications, and that they can be integrated with pharmacological approaches to management. The problem of long-term adherence to treatment still needs to be examined in detail, and this may be aided by investigating the cognitive and mood changes that accompany successful therapy. The material collected in these chapters will help to promote the behavioural management of hypertension, and we hope that it will also benefit the vast numbers of people afflicted with this serious disorder.

REFERENCES

Brauer, A. P., Horlick, L., Nelson, E., Farquhar, J. W. and Agras, W. S. (1979). Relaxation therapy for essential hypertension; A Veterans Administration out-patients study. *Journal of Behavioral Medicine*, **2**, 21–29.

Patel, C. and North, W. R. S. (1975). Randomised controlled trial of yoga and biofeedback in the management of hypertension. *Lancet*, **II**, 93–99.

6

Can Psychophysiological Changes Explain the Blood Pressure Lowering Effect of Relaxation Training?

J. Vinck,* M. Arickx,* M. Hongenaert,† P. Grossman,‡
H. Vertommen§ and J. Beckers‖

*Limburgs Universitair Centrum, Diepenbeek, Belgium
†Limburgs Universitair Centrum, Diepenbeek, Belgium (now at Catholic
University, Leuven, Belgium)
‡N.I.A.S., Wassenaar, The Netherlands (now at Freiburg University, Freiburg,
FRG)
§Catholic University, Leuven, Belgium
‖Centrum Geestelijke Gezondheidszorg, St Truiden, Belgium

INTRODUCTION

There is accumulating evidence that stress leads to an increase of blood pressure (BP) and that, eventually, this effect may lie at the origin of chronic essential hypertension (EHT) (Henry and Cassel, 1969; Johnston, 1986a). If this is true, techniques that reduce the person's reaction to stress situations, or that help the person to react differently in such situations, should lead to reductions of BP and should, therefore, reduce the risk of EHT. For a number of years it has been known that in hypertensive patients moderate reductions of BP are produced by relaxation training (Jacob et al., 1977; Agras, 1982; Shapiro and Goldstein, 1982). In this contribution we will focus on the fact that these reductions are moderate in size and, thus, not always clinically significant (Vaitl, 1982), on the possible explanations for this fact, and on ways in which the effects of relaxation training might be strengthened. The basic hypothesis is that the modest effects of relaxation training on BP are due to the complexity of both BP and relaxation training. Blood pressure is clearly controlled by many factors other than stress (Shapiro and Goldstein, 1982; Vaitl, 1982). The relative weight of these different factors is different in different subjects, so that stress and relaxation training are inevitably more relevant for the BP control of some

91

subjects than for others. If this is true, the somewhat small mean reductions of BP after relaxation training may mask important individual differences. On the other hand, relaxation training itself is also a complex technique, as is the relaxation response it elicits. Here also some components may have more impact on BP than others. Furthermore, there may be individual differences in the relaxation response, possibly helping to account for the fact that BP is differentially affected by relaxation training in different subjects.

These hypotheses suggest ways of enhancing the effects of relaxation training on BP. The first of these possibilities only will be mentioned here. As far as BP being variably affected by stress and relaxation training in different subjects is concerned, it is of course important to develop methods for identifying those people whose BP is related to stress and who can be expected, therefore, to have their BP reduced by relaxation training (Vinck et al., 1987).

Our primary concern in this chapter will be with a second, and complementary, possibility. At present we do not know very much about the mechanisms through which relaxation training results in a reduction of BP (Johnston, 1986b). A task of primary importance then is to explore these mechanisms. In setting out on this enterprise, several lines of reasoning present themselves. One of these is to look at the possibility that the BP response to relaxation training is mediated by some element of the global relaxation response. At least two groups of sub-effects of relaxation training are reasonable candidates in this respect: on the one hand, relaxation training can bring about a number of behavioural changes which could be related to a reduction of BP; on the other, relaxation training is known to lead to a number of physiological changes which could reasonably explain the BP response.

On the behavioural side, there are a number of more-or-less direct effects of relaxation training which may be related to blood pressure, such as adopting an altered lifestyle, changing coping behaviour or developing a feeling of subjective calmness.

In this study, however, we will be particularly concerned with the possibility that the effect on BP is primarily mediated by physiological components of the relaxation response. Three physiological components of the relaxation response are promising in this respect because it is well established that they are produced by relaxation training and, at the same time, because they may be specifically trained. These are muscle relaxation, peripheral vasodilation resulting in increased peripheral temperature, and a reduction of respiratory rate.

A reduction of muscle tonus has always been conceived of as one of the most obvious and important aspects of relaxation, and it is also the crucial factor in one of the most frequently used forms of relaxation training, progressive relaxation. In a number of studies the effects of progressive relaxation on BP were as good as those of other active techniques (Taylor et al., 1977; English and Baker, 1983).

Peripheral temperature increases as a consequence of general relaxation. The question of the clinical significance of peripheral temperature control (as in the treatment of migraine) is, however, far from resolved (Reading, 1986). As far as the control of BP is concerned, McCaffrey and Blanchard (1985) reported preliminary results showing that training to increase finger temperature resulted in greater reductions of BP than progressive relaxation. Our understanding of this effect is, however, very poor.

There are some hypotheses, finally, to explain how respiratory training could lead to a reduction of BP, especially in hypertensives. The increased oxygen consumption, cardiac output, and heart rate as well as the disturbed sinus arrhythmia which are all typically found in early labile hypertensives, may well be the consequence of a chronically rapid breathing pattern. Increased respiratory rate is known to be a possible response to stress and anxiety provoking situations. Thus 'it seems plausible that respiratory processes may at least partially mediate the relationship between stress and hypertension in predisposed individuals' (Grossman and Defares, 1984). When relaxation training leads to a reduction of BP, it might be that it does so via changes of the respiratory pattern. Moreover, it is known that relaxation training has a reduction of respiratory rate as one of its possible consequences.

In this study we explored the possibility that BP reduction after relaxation training is mediated by a decrease of muscle tonus, an increase of peripheral temperature or a reduction of respiratory rate. All these may follow relaxation training and therefore explain the BP lowering effects of such training. If it could be shown that one of these is more directly involved than others, the strength of the technique could be enhanced by directly training that element of relaxation.

We used two strategies to study this question. The first was to give groups of subjects relaxation training with special emphasis on one of the potentially relevant physiological changes and to see whether this had a specific effect on BP; the second was to look for correlations between changes during relaxation in one of the hypothetically important functions and changes in BP.

METHOD

Subjects

Subjects came from a pool of 86 male and 51 female second-year medical students in the age range between 19 and 21. They had no health problems at the time of training and took no medication. Independently of this study, these students had been assigned to six groups of 12 to 27 people.

Conditions

These groups were randomly assigned to the following conditions:

Muscle training (MUSC): this group was trained to focus on muscle tension and relaxation, as in regular progressive relaxation.
Temperature training (TEMP): these subjects were trained to focus on body temperature and to make this go up, as is routinely done in one of the stages of autogenic training.
Respiratory training (RESP): these subjects were trained to focus on their breathing and to try to slow down the rate of their respiration, especially to lengthen the expiratory phase of respiration.
Combined training (COMB): in this group elements of the three other conditions were combined, making this condition resemble what is usually done in clinical practice.
Wait list (WAIT): after completion of the pre-training assessment this group was told that they were on a wait list and that they would receive relaxation training during the next trimester.
Placebo (PLAC): subjects in this group were led to believe that they too received relaxation training, by treating them in exactly the same way as their fellow students, except for the intended peculiarity that they merely had to learn to 'yield' to the relaxing atmosphere, built up by a perfumed but fake hormonal preparation (said to be an hormonal agent blocking the production of adrenaline and sprayed in the training room) and by chamber music.

Training procedures were carefully planned so that, apart from the specific training mode, the five training groups were treated as identically as possible. In PLAC, for example, subjects were regularly invited to discuss their progress, as was done in the active conditions. Training was given in six group sessions of 1 hour over a 6-week period.

The only differences between conditions were that PLAC subjects were allowed some quiet activity like reading which was not allowed in the other conditions, and that subjects in TEMP laid down while in the other conditions subjects were sitting.

Table 1 shows the numbers of subjects in the different groups and their mean pretreatment BP values. Analysis of variance showed that, unfortunately, groups differed significantly on systolic BP (SBP, $F = 2.56$, $p < 0.05$ with d.f. 5, 93), with WAIT scoring higher and MUSC scoring lower.

Data collection

About 1 week before the start of training all subjects were asked to fill out a battery of psychological questionnaires, the results of which will not be considered in this article. Immediately after finishing the questionnaires they

Table 1. Means and SDs of initial systolic and diastolic BP measured prior to training in each condition.

Conditions	Systolic BP			Diastolic BP		
	Mean	SD	n*	Mean	SD	n
WAIT	135.4	18.1	22	75.1	8.5	22
PLAC	131.8	16.7	21	72.6	11.7	20
MUSC	119.5	12.8	17	68.7	9.7	17
TEMP	128.5	18.0	13	70.8	8.4	13
RESP	125.1	9.9	12	65.4	11.0	12
COMB	122.0	18.1	14	70.7	7.2	14
All conditions	127.9	16.6	99	71.2	9.8	98

*Numbers in conditions may vary due to missing observations.

were weighed and were invited to lie down and rest while their BP (systolic and diastolic) and heart rate (HR) were measured after about 3 minutes, and once more after about 10 minutes rest in the same posture. All these measurements were taken with Spengler electronic sphygmomanometers with digital readout of systolic and diastolic BP in mmHg and of heart rate in beats per minute (Spengler Sphygmodigital 4000).

Upon completion of the last training session all subjects made an appointment for an individual post-treatment test session. In order to minimize test anxiety and to facilitate psychological and physiological adaptation to the unusual test situation, the purpose of every electrode and of every sensor was explained while it was being attached. Muscle tension was recorded from the right biceps using the Enting Myotron 2000. Finger temperature was derived from a thermistor element attached to the index finger of the right hand. A tubular belt was placed around the waist and connected to a pressure gauge, enabling us to monitor respiration. Three large plate electrodes to derive the electrocardiogram (ECG) were connected to both wrists and to the left ankle. The respiration curve was registrated simultaneously with the ECG signal so that it was possible to determine differences in respiratory sinus arrhythmia. BP, finally, was taken from the left upper arm with the Spengler Sphygmodigital 4000.

Subjects were required to lie down on a laboratory-type bed and were told that the first part of the test was a 10-minute adaptation period during which no attempts toward relaxation were to be undertaken. After about 10 minutes subjects were instructed to make use of whichever technique they had learned to produce as deep a state of relaxation as possible for the next 10 minutes. Subjects from the control conditions (WAIT and PLAC), who had not learned a proper relaxation technique, were instructed to use their imagination to produce this effect. After about 10 minutes of voluntary relaxation the subject was asked to stop relaxing but to remain quiet for another 3 minutes to allow the collection of some final data. Finally, the transducers were removed and subjects were invited to describe their subjective experiences by means of a short checklist.

A two-channel polygraph was used to record three samples, each about 3 to 4 minutes long, of the respiration curve and, synchronous with it, the ECG signal. The first and shortest sample was recorded at the onset of the adaptation period, from minute 0 to minute 3. The second sample was taken from the end of adaptation through the onset of relaxation, from minute 8 to minute 12. The third and last sample was taken from the end of relaxation to the end of the test, from minute 18 to minute 22. All other non-continuous measurements, i.e. integrated EMG activity, finger temperature, BP (systolic and diastolic), and pulse were collected by the experimenter on five occasions at intervals of about 5 minutes, at minute 3, 7, 12, 17, and 22. The first two measurement points cover beginning and ending of the adaptation period. The next two points cover the start and finish of the relaxation period, and the last point marks the return to normal resting.

About 1 week after the sixth and final training session all subjects were asked to fill out for the second time the whole battery of questionnaires, enabling us to measure concomitant changes in behavioural coping style and in the amount of anxiety, stress, and other negative emotions that were experienced.

RESULTS

The aim of our study was to find out if any of the physiological functions under consideration could mediate the BP reducing effect of relaxation training. Before the BP data are considered, it is necessary to determine whether our training was effective, and whether our subjects really learned what was required.

Table 2. Differences between treatment groups on the three parameters focused upon in relaxation training: using electromyogram (EMG) activity (in microvolts), finger temperature (in degrees centigrade), and respiration frequency (in breaths per minute) as indices of the intended effects. Table entries are mean differences between measurements taken on minute 17 and on minute 3 of the post-treatment test session.

Conditions	EMG activity Mean	n	Finger temperature Mean	n	Respiration frequency Mean	n
WAIT	−0.22	(26)	1.40	(26)	−3.11	(27)
PLAC	−0.42	(23)	2.12	(23)	−0.87	(23)
MUSC	−0.19	(17)	1.34	(17)	−0.94	(17)
TEMP	−0.29	(17)	1.41	(18)	−1.12	(16)
RESP	−0.14	(12)	2.15	(12)	−8.33*	(12)
COMB	−0.26	(17)	−0.05	(17)	−3.20	(15)
All groups	−0.26*	(112)	1.43*	(113)	−2.60*	(110)

*$p < 0.001$.

Table 2 shows the changes in EMG activity, finger temperature, and respiration over the test session (min 17 – min 3) for the different conditions. It can be seen that, when all conditions were combined, the physiological changes that might be expected during relaxation did in fact occur: EMG fell by $-0.26 \mu V$ ($t = 5.93$, $p < 0.001$), finger temperature increased 1.43 degrees Celsius ($t = 5.16$, $p < 0.001$), and respiration slowed down by 2.6 breaths per minute ($t = 7.1$, $p < 0.001$). This general relaxation was also reflected in a significant decrease in heart rate from min 3 to min 17 (-3.17 bpm, $p < 0.001$) and in the ratings of subjective relaxation.

As far as the comparison between the groups is concerned, however, analysis of variance indicated that groups were not performing differently for EMG activity ($F = 0.79$, NS with d.f. 5, 106) or finger temperature ($F = 1.22$, NS with d.f. 5, 107). So the MUSC or TEMP groups did no better on the function they were trained for than relaxing students in general (without any training or with another training). The anticipated effect of training was found for respiration, since the RESP group clearly performed differently from other groups ($F = 11.03$, $p < 0.001$ with d.f. 5, 104). So, while it is clear that our subjects did relax and that this was reflected in physiological changes, we do not find specific training effects, except for RESP.

Did training, then, significantly affect BP, and were differences between the various conditions found in this respect? For diastolic BP, there were no significant effects, either overall or in any of the conditions studied. These data will not therefore be discussed any further. As was noted above, experimental groups differed significantly in their pre-treatment systolic BP. At the beginning of the post-treatment test session, groups again differed in systolic BP ($F = 3.14$, $p < 0.05$ with d.f. 5, 105). The systolic BP of the TEMP group was much higher than in other conditions, as can be seen from Table 3. In comparison with the pre-training level, the mean pressure of TEMP remained constant (128.5 and 128.2, respectively), while the mean pressure levels for the other conditions decreased significantly. So

Table 3. Mean BP at beginning of post-training test session (min 3) and BP changes over the test session (difference min 17 – min 3).

Conditions	n	Systolic BP min 3	Systolic BP min 17 – min 3	Diastolic BP min 3	Diastolic BP min 17 – min 3
WAIT	26	121.73	$-3.31**$	70.23	0.54
PLAC	20	122.29	$-5.20***$	69.67	-0.90
MUSC	17	111.59	-1.24	69.00	-0.06
TEMP	17	128.18	$-4.76***$	67.59	0.06
RESP	13	118.23	-1.38	67.46	-1.15
COMB	17	117.41	$-3.62*$	68.65	0.12
All conditions	110	120.20	$-3.38***$	68.96	-0.17

$*p < 0.05$, $**p < 0.01$, $***p < 0.001$.

the long-term effect of the TEMP condition on SBP appears to be rather negative, while the other conditions do not differ among each other in this respect.

When the changes in SBP over the post-training test session are considered, it can be seen from Table 3 that, overall, the SBP was reduced slightly but significantly (-3.38 mmHg, $t = 5.57$, $p < 0.001$). When the different conditions were evaluated separately, significant reductions of SBP were found in the TEMP and COMB conditions and also in the WAIT and PLAC groups but not in the MUSC and RESP conditions. This surprising result is corroborated by the lack of difference between the combined active training and control groups in SBP decrease. Analysis of variance accordingly showed that our experimental groups were not different in terms of the amount of SBP decrease over the test session ($F = 1.16$, NS with d.f. 5, 103).

It appears therefore that SBP decreased whether or not subjects had learned a specific relaxation technique. Thus we cannot conclude from these results that the training of any of these functions led to an enhancement of the effect of relaxation training on BP. For the respiratory training group, this failure was found in spite of the fact that subjects had apparently learned a specific skill in reducing their respiratory rate. For the muscle relaxation and the finger temperature groups, the possibility that failure to achieve recognizable skills was responsible for this result cannot be excluded.

The second strategy for finding out whether BP changes were mediated by one of the physiological parameters under consideration was to look at correlations between these functions and BP. Such an analysis can only be carried out when subjects are really relaxing. Although it is not possible to maintain that training was very specific, it appeared from Table 2 that subjects were, as a group, really relaxed. Even control conditions did remarkably well in this respect. Nevertheless, when the correlations between changes over the post-training test session in muscle tension, finger temperature, and respiratory rate and in SBP and DBP were computed, no relationship between changes in one of the parameters which were thought to be potentially important and variations in BP was observed. So the negative conclusion we arrived at with the group comparison is reinforced by the results of the correlational analysis.

It may be noted, parenthetically, that there was a striking overall lack of correlation between parameters in these data. There was only a small but significant correlation between changes in SBP and changes in DBP ($r = 0.28$, $p < 0.01$). In this study we clearly did not find evidence for a relaxation response that was reflected simultaneously in several different physiological parameters.

DISCUSSION

On the basis of these results it is impossible to maintain that BP changes after relaxation training are mediated by changes in muscle tension, peripheral temperature or respiration rate. When confronted with this conclusion, it is necessary to consider two further questions: Did we examine our hypothesis correctly? Did we formulate the right hypothesis?

As far as the first question is concerned, the possibility has to be considered that we did not find stronger BP reductions because we used normotensive subjects in a state of minimal arousal: the low initial levels could have prevented stronger effects of the training, possibly obscuring existing relations with mediating variables. Furthermore, it has already been mentioned that the muscle relaxation training and the finger temperature training did not succeed in establishing specific and observable skills in the subjects involved. Also, the active training groups did not achieve greater reductions of their BP than the control groups. These weaknesses may be the result of the fact that training was not sufficiently intense. A more intensive training programme might have resulted in larger BP reductions in the active training groups as compared to the control groups. It is also possible that, for the muscle relaxation and the finger temperature training groups, the inclusion of biofeedback would have facilitated the acquisition of specific skills. Indeed it seems obvious that it is easier to monitor respiration directly than low level muscle tension or finger temperature. In a subsequent study, which has not yet been concluded, we have collected some data supporting this hypothesis, showing that EMG feedback results in specific effects at the muscular level and in greater reductions of SBP, and that temperature feedback has no such effects. The difficulty of the task with which the TEMP and MUSC groups were confronted may even have induced more test anxiety in these individuals than in other groups.

These factors weaken the strength of the group comparison. We do not think, however, that the design was rendered totally invalid for addressing the basic research question. Subjects were definitely relaxing, and the subjects in the respiratory condition clearly developed a specific skill. In addition, these weaknesses are hardly relevant to the correlational analysis which led, nevertheless, to the same negative result.

This leaves the possibility that the wrong hypothesis may have been formulated. Perhaps other physiological parameters mediate the effect of relaxation training on BP. Alternatively, the effect of relaxation training on BP may be mediated by some of the behavioural changes mentioned in the introduction. We have collected some data on the possible role of changes in coping behaviour, in general attitudes toward the environment, and in subjective relaxation in order to study this issue, but these results have not yet been analysed.

The conclusion to emerge from this study is cautiously negative. As far as we can tell, the effects of relaxation training on BP are not mediated via changes in muscle tension, peripheral temperature or respiratory rate. It is necessary therefore to await more positive answers if we wish to enhance the strength of relaxation training in the treatment of EHT by focusing on more active components of the technique.

REFERENCES

Agras, W. S. (1982). Weight reduction and blood pressure management: the generalised and enduring effects of two behavior-change procedures. In Stuart, R. B. (Ed.), *Adherence, Compliance and Generalization in Behavioral Medicine*. Brunner-Mazel, New York.

English, E. H. and Baker, T. B. (1983). Relaxation training and cardiovascular response to experimental stressors. *Health Psychology*, **2**, 239–259.

Grossman, P. and Defares, P. B. (1984). Breathing to the heart of the matter. Effects of respiratory influences upon cardiovascular phenomena. In Spielberger, C. D. and Sarason, I. (Ed.), *Stress and Anxiety*, vol. 10, Hemisphere, Washington, D.C.

Henry, J. P. and Cassel, J. C. (1969). Psychosocial factors in essential hypertension. Recent epidemiological and animal experimental evidence. *American Journal of Epidemiology*, **90**, 171–200.

Jacob, R. B., Kraemer, H. C. and Agras, W. S. (1977). Relaxation therapy in the treatment of essential hypertension. *Archives of General Psychiatry*, **34**, 1417–1427.

Johnston, D. W. (1986a). The treatment of hypertension by relaxation training. In Vinck, J., Vandereycken, W., Fontaine, O and Eelen, P. (Eds), *Annual Review of European Research in Behavior Therapy, vol. I, Topics in Behavioral Medicine*. Swets & Zeitlinger, Lisse.

Johnston, D. W. (1986b). How does relaxation training reduce blood pressure in primary hypertension? In Schmidt, T. H., Dembroski, T. D. and Blumchen, C. (Eds), *Biological and Psychological Factors in Cardiovascular Disease*. Springer, Berlin-Heidelberg.

McCaffrey, R. J. and Blanchard, E. B. (1985). Stress management approaches to the treatment of essential hypertension. *Annals of Behavioral Medicine*, **7**(1), 5–12.

Reading, C. (1986). Psychophysiology and the treatment of headache. In Vinck, J., Vandereycken, W., Fontaine, O. and Eelen, P. (Eds), *Annual Review of European Research in Behavior Therapy, vol. I, Topics in Behavioral Medicine*, Swets & Zeitlinger, Lisse.

Shapiro. D. and Goldstein, I. B. (1982). Biobehavioral perspectives on hypertension. *Journal of Consulting and Clinical Psychology*, **50**, 841–858.

Taylor, C. B., Farquhar, J. W., Nelson, E. and Agras, W. S. (1977). The effects of relaxation therapy and high blood pressure. *Archives of General Psychiatry*, **34**, 339–342.

Vaitl, D. (1982). *Essentielle Hypertonie. Psychologisch-medizinische Aspekte*. Springer, Berlin-Heidelberg–New York.

Vinck, J., Arickx, M. and Hongenaert, M. (1987). Predicting interindividual differences in blood pressure response to relaxation training in normotensives. *Journal of Behavioral Medicine*, **10**(4), 395–400.

Behavioural Medicine in Cardiovascular Disorders
Edited by T. Elbert, W. Langosch, A. Steptoe and D. Vaitl
©1988 John Wiley & Sons Ltd

7

Efficiency of Behavioral Intervention in Hypertension

Burkhard Walter, Heinz Rüddel* and August Wilhelm von Eiff

Department of Medicine, University of Bonn, FRG

SUMMARY

Clinical casual blood pressure in patients with mild essential hypertension decreased during and after participation in a stress management seminar based on cognitive behavior modification and relaxation therapy. The mechanisms of these behavioral interventions to lower blood pressure are only poorly understood. To exclude that patients had only learned to be less aroused when blood pressure is taken in the physicians's office we assessed clinical casual blood pressure, self-recorded home blood pressure, and ambulatory blood pressure at work and at home, as well as behavioral patterns, coping strategies, and personality traits before and after a group seminar in patients with mild essential hypertension and in a control group of patients on effective antihypertensive monotherapy. The results show that in addition to a decreased clinical casual blood pressure, self-recorded and automatically recorded blood pressure are within the normotensive range. This demonstrated that patients effectively changed life-style and/or the physiologic responses to mental challenge and really had learned to control blood pressure throughout the day. This was also reflected by changes in questionnaire-assessed behavioral characteristics. We suggest that behavioral interventions should be integrated into all antihypertensive regimens if the patients are motivated to participate.

INTRODUCTION

In our first large interdisciplinary prospective study (1957–1964), we demonstrated that clinical casual blood pressure (BP) could temporarily be lowered in a subset of patients with essential hypertension during long-term psychoanalytical therapy (von Eiff, 1967).

*Correspondence to: Dr H. Rüddel, Department of Internal Medicine, Sigmund-Freud-Str. 25, D-5300 Bonn 1, FRG.

During the last decade different groups have published behavioral programs to lower BP. Most of them are based on the assumption that stress is involved in the etiology of hypertension (von Eiff, 1984). These methods have tried to improve strategies for coping with stress (Kalinke *et al.*, 1982; Charlesworth *et al.*, 1984). A wide spectrum of very different treatments has been implemented in regard to the improvement of stress coping, though problems remain with differences in standardization, duration, and extent of treatment, as well the variety of samples (inpatient–outpatient) used, together with medication and other factors (Seer, 1979; Linden, 1983). It has also been demonstrated that it is possible to lower clinical casual BP with biofeedback methods (Patel *et al.*, 1981 and 1985; Engel *et al.*, 1983).

All these regimens have in common an uncertainty concerning which group of patients are respard and which changes are brought about by what sort of treatment. It remains to be seen which mechanisms really produce reductions in blood pressure and which interventions are both effective and economical (Kaluza *et al.*, 1980; Nitsch, 1981). Although short and even long-term lowering of BP has been reported, it has not yet been demonstrated that these interventions lower BP in everyday life (World Health Organization, 1983).

However, BP recorded throughout the day is the best predictor of cardiovascular damage (Perloff *et al.*, 1983; Sokolov *et al.*, 1966; Pickering *et al.*, 1985). Ambulatory BP values are difficult to predict from clinical casual BP (Floras *et al.*, 1981; Harshfield *et al.*, 1982; des Combes *et al.*, 1984). We therefore used a portable automatic BP system to examine BP reductions throughout the day.

We have developed a training program of nine sessions (2 hours each) concentrating on a change of stress coping in everyday life, and this is tailored to the individual needs. After effective pharmacological monotherapy had been withdrawn, the behavioral treatment was initiated when BP had increased over 160/95 mmHg. According to our examinations it is to be expected that 22 weeks after withdrawal of medication, 75% of all patients will demonstrate clinical casual BP values in the hypertensive range again (Schmieder *et al.*, 1985). We therefore examined whether or not our behavioral intervention could effectively lower BP throughout the day. We postulated that:

> The stress management training improves the efficiency of coping strategies and reduces BP values in everyday life into the normotensive range.

This assumption was based on our clinical experience that hypertensive patients can be considered to have inefficient stress-coping strategies that either increase stress or lead to denial. Both strategies may be supposed to increase BP in the long run.

Table 1. Age (in years) and blood pressure (BP) (in mmHg) of the patients in the experimental and control group. No significant differences were observed between the two groups except for a higher diastolic BP in the experimental group before initiation of the stress–management training ($p < 0.01$).

		Experimental group ($n = 9$)	Control group ($n = 8$)
Age	x	43	48
	SD	7	3
Blood pressure screening	x	158/104	151/96
	SD	19/16	13/6
1st clinical casual BP before medical	x	146/101	150/99
treatment	SD	14/14	16/8
Last clinical casual BP before stress–	x	141/98	139/87
management training	SD	10/11	11/9

METHODS

Sample

Male executives were screened for elevated BP. Those who were diagnosed as essential hypertensive for the first time were treated either with beta-blockers or calcium antagonists, leading to reductions in clinical casual BP to below 140/90 mmHg for at least 6 months. After that, all drugs were withdrawn. If casual BP increased after withdrawal of pharmacotherapy, patients were either again put on the drugs that were known to be effective in these individuals (control group, $n = 8$) or they participated in a behavioral modification program ($n = 9$). To control for other factors, patients in both groups were selected to be males only, within the age bracket of 30–50 years, and none had hypertension-related target organ damage (WHO Stage I). Patients in the behavioral treatment group were somewhat younger and showed a higher clinical casual BP before the initiation of therapy (see Table 1).

Study design

Ambulatory BP values throughout the day were assessed in both groups at the end of the regimen. Clinical casual BP was measured before, during, and after therapy. Questionnaires were handed out to the members of both groups after the experimental period and in addition at the beginning of therapy to the experimental group (see details in Figure 1).

BP recordings

We assessed:

1. Clinical casual BP with a random-zero-sphygmomanometer after a 5-minute rest, in the seated position.

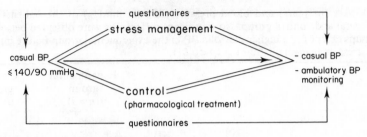

Figure 1. Design of the study.

2. Home BP recordings from the beginning to the end of therapy (three times a day: before breakfast, after coming home from work, before going to bed), mainly for its therapeutic value (Vaitl, 1978; Agras *et al.*, 1982; Goldstein *et al.*, 1984).
3. Ambulatory BP monitoring with a portable automatic system (Physioport, Par Electronics, Langewitz *et al.*, 1985, 1987) between 9:00 am and 6:00 pm. BP was recorded at random time intervals of approximately 15 minutes.

Psychometric tests

Most of the reported methods of assessing coping strategies have not been validated as yet (Nitsch, 1981; Prystav, 1981). Therefore, we put together a battery of tests, which covered most of the hypertension-related behavioral

Table 2. Questionnaires used to assess an impact of the behavioral intervention on psychological parameters

---

Moods
  Spielberger: state/trait anxiety (Laux *et al.*, 1981)
  v. Zerssen: Befindlichkeits-Skala (self + spouse's rating) (von Zerssen, 1976a)
              'Beschwerden'-Liste (von Zerssen, 1976b)

Type A
  Thurstone: type A scale
  Framingham: type A scale (Rüddel *et al.*, 1986)

Social skills
  Ullrich and Ullrich: 'Unsicherheitsfragebogen' (5 subscales) (Ullrich and Ullrich, 1979)

Frustration–aggression
  Rosenzweig: Picture Frustration Test (Rauchfleisch, 1979)

Coping strategies
  'Streßverarbeitungsbogen' (SVF), 5 subscales (Janke *et al.*, 1981) (form hab 5 s 144 i 24 k)
  'Means-End-Problem-Solving Procedure' (Platt and Spivack, 1975; Braukmann *et al.*, 1980)

---

problems (Rüddel *et al.*, 1980) and at the same time were also sensitive to changes over a relatively short period of time. This included the Rosenzweig PFT, a standardized thematic projective test, which is intended to record individual reactions to emotional stress (see Table 2).

Stress-management training

We tried to develop an efficient and economical group therapy program in which the patients were to acquire the skill of handling everyday stress and be able to relax. We also defined the following therapeutic goals: to change destructive lifestyles, approach and solve personal problems, and discover more joy in life.

The methodological orientation is mainly based on Meichenbaum (1979), e.g. stress-inoculation training, self-instructional approach to stress management or cognitive restructuring, at the same time implementing rules from group therapy and Rogerian therapy too. All patients were taught autogenic training (AT, Schulz, 1976) with various additional exercises plus visual imaginations. Details are published in Walter (1988). Besides, information was given on the impact of nutrition, exercise, lifestyle, and stress on elevated BP (WHO, 1983). A biographical history was taken from each patient prior to group therapy. Thus, we were able to focus on the individual problems in the training sessions. We also included the spouses of the patients in the program. A timetable itemizes the schedule in Figure 2.

Particular attention was paid to issues such as recreation, behavioral attitudes toward work and family, perception through the spouse and peer group, as well as to self-esteem. In cases where people had alcohol or marital problems, further individual therapy sessions were instituted.

Results

Before therapy patients in both groups did not differ significantly, either in BP levels (see Table 1) or in psychometric results. The hypertensive patients being

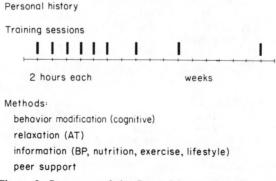

Figure 2. Summary of the Stress Management Program.

Table 3. Blood pressure in the experimental group (behavioral intervention) and the control group (effective longtime pharmacologic therapy) after 3 months of therapy.

		Experimental group	Control group	Difference between the groups	Level of significance (p)
Average blood pressure during the day (mmHg)	x SD	125/90 4/7	135/90 8/8	− 10 systolic BP − 5 diastolic BP	<0.05 0.25
Mean of the three lowest blood pressure readings during the day (mmHg)	x SD	111/77 6/10	122/85 7/8	− 11 systolic BP − 8 diastolic BP	<0.05 0.22
Clinical casual blood pressure (mmHg)	x SD	131/86 8/5	139/87 11/9	− 8 systolic BP − 1 diastolic BP	0.15 —

Table 4. Comparison of blood pressure values and psychometric variables before and after the behavioral intervention.

		Before therapy	After therapy	Difference after therapy	Level of significance (p)
Clinical casual blood pressure (mmHg)	x SD	138/94 17/6	131/86 8/5	− 7 systolic BP − 7.6 diastolic BP	0.22 0.04
Average of self-reported blood pressure over a period of 1 week (mmHg)	x SD	136/88 15/13	129/88 9/2	− 7.6 systolic BP + 0 diastolic BP	0.2
State anxiety (aU)	x SD	41 11	31 6	− 10.4	0.007
Befindlichkeit (aU)	x SD	16 6	9 5	− 7	0.028
Coping strategies (aU) aktionale Situationskontrolle kognitive Situationskontrolle Entspannungsversuche		16.3 11.9 12.6	18.8 15.4 16.3	+ 2.66 + 3.6 + 3.7	0.025 0.063 0.023

studied appeared to lie in normal range in regard to the psychological parameters. State anxiety, however, was somewhat elevated and these patients seemed more demanding, demonstrated a lack of calmness, and seemed to avoid conflicts.

After the behavioral intervention the experimental group showed lower BP levels throughout the day in comparison with the control group. BP values in both groups, however, were within the normotensive range (Table 3). As to the systolic BP these differences were statistically significant.

After behavioral therapy patients in the experimental group used more relaxation techniques than patients on drugs (SVF; 17 ± 3 vs 13 ± 3, $p = 0.03$), showed more initiatives on their own (PFT: i; 6 ± 1.6 vs 4 ± 1.6, $p = 0.03$), showed a tendency for trying to solve problems (PFT: N-P; 6.5 ± 1.8 vs 4.6 ± 2.4, $p = 0.11$) and appeared less anxious (state anxiety: 31 ± 6 vs 37 ± 7, $p = 0.06$).

Throughout the non-pharmacological intervention anxiety and type-A behavior pattern decreased while well-being and relaxation increased as well as the feeling of having managed problems oneself (see Table 4).

The PFT results were in the expected direction. We observed:

1. a reduction in the tendency for denial of social conflicts and an impediment in ability to express emotion;
2. an improvement in making light of conflicts;
3. a more adequate self-criticism;
4. a reduction of denial guilt;
5. a development of more outwardly-directed aggression into the normal range;
6. a small decrease in feeling of guilt.

In summary, after application of behavioral intervention methods the patterns of subscales of the PFT, which assessed reactions towards frustration, tended to be within the normal range, whereas the PFT showed low or high values before therapy.

We found hardly any correlation between the BP values throughout the day and the casual and self-measured BP measurements. However, numerous correlations with psychometric scores were observed. In brief, low BP values were associated with positive feelings about coping with stress:

1. actively by doing something or by cognitive positive self-instruction;
2. by facing conflicts;
3. by relaxing well and often;
4. by having enough aggression against others and self;
5. by expressing emotions more frequently;
6. by being less compliant and expressing one's point of view;
7. by showing type-A behavior pattern less frequently;
8. by having the courage to decline or neglect responsibilities when needed;
9. by demonstrating less anxiety.

DISCUSSION

The most important finding in this study, albeit with a small sample was the fact that in patients with behavioral therapy, clinical casual BP and BP throughout the day could be effectively lowered into the normotensive range. Furthermore, ambulatory systolic BP in the experimental group was even lower than BP in patients on effective drug therapy. This result demonstrates that patients who participate in behavioral intervention programs do not only learn to lower BP when BP is measured in the physician's office but that BP is lower throughout the entire work day.

Technical and methodical difficulties impose potential problems on ambulatory BP monitoring. Some patients are not willing to work with the automatic unit, since they feel stigmatized as a 'patient'. Also, all available units restrict the patient in everyday activities like sports, etc. (Mancia, 1983). A relatively high percentage of all BP recordings are artefacts which have to be subtracted before analyzing the data (Messerli, 1984).

With reference to the psychometric tests there remains one problem to be solved (Arndt-Page et al., 1983). It concerns the validity of the instruments used since they might not assess coping strategies adequately. In view of this problem we attempted to cover a wide range of behavioral patterns by different methods such as projective tests, questionnaires on coping, well-being, anxiety and self-esteem.

Along with the decrease of BP most of the negative behavioral conditions, favorable for elevated BP (e.g. anxiety, tenseness, loss of control) were changed by the experimental treatment, at least temporarily. Long-term follow-up of these patients has not yet been concluded.

The participants of the experiment were not randomly allocated into the experimental behavioral therapy and control groups, because some patients were no longer willing to take any drugs, while others refused to participate in the time-consuming behavioral intervention or a therapeutic group setting. The results can therefore be considered only provisional.

Our results demonstrate that no general 'hypertensive' personality can be identified. However, the behavioral pattern of each of the patients is heterogenous (von Eiff, 1967; Linden, 1983). None of our patients appeared to lie in the 'normal' range on psychometric variables, even though as a group the hypertensive patients did not significantly differ from the normotensive population. This fact stresses the need for more single case studies, and gives support to our therapeutic approach in which we try to individualize interventions within the group session.

Nevertheless, the results of this pilot study demonstrate that behavioral intervention can be an effective part of antihypertensive regimens if the patient is motivated to participate.

REFERENCES

Agras, W. S., Horne, M. and Taylor, C. B. (1982). Expectation and the blood-pressure-lowering effects of relaxation. *Psychosomatic Medicine*, **44**, 389–395.

Arndt-Page, B., Geiger, E., Koeppen, M. and Künzel, R. (1983). Klassifizierung von Copingverhalten. *Diagnostica*, **24**(2), 183–189.

Braukmann, W., Filipp, S.-H., Ahammer, I., Angleitner, A. and Olbrich, E. (1980). *Zur diagnostischen Erfassung von sozialer Kompetenz: Entwicklung einer deutschen Version des "Means-Ends Problem-Solving Questionnaire" (MEPS) von Platt & Spivack*. Forschungsbericht Nr. 5 aus dem Projekt "Entwicklungspsychologie des Erwachsenenalters". Trier.

Charlesworth, E. A., Williams, B. J. and Baer, P. E. (1984). Stress management at the worksite for hypertension: compliance, cost-benefit, health care and hypertension-related variables. *Psychosomatic Medicine*, **46**(5), 387–397.

des Combes, B., Porchert, M., Waeber, B. and Brunner, H. R. (1984). Ambulatory blood pressure recordings. Reproducibility and unpredictability. *Hypertension*, **6**, 110–114.

von Eiff, A. W. (1967). *Essentielle Hypertonie*. Thieme, Stuttgart.

von Eiff, A. W. (1984). Pathophysiologie und Ätiologie der essentiellen Hypertonie. *MMW*, **126**, 165–170.

Engel, B. T., Glasgow, M. S. and Gaarder, K. R. (1983). Behavioral treatment of high blood pressure: III. Follow-up results and treatment recommendations. *Psychosomatic Medicine*, **45**, 23–30.

Floras, J. S., Hassan, M. O., Seuer, P. S., Jones, J. U., Ossikowska, B. and Sleight, P. (1981). Cuff and ambulatory blood pressure in subjects with essential hypertension. *Lancet*, **2**, 107–109.

Goldstein, I. B., Schapiro, D. and Thananopavaran, C. H. (1984). Home relaxation techniques for essential hypertension. *Psychosomatic Medicine*, **46**, 389–414.

Harshfield, G. A., Pickering, T. G., Kleinert, H. D., Blank, S. and Laragh, J. H. (1982). Situational variations of blood pressure in ambulatory hypertensive patients. *Psychosomatic Medicine*, **44**, 237–245.

Janke, W., Erdmann, G. and Boucsein, W. (1981). Streßverarbeitungsbogen Form hab 5s 144i 24k. Düsseldorf: unpublished.

Kalinke, D., Kulick, B. and Heim, P. (1982). Psychologische Behandlungsmöglichkeiten bei essentiellen Hypertonikern. In Köhle, K. (Ed.), *Zur Psychosomatik von Herz-Kreislauf Erkrankungen*, Springer, Berlin.

Kaluza, K., Lehnert, H. and Dorst, K. (1980). Klinisch-psychologische Therapie der essentiellen Hypertonie. In Hautzinger, M. and Schulz, W. (Eds), *Klinische Psychologie und Psychotherapie*, vol. 3, Kongressbericht Berlin 1980. DGVT, Tübingen, pp. 327–336.

Langewitz, W., Zünkler, B., Otten, H. Rüddel, H. and von Eiff, A. W. (1985). First experiences with a new automatic ambulatory recording device for blood pressure, heart rate, EMG, and respiratory rate: Physioport. *Psychophysiology*, **22**, 500 (abstract).

Langewitz, W., Rüddel, H., Dähnert, A. (1987). Zur Validität der Blutdruckmessung eines neuen tragbaren automatischen Blutdruckmefsgerätes (Physioport). *Medizinische Welt*, **38**, 1–6.

Laux, L., Glanzmann, P., Schaffner, P. and Spielberger, C. D. (1981). *Das State-Trait-Angstinventar*, Theoretische Grundlagen und Handanweisung, Beltz, Weinheim.

Linden, W. (1983). *Psychologische Perspektiven des Bluthochdrucks*. Ursprung, Verlauf und Behandlung. Karger, Basel.

110 BEHAVIOURAL MEDICINE

Meichenbaum, D. (1979). *Kognitive Verhaltensmodifikation*. Urban & Schwarzenberg, München.

Messerli, F. H. (1984). Continuous noninvasive automatic blood pressure recording. Value and limitations in clinical practice. *Postgraduate Medicine*, **75** (4), 115-124.

Nitsch, J. R. (Ed.) (1981). *Streß*. Theorien, Untersuchungen, Maßnahmen. Huber, Bern.

Patel, C., Marmot, M. G. and Terry, D. J. (1981). Controlled trial of biofeedback-aided behavioral methods in reducing mild hypertension. *British Medical Journal*, **282**, 2005-2008.

Patel, C., Marmot, M. G., Terry, D. J. Carruthers, M., Hunt, B. and Patel, M. (1985). Trial of relaxation in reducing coronary risk: four years follow up. *British Medical Journal*, **290**, 1103-1106.

Perloff, D., Sokolov, M. and Cowan, R. (1983). The prognostic value of ambulatory blood pressures. *Journal of the American Medical Association*, **249** (20), 2792-2798.

Pickering, T. G., Harshfield, G. A., Devereux, R. B. and Laragh, J. H. (1985). What is the role of ambulatory blood pressure monitoring in the management of hypertensive patients? *Hypertension*, **7**, 171-177.

Platt, J. J. and Spivack, G. (1975). *Manual for the Means-End-Problem-Solving Procedure (MEPS)*. A Measure of inter-personal cognitive problem-solving skill. Hahnemann Medical College and Hospital, Philadelphia (unpublished).

Prystav, G. (1981). Psychologische Copingforschung. Konzeptbildungen, Operationalisierungen, Meßinstrumente. *Diagnostica*, **27**, 189-214.

Rauchfleisch, U. (1979). *Handbook zum Rosenzweig Picture-Frustration Test (PFT)*, vol. 2. Huber, Bern.

Rüddel, H. (1980). Psychophysiologische Voraussetzungen bei der Entstehung der essentiellen Hypertonie. In Hautzinger, M. and Schulz, W. (Eds), *Klinische Psychologie und Psychotherapie*, vol. 3, Kongressbericht Berlin 1980, DGVT, Tübingen, pp. 297-309.

Rüddel, H., Schmieder, R., Neus, J., Neus, H., Otten, H., Langewitz, W. and Eiff v., A. W. (1986). Bio-behavioral effects of monotherapy with oxprenolol and nitrendipine. In Dembrowski, T., Schmidt, T. and Blümchen, G. (Eds), *Biological and Psychological Factors in Cardiovascular Disease*, Springer, Berlin, pp. 584-593.

Schmieder, R., Rüddel, H., Neus, J., Eiff, v., A. W. (1985). Blutdruckverhalten nach Absetzen einer 6-monatigen anti-hypertensiven Therapie. *Herzmedizin*, **6**, 220-225.

Schultz, I. H. (1976). *Das autogene Training*, 15th edn. Thieme, Stuttgart.

Seer, P. (1979). Psychological control of essential hypertension: review of the literature and methodological critique. *Psychology Bulletin*, **86**, 1015-1043.

Sokolov, M., Werdegar, D., Kain, H. K. and Hinman, A. T. (1966). Relationship between level of blood pressure measured casually and by portable recorders and severity of complications in essential hypertension. *Circulation*, **34**, 279-298.

Ullrich, R. and Ullrich, R. (1979). *Der Unsicherheitsfragebogen*. Testmanual U. Anleitung für den Therapeuten Teil 2, 2nd edn. Pfeiffer, München.

Vaitl, D. (1978). Medikamentöse Behandlung der Hypertonie und Motivation der Patienten zur Dauerbehandlung. In Bundesvereinigung für Gesundheitserziehung, e.V. (Eds), *Auf den Blutdruck achten*. Universitäts-Buchdruckerei, Bonn.

Walter, B. (1988). Zur Effektivität einer verhaltensmedizinischen Therapie in der antihypertensiven Therapie. Medical Dissertation, University of Bonn (in preparation).

World Health Organization, Report of a WHO scientific group (1983). *Primary prevention of essential hypertension*. WHO Technical report series 686, Geneva.

Zerssen, von D. (1976a). Klinische Selbstbeurteilungs-Skalen (KSb-S) aus dem Münchener Psychiatrischen Informationssystem (PSYCHIS München). *Die Beschwerde-Liste—* Parallelformen B-L und B-L'—Ergänzungsbogen B-L,—Manual. Beltz, Weinheim.
Zerssen, von D. (1976b). Klinische Selbstbeurteilungs-Skalen (KSb-S) aus dem Münchener Psychiatrischen Informationssystem (PSYCHIS München). *Die Befindlichkeits-Skala-* Parallelformen Bf-S und Bf-S'—Manual, Beltz, Weinheim.

Behavioural Medicine in Cardiovascular Disorders
Edited by T. Elbert, W. Langosch, A. Steptoe and D. Vaitl
© 1988 John Wiley & Sons Ltd

8

Behavioral Therapies in Essential Hypertensives: A Controlled Study

*E. Richter-Heinrich, V. Homuth, B. Heinrich, U. Knust,
K. H. Schmidt, R. Wiedemann and H. R. Gohlke
*Central Institute of Cardiovascular Research,
Academy of Sciences of the German Democratic Republic*

INTRODUCTION

The present study is based on previous investigations (Richter-Heinrich *et al.*, 1971, 1974, 1976) in which we demonstrated that, compared to normotensives, hypotensives, and cardiophobics, essential hypertensives show in the early stages of disease:

1. higher *sensitivity* during stimulus input (lower absolute acoustic thresholds);
2. higher physiological *reactivity* in a mental load test and during the acquisition of a backward conditioned electrodermal reflex;
3. less *adaptation* to an acoustic signal (signal detection experiment)

The question arises whether these physiological patterns are correlated with special personality traits. Attempts to find a specific hypertensive personality have failed. Recently, attempts have been made to characterize behavior traits often observed in hypertensives in a social context, such as social anxiety, lack of self-assertiveness, suppressed hostility, drive for perfectionism, lack of emotional expression, leading to overtly adapted behavior and repressive, defensive, stress coping styles (Linden, 1984; Richter-Heinrich, 1983).

Therefore, recently, we evaluated the stress coping styles of hypertensives using the stress coping questionnaire (SVF) of Janke *et al.* (1985). This self-report instrument contains 19 'habitual' coping styles each of them including six items, measured by a five-point Likert-type rating. We performed a cluster analysis over these 19 coping styles in 75 hypertensive patients.

*Address for correspondence: Central Institute of Cardiovascular Research, Academy of Sciences of the German Democratic Republic, Wiltbergstr. 50, Berlin, GDR-1115.

Table 1. Cluster analysis of the 19 stress-coping strategies of the SVF (Janke *et al.*, 1985) in 75 essential hypertensives.

Clusters	1	2	3	4	5
Main coping strategies within the single clusters	imaginary carrying on (60)	need for social support (56)	drug taking (60)	aggression (55)	positive self-instruction (61)
	self-accusation (58)	efforts to reaction control (54)	substitutional satisfaction (60)	imaginary carrying on (50)	bagatellization (60)
Numbers in parenthesis: Average T-scores	aggression (57)	positive self-instructions (53)	need for social support (56)		efforts to reaction control (57)
	resignation (55)	efforts to situation control (51)	aggression (56)		distraction (56)
	social seclusion (55)	aggression (51)			
More positive (+) and more negative (−) strategies	−	+	−	−	+/−
Percentage of the sample	21.4	20.0	26.6	13.4	18.6

Results, given in Table 1, revealed that only 20% of hypertensives seem to prefer active effective coping styles such as reaction control, situation control, positive self-instructions (see cluster 2), 18.6% showed a mixture of active coping and denial (see cluster 5) while the other 61.4% of the patients had their highest T-scores in strategies such as aggression brooding, resignation; or compensative activities such as drug taking and substitutional satisfaction (see clusters 1, 3, and 4). Aggression, which is often reported in the literature as a typical behavior trait of hypertensives, is represented in 4 of the 5 clusters, indicating that it is a frequently used coping behavior in hypertensives.

Thus essential hypertensives are characterized physiologically by highly sensitive activating systems, and psychologically by a deficiency in reacting adequately to the challenges of the environment. Therefore, we developed a non-pharmacological behavioral treatment program pursuing the following aims:

1. Somatically, to modify the heightened arousal level of hypertensives, their heightened reactivity, and their lowered adaptivity, especially of the cardiovascular system.
2. Psychologically, to modify maladaptive attitudes and behavior patterns.

The following therapeutic methods are used:

1. *Breath-relaxation training* (a modified technique after Benson *et al.*, 1974) supported during the first sessions by biofeedback of systolic blood pressure (BP) and muscle relaxation training aimed at decreasing the heightened tonic arousal level and the reactivity to daily life events. The patients were instructed to train for 20 minutes daily and to use the method occasionally for a few minutes in stressful daily life situations.
2. *Daily self-measurements* of BP to make the patient aware of the variability of BP and of the situations leading to BP increases (three measurements after getting up, three after work, and three before sleeping).
3. *Individual psychotherapeutic interventions* and/or psychological group *stress management training* aimed at learning:
   (a) perception and control of individual physiological stress patterns;
   (b) perception and control of individual psychological stress patterns;
   (c) stress-reducing behavior patterns by modifying stress related appraisals and attitudes (Lazarus and Launier, 1978) by a social skill training and specific stress coping techniques such as thought stopping, etc. (see Birbaumer, 1977).

Throughout training we tried to make the patients sensitive to their own role in generating stress, by analyzing the vicious circle: automatic appraisal of a situation as threatening→somatic and emotional strain→negative stress augmenting thoughts and self-verbalizations→stress behavior (see Kallinke *et al.*, 1982).

As it is routine in pharmacotherapy, prior to practical application the therapeutic efficacy of behavioral methods has to be thoroughly tested (Shapiro *et al.*, 1977).

The two main steps of testing are (Vaitl, 1975):

1. *Proving their effectiveness in decreasing BP and studying underlying mechanisms.*
   In previous experiments we have evaluated the effectivity of relaxation and biofeedback methods, examined hemodynamic changes during these forms of training, correlated success in training with personality traits, assessed breathing patterns of good and less good performers, etc. The quintessence of these studies was that compared with biofeedback, the relaxation methods appeared to be more effective for practical use. Relaxation training was easier to learn, had broader physiological effects, and could be used at home without special devices; furthermore, success in lowering BP was not related to personality while in biofeedback training neurotic patients showed smaller BP decreases than others (Richter-Heinrich *et al.*, 1982).
2. *Proving their therapeutic efficacy in clinical long-term studies, evaluating the results by comparisons with appropriate pharmacological and other control groups.*

Our long-term studies were performed in three parts. In this chapter we refer particularly to results assessed in part I because we have only preliminary results in parts II and III at present.

PART I

Part I comprises 64 essential hypertensives, at the clinical stage I (WHO), aged 18 to 48 years, mean age 34 years. They were allotted to the following three groups:

1. Behavioral therapy group I ($n = 20$). These patients stayed in hospital for about 3½ weeks, undergoing in the first 8 (± 3) days clinical and psychophysiological diagnostics and being taught self-recording of BP. Then they received the above described behavioral treatments over 14 days. The self-recordings of this treatment period were used as baseline and compared in a first step with the self-recordings in the last 14 days of a 3-month therapeutic interval. During stay in hospital patients had to practice the relaxation twice a day in the laboratory and additionally once a day for 20 minutes in their bedroom. During the control sessions in the laboratory BP was measured automatically in an adjoining room each minute (5 minutes before, 20 minutes during, and 5 minutes after training). After each session the BP protocol was discussed with the patients. In four sessions the relaxation training was combined with feedback of systolic BP.

Furthermore, patients were given circulatory and respiratory gymnastics (eight times) and muscle relaxation training (six times). (For details see Richter-Heinrich *et al.*, 1981.) Psychotherapy was given individually. These patients have been followed up for more than 4 years.

2. Control group I ($n = 24$). These patients had in the first phase only to perform self-monitoring of BP over 3 months, during the first 14 days of which they were also in a hospital ward. They were instructed that the information they gathered during the daily self-recordings of their BP might be sufficient to control BP effectively and that after 3 months a decision would be made whether additional therapy would be necessary.

Twenty of these patients (behavioral therapy group II) received in the second phase of the cross-over design a variation of the above described psychological 'treatment package'. A rationalized, i.e. a cost and time-saving, therapy variant was used. Unlike group I the patients of group II were outpatients from the very beginning of treatment and underwent group stress management training. Additional individual therapy was only given when necessary.

3. Pharmacological control group II ($n = 20$). These patients were treated with beta-blocker monotherapy in the first 3 months (10 patients with talinolol, 10 with propranolol). After this they were followed up for another 9-month period with combined drug therapy, usually a diuretic and/or a vasodilator in addition to the beta-blocker.

All three groups were matched with respect to age, sex, and body mass. Behavioral therapy groups I and II were without medication over the entire treatment period.

The therapeutic effectiveness was analyzed on four different data levels:

1. casual recordings of BP by the physician;
2. self-recordings of BP;
3. pre- and post-treatment data of a psychophysiological mental load test;
4. psychological trait and state inventories.

Some major findings

Self-recordings of BP

The comparison between the daily self-recordings (mean values of nine measurements each) of the first 14 days of therapy and the same number of self-recordings at the end of the first 3 months of therapy using Cox and Stuart's (1978) Trendtest yielded the following results in the psychologically treated groups. In therapy group I most of the patients had significant systolic and/or diastolic BP decreases, whereas the 3 months of self-recordings in the 24 patients without special therapeutic interventions caused significant decreases in only

Table 2. Trends (assessed by the Trendtest of Cox and Stuart) of 3 months' self-monitoring of blood pressure in the behavioral therapy group I, the self-monitoring control group and the behavioral group II.

Significant blood pressure changes (%)	Behavioral therapy I ($n = 20$)	Controls Self-monitoring ($n = 24$)	Behavioral therapy II ($n = 20$) cross-over
Decreases	75	16.7	69.9
No change	10	33.3	20.6
Increases	15	50.0	9.5

16.7% of the patients and increases in half of the patients. The cross-over to the outpatient stress management training resulted in significant BP decreases in the majority of these patients, too (see Table 2; Richter-Heinrich et al., 1981).

Casual recordings of BP by the physician

In comparing the psychological therapy group I with the pharmacological control group the casual recordings made by the physician in the course of a year were used, since the pharmacological group did not take any self-measurements. Therapy group I and the beta-blocker group had identical mean initial values of 166/104 mmHg and 164/104 mmHg and after 3 months of therapy BP decreases of 15/11 and 14/8 mmHg. The decreases in systolic BP were significant for both groups, but only the behavior therapy group showed a significant reduction in diastolic BP. In the following 9 months the pharmacological group was given additional drugs. The t-tests for paired samples showed that over these 9 months the two groups did not differ significantly in their mean values. After 1 year the mean decreases in the psychologically treated group were 16/11 mmHg, those of the pharmacologically treated group 20/11 mmHg, and the mean values of both groups were in the borderline hypertensive range (Table 3). Because of drop-outs in both groups at 6 and 12 months follow-up, we performed a second analysis using only the 14 patients remaining in both groups for 1 year. Starting from the initial values of 165/103 mmHg, the behavior therapy group showed significant decreases of 16/11 mmHg. The drug therapy group had initial values of 163/102 mmHg and significant decreases of 20/11 mmHg. Differences between groups were significant only after 3 but not during the following 9 months. Thus both showed the same pattern as the whole sample, referred to in Table 3. Therapy group II has been followed up for 2 years and shows the same trend.

Therapy group I has been followed up for 4 years. A total of 60% of the patients have continued treatment without medication. Their BP values are in the normotensive or borderline range. Twenty percent have dropped out for reasons of compliance. In 20% high BP has required drug administration.

Table 3. Mean casual blood pressure of the drug and behavioral therapy groups over 1 year.

Duration of therapy		Before		3 months		6 months		12 months	
Blood pressure (mmHg)		Systolic	Diastolic	Systolic	Diastolic	Systolic	Diastolic	Systolic	Diastolic
Behavioral Therapy Group	Mean	166	104	151	93	155	94	150	93
	SD	18.7	10.9	14.0	8.7	13.4	8.8	17.0	1.0
	n		20		20		16		14
Drug Therapy Group	Mean	164	104	152	96	150	96	144	93
	SD	19.9	12.2	19.9	12.9	15.1	11.9	11.8	9.8
	n		20		19		18		14
Medication		—		beta-blocker		beta-blocker + diureticum and/or vasodilator			

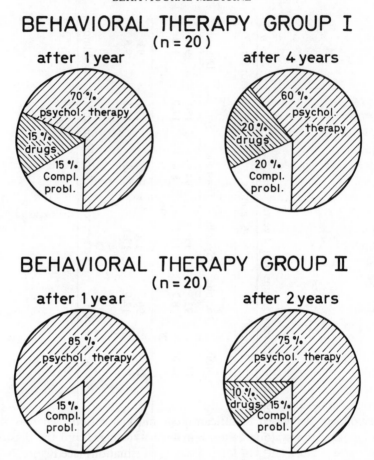

Figure 1. Percentage of patients who (1) continued non-drug therapy; (2) needed additional drugs and (3) dropped out by lack of compliance.

The patients of therapy group II confirm this trend since after 2 years 75% of the patients are still being treated without medication (see Figure 1).

Differentiation of responders and non-responders

An essential point is to find criteria for identifying therapy responders and non-responders, for which purpose we have used the self-recorded BP data of the patients after 3 months of therapy. Accordingly, the patients were divided into two groups:

Responders: patients with distinct positive effects, i.e. their BP decreased significantly to values < 145/95 mmHg.

Non-responders: patients with no or insufficient therapy effects, i.e. their BP decreased but only to levels > 145/95 mmHg, remained unchanged or even increased significantly.

This might be considered a somewhat arbitrary criterion. It was, however, chosen because patients with BP levels below 145/95 mmHg were able to continue treatment without medication. Among the non-responders those patients who had already reached low BP levels in the first 14 days of therapy and thereafter produced no further decrease in the following 3 months of therapy, did not require medication either. But it was not possible to decide whether their decreases in BP were due to our therapeutic intervention or to spontaneous relaxation. Details are given elsewhere (Richter-Heinrich *et al.*, 1981). It should, however, be mentioned that after a longer time of therapy the number of responders increased.

Separate analysis of the two non-pharmacological therapy groups I and II yielded the same data with regard to all criteria of efficacy so that in the following discussion both groups are taken together as one.

A number of meaningful differences between responders ($n = 18$) and non-responders ($n = 22$) were observed:

1. Non-responders had a higher incidence of family history of hypertension than responders (63.6% vs. 33.3%).
2. In the mental load test the two groups did not differ significantly before therapy in their systolic and diastolic BP, and heart rate in the seven test situations. After 3 months of therapy the systolic and diastolic BP of responders decreased significantly in most situations whereas in non-responders the systolic values remained unchanged and the diastolic BP increased significantly in four of the seven situations (see Figure 2). It is of interest that the BP difference scores between initial rest and mental arithmetic did not differ significantly in both responders and non-responders either before or after therapy. Before therapy both groups showed rises of 28 mmHg in systolic BP. Diastolic BP rose in responders by 18 mmHg, and in non-responders by 14 mmHg, but these differences were not significant. During post-therapeutic test-application both groups lowered their difference scores to 22/14 mmHg.
3. Non-responders tended more to neurosis, i.e. in the Freiburger Persönlichkeits-Inventar (FPI) (Fahrenberg and Selg, 1970) and in the anxiety scale (Spreen, 1961) their standard values were significantly higher with regard to nervousness, aggressivity, dominance, and anxiety (Figure 3).
4. These findings seem to indicate more pronounced type A behavior in non-responders. This was verified by results of the Jenkins Activity Survey: 66.7% of non-responders were classified as type A compared to only 35.3% of the responders.

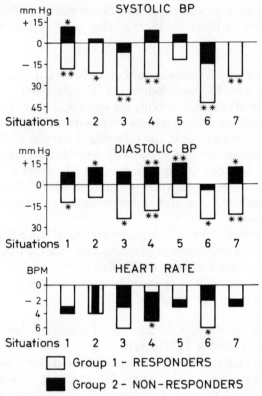

Figure 2. Differences between the absolute mean levels of the pre- and post-treatment sessions in the mental load test. Each test situation lasts 2 minutes. The test consists of seven different situations:
1 Rest I (last 2 min of a 10 min rest period)
2 Anticipation I (announcement of mental arithmetic tasks)
3 Mental arithmetic (multiplication of two-digits)
4 Rest II
5 Anticipation II (announcement of sentence-completion tasks)
6 Sentence completion (sentence with 5 words with the same given initial letters)
7 Rest III
$*p < 0.5$, $**p < 0.1$

5. Non-responders tended to prefer further 'ineffective' stress-coping styles such as self-pity, imaginary carrying on, resignation, drug taking (i.e. sleeping pills, alcohol, etc.), aggression, social seclusion, a tendency to escape, etc. Responders preferred more efficient coping styles such as positive self-instruction, efforts at controlling reactions, etc. All of these were registered by the Janke questionnaire.
6. With respect to cardiovascular complaints, comparisons between the pre- and post-therapeutic scores of a symptom checklist (12 items, 5-point

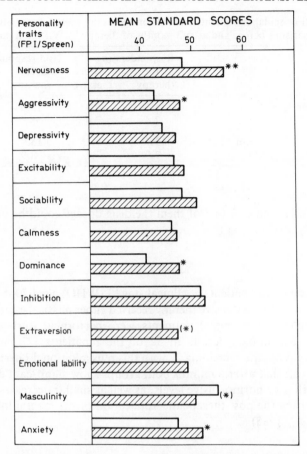

Figure 3. Mean standard scores on the Freiburger Personality Inventory and the Anxiety Scale. White column: responders ($n = 18$); hatched columns: non-responders ($n = 22$). $*p < 0.5$, $**p < 0.1$.

Likert-type rating) revealed no changes in non-responders, but significantly fewer complaints in responders after therapy (see Table 4).

Tension scores (8 items), however, were lowered significantly in both groups after therapy.

PART II

Part II comprises 33 essential hypertensives, clinical stages II or III (WHO). They received antihypertensive drugs, but as their BP was difficult to control behavioral treatment was added. Preliminary results indicate that 7 patients out of 15, who were all treated with this combination over 18 months, lowered their

Table 4. Cardiovascular complaints and tension scores in hypertensives patients, within-subjects comparisons before and after 3 months of therapy by Wilcoxon rank sum tests.

| | | Responders ($n = 18$) | | Non-responders ($n = 22$) | |
		Before therapy	After therapy	Before therapy	After therapy
Cardiovascular	Mean	11.5	6.3*	13.0	12.2
Complaints	SD	7.4	7.0	8.7	9.8
Tension	Mean	13.7	9.2*	15.7	11.7
	SD	7.0	7.4	8.9	6.8

*$p < 0.05$.

BP significantly, and that in 5 of them the drug dosage could be also lowered (Knust *et al.*, 1987).

PART III

Another group of 160 patients at clinical stage I (WHO) aged 20–50 years and with or without antihypertensive therapy received either physical exercise training and/or behavioral training. Treatments were performed during stay in a Sanatorium. Preliminary results in 52 of these patients (27 patients with behavioral training, the remaining 27 with this plus additional physical exercise training) reveals that after 6 months both groups show significant decreases in BP to borderline or normotensive levels, as well as similar decreases of BP and heart rate during the post-therapeutic application of the mental load test (see Heinrich *et al.*, 1985).

CONCLUSIONS AND PROSPECTIVES

The results suggest that in certain patients with mild hypertension a behavioral treatment may substitute for a pharmacological approach. The data indicating that non-responders more often had a positive family history of hypertension and increases in diastolic BP in the mental load test suggests that genetically predisposed patients who perhaps already have morphologically damaged vessels cannot be treated solely by psychological methods. Consequently, for patients with higher stages of hypertension, these approaches appear to be an adjunct only to drug treatment. In this context however they may be effective in reducing the drug dosage or improving BP adjustment, as was shown in our pilot study (part II), and by Patel (1977).

There is considerable interest in the literature at present in the relationship between stress-induced hyper-reactivity and hypertension and cardiovascular disease (Weiss *et al.*, 1984). In our study both groups, responders and non-responders, showed an equal decrease in short-term reactivity (i.e. rest/stress difference scores) after therapy. This suggests that in our test, difference scores seem to be indicators of actual activation, whereas changes in tonic BP levels over all the test situations seem to be good indicators of how the patients cope with stress (Ursin, 1982).

The negative outcome in the control group (self-monitoring only) indicates that the BP decreases of the behavioral treatment groups were due to the psychological treatment package provided. But within the treatment package it is not possible to tell which factors contribute to the outcome of the therapy. It seems that for most of the patients, regular relaxation training at home is necessary to maintain BP decreases. In 7 out of 10 patients who were instructed to stop training after 2 years, BP rose but went down after taking up training again. During training a shift from ergotrophic to trophotrophic patterns was produced, i.e. reductions of BP, heart rate and electrodermal activity (Richter-Heinrich *et al.*, in press), and decreases in stroke volume and cardiac output have also been recorded (Richter-Heinrich *et al.*, unpublished).

With respect to the effectiveness of the stress management training *per se* we do not have any precise data. Behavior changes that were often reported by patients include: acting in a less hectic way, avoiding useless brooding over problems, and thinking a situation over before starting actions. It was more difficult in certain patients with type A behavior to overcome their drive for perfectionism and their tendency to feel responsible for nearly everything in their daily lives. These reports are not just the results of self-assessments but have been confirmed by family members and colleagues at work.

The fact that therapy responders seem to have more efficient stress coping strategies underlines that proper assessment of situations and adequate coping strategies may have positive health effects. Neurotic patients are in need of additional individual psychotherapy.

The daily self-recordings of BP offer not only an opportunity to control the course of therapy but provide exact information about the variability of BP, and about situations in which BP rises. Thus they strengthen the patient's motivation for therapy and sense of responsibility. From the very beginning we tell patients that they are active participants in their own therapy and that our role as therapists is to be a partner in this enterprise.

Intervention programs on a community level have been started now on the basis of these results. During 'cures', patients will receive non-pharmacological therapy consisting of physical training, behavioral treatments, and a dietary regimen. They will be followed up by their local cardiologists and psychologists over subsequent years. Pharmacological and other control groups are included. Thus we hope to gather further knowledge about the possibilities and frontiers of non-pharmacological treatment.

REFERENCES

Benson, H., Beary, J. F. and Carol, M. P. (1974). The relaxation response. *Psychiatry*, 37, 37–46.

Birbaumer, N. (1977). Psychophysiologie der Angst, 2. Aufl., Urban & Schwarzenberg, München, Wien, Baltimore.

Cox, W. and Stuart, B. (1978). Verteilungsfreie Methoden in der Biostatistik, Band 2, Lienert, G. A. (Ed.). Verlag Anton Stain, Meisenhaim.

Fahrenberg, J. and Selg, J. (1970). Das Freiburger Persönlichkeitsinventar (FPI). Handanweisungen für die Durchführung und Auswertung, Göttingen.

Heinrich, B., Heil, J., Richter-Heinrich, E., Priebe, U. and Grosse, W. (1985). Zur Effektivität der nichtmedikamentösen, psychophysiologisch orientierten Therapie bei Hypertonikern während Kuren. Paper Kolloquium '14. Rostocker Gespräch über Fragen der Hypertonietherapie', Ahrenshoop, 14–16.4.

Janke, W., Erdmann, G. and Kallus, W. (1985). Streßverarbeitungsfragebogen (SVF) nach W. Janke, G. Erdmann and W. Boucsein. Handanweisung. Verlag für Psychologie—Dr C. J. Hogrefe, Göttingen, Toronto, Zürich.

Kallinke, D., Kulick, B. and Heim, P. (1982). Psychologische Behandlungsmöglichkeiten bei essentiellen Hypertonikern. In Köhle, K. (Ed.), *Zur Psychosomatik von Herz-Kreislauf-Erkrankungen*, Springer-Verlag, Berlin, Heidelberg, New York.

Knust, U., Homuth, V. and Richter-Heinrich, E. (1987). Pilotstudie zur Effektivität einer kombinierten medikamentösen und psychophysiologisch orientierten Therapie bei essentiellen Hypertonikern. *Zeitschrift für Klinische Medizin*, 42/13, 1115–1117.

Lazarus, R. S. and Launier, R. (1978). Stress-related transactions between person and environment. In *Perspectives in Interactional Psychology*, Pervin, L. A. and Lewis, M. (Eds). Plenum Press, New York, London, pp. 287–327.

Linden, W. (1984). *Psychological Perspectives of Essential Hypertension*. Karger, Basel.

Patel, C. H. (1977). Biofeedback-aided relaxation and meditation in the management of hypertension. *Biofeedback Self-Regulation*, 2, 1–41.

Richter-Heinrich, E., Borys, M., Sprung, H. and Läuter, J. (1971). Psychophysiologische Reaktionsprofile von Hypo- and Hypertonikern, *Deutsches Gesundheitswesen*, 26, 1481–1489.

Richter-Heinrich, E., Borys, E., Kreihs, W., Curio, I. and Läuter, J. (1974). A contribution to diagnostic differentiation of certain pathological groups by multivariate psychophysiological tests. *Studia Psychologica, Bratislava*, 16, 51–55.

Richter-Heinrich, E., Knust, U., Sprung, H. and Schmidt, K. H. (1976). Psychophysiologische Untersuchungen zur Streßsensibilität von arteriellen essentiellen Hypertonikern. *Therapiewoche*, 26, 84–92.

Richter-Heinrich, E., Homuth, V., Heinrich, B., Schmidt, K. H., Wiedemann, R. and Gohlke, H. R. (1981). Long term application of behavioral treatments in essential hypertensives. *Physiology Behaviour*, 26, 915–920.

Richter-Heinrich, E., Lori, M., Knust, U. and Schmidt, K. H. (1982). Comparison of blood pressure biofeedback and relaxation training in essential hypertensives. In Richter-Heinrich, E. and Miller, N. E. (Eds), *Biofeedback—Basic Problems and Clinical Applications*. VEB Deutscher Verlag der Wissenschaften, Berlin, pp. 107–120.

Richter-Heinrich, E. (1983). Psychophysiologisch orientierte Therapieverfahren bei arteriellen essentiellen Hypertonikern. In Faulhaber, H.-D. (Ed.), *Die Therapie der arteriellen Hypertonie*, Fischer-Verlag, Jena, pp. 169–179.

Richter-Heinrich, E., Doil, R., Enderlein, J., Heinrich, B., Knust, U. and Schmidt, K. H. (in press). Physiological and psychological mechanisms of a breath relaxation training. In International Series *Systems Research in Physiology*.

Shapiro, A. P., Schwartz, G. E., Ferguson, D. C. E., Redmond, D. P. and Weiss, St.M. (1977). Behavioral methods in the treatment of hypertension. A review of their clinical status. *Annals of Internal Medicine*, **86**, 626–636.

Spreen, D. (1961). Konstruktion einer Skala zur Messung der manifesten Angst in experimentellen Untersuchungen. *Psychologische Forschung*, **26**, 205–223.

Steptoe, A. (1978). New approaches to the management of essential hypertension with psychological techniques. *Journal of Psychosomatic Research*, **22**, 339–354.

Ursin, H. (1982). The search for stress markers. *Scandinavian Journal of Psychology*, suppl. 1, 165–169.

Vaitl, D. (1975). Zur Problematik des Biofeedback, dargestellt am Beispiel der Herzfrequenzkontrolle, *Psychologische Rundschau*, **26**, 191–211.

Weiss, S. M., Matthews, K. A., Dettre, T. and Graeff, J. A. (1984). *Stress, Reactivity, and Cardiovascular Disease*. Proceedings of the working conference, NIH Publication, No. 84-2698.

Behavioural Medicine in Cardiovascular Disorders
Edited by T. Elbert, W. Langosch, A. Steptoe and D. Vaitl
©1988 John Wiley & Sons Ltd

9

Group Treatment with Obese Essential Hypertensive Patients in a General Practice Setting: Results of Six Years' Research

Heinz-Dieter Basler

Institut für Medizinische Psychologie, Bunsenstraße 3, 3550 Marburg, FRG

SUMMARY

In a series of studies with obese essential hypertensive patients in a general practice setting, we tested the hypothesis that group work on a behavioural basis might be an effective way to improve patient care and to lower blood pressure values in addition to pharmacological treatment. Our treatment goals—reduction of weight, changing of health behaviour including salt consumption, improvement of stress coping mechanisms, and finally, stabilization of blood pressure values at a lower level, together with a reduction of antihypertensive medication—were realized in three studies with a total of 900 patients, all of them being pharmacologically treated with antihypertensive agents at the beginning of group work. Both medical psychologists and other practice staff worked as group leaders in the doctors' offices, applying a standardized therapy programme, with little difference in the outcome. As results are encouraging, the project is being continued in cooperation with an industrial company on a nationwide basis.

INTRODUCTION

In a series of studies carried out over recent years in general practice settings, we have tried to clarify if and under what conditions group therapy on a behavioural basis is an effective method of reducing the blood pressure values of obese hypertensive patients, all of whom have been treated pharmacologically for at least one year. When we started our project in the late 1970s, the first reports on effective behavioural treatments of hypertensive patients in clinical settings had been published. There was a focus on relaxation training

(Blackwell *et al.*, 1976; Benson *et al.*, 1977; Beiman *et al.*, 1978; Brauer *et al.*, 1979), on self-monitoring of blood pressure sometimes combined with stress-management (Benson *et al.*, 1971; Carnahan and Nugent, 1975; Blanchard *et al.*, 1979), on information processing (Sackett *et al.*, 1975; Levine *et al.*, 1979), and, in obese patients, on weight reduction (Basler and Schwoon, 1977; Pudel, 1978). We made the assumption that psychological methods only have a chance of being integrated into basic medical care if two conditions can be fulfilled: Firstly, they have to prove their effectiveness not only in a clinical setting, but also in a context of the general practitioner's work, and, secondly, these methods have to be accepted not only by the practitioners but by their patients as well.

Our first step in this research was to test the effectiveness of different psychological treatments in an outpatient setting and to get feedback by the doctors and by the patients themselves.

STUDY I: COMPARISON OF DIFFERENT TREATMENT METHODS

As we didn't know which of the treatments discussed in the literature would prove effective in basic medical care units, we studied the differential effects of these methods (Basler *et al.*, 1982a,b). Since there is no doubt about the benefits of weight reduction in obese hypertensive patients, all of our therapy groups were trained in the self-control of eating habits. Three different behavioural treatments were offered to the patients:

Treatment I: a weight reduction programme to strengthen the self-control of eating habits.
Treatment II: in addition to weight control (TI) training in self-monitoring of blood pressure in order to recognize the typical variation of blood pressure values with the stress-inducing events of everyday life, combined with training in stress-management using role-play.
Treatment III: in addition to weight control (TI) training in relaxation according to Jacobson (1938).

We tested these methods against two different control conditions. Our first control group received intense counselling on the need for behaviour modification but were given *no* behavioural training as put forward in the experimental groups. Special emphasis was laid on activating the patients and giving support to all self-help endeavours. Time spent with the patients was identical in experimental groups and control group 1. The second control group was not given any additional psychological treatment, and thus served as a waiting control group.

All these procedures were carried out by medical psychologists according to a standardized therapy manual in the doctor's waiting room. Eight general practitioners in the city of Hannover participated in the study. Each of them selected up to 30 patients, who were divided into a treated group and a waiting control group, in such a way that a total of eight patient groups was formed. Thus, each experimental condition as well as control condition 1 could be studied in two different practices. For each group there were 12 sessions lasting 1½ hours at weekly intervals.

Before the intervention and again 5 to 6 months after the conclusion of the intervention, the patients were questioned on their health behaviour by means of a standardized interview. In addition, blood pressure readings taken by the physicians during the year before the intervention and half a year after the intervention were analysed.

A total of 209 obese, pharmacologically treated, essential hypertensives (at least 10% overweight according to Broca) were included in the study. Therapy group I consisted of 25 patients, group II of 27 patients, group III of 27 patients, control group I of 28 patients and control group II of 102 patients.

The main result was that, although the treatment groups clearly differed from the waiting-control group in blood pressure and weight reduction, the differences between the individual therapeutic procedures were slight. Moreover, a covariance analysis in which the three treatment groups were compared to control group 1 yielded no significant differences among groups either for weight reduction or for lowering of systolic and diastolic blood pressure. Hence, a differential effect between the various experimental conditions and control condition 1 on weight or blood pressure could not be demonstrated with any certainty.

Differences in blood pressure and weight reduction as reported by the doctors, however, were impressive. Data taken in a period of 3 months preceding group treatment and 4 to 6 months after the treatment indicate a mean weight reduction of 4.2 kg and a mean blood pressure reduction of 16/8 mmHg in the experimental groups. Medication was withdrawn or reduced in 17% of the patients.

Considering the fact that there was no differential effect between experimental groups and control group 1, we put forward the hypothesis that the effective agent was not the treatment method itself, but the motivation to change behaviour, and that this might emerge through various methodological routes. This hypothesis seemed reasonable, since control group 1 reported changes in health behaviour to the same extent as the experimental groups. Presumably, focusing on information and self-help was an effective way of influencing blood pressure values.

The acceptability of the group method proved to be rather high. Although about one-quarter of the patients dropped out of group treatment, those who attended the sessions up to the end were very satisfied with their results. High satisfaction was also reported by the practitioners, all of which decided to continue group work in their practice. A severe problem arose in trying to finance the work of the psychologists outside the research setting.

STUDY II: PRACTICE STAFF AS GROUP LEADERS

On the basis of these results, we modified our therapy programme as well as the contextual framework of group treatment in general practice. In a second study, we explored whether group treatment can also be effectively done by practice staff (doctor's assistants) working within a highly structured group therapy programme (Basler *et al.*, 1985a,b).

This programme aimed at combining the treatment methods of our previous study. The following therapy goals were set:

1. weight reduction through self-control of eating habits;
2. reduction of salt consumption;
3. improvement of stress coping mechanisms.

Special emphasis was given to weight reduction. We utilized behavioural programmes tested for effectiveness (e.g. BZgA, 1980; Wilson, 1980). Self-monitoring of blood pressure was carried out in order to improve patients' awareness that blood pressure varies with the occurrence and absence of stress. Social competence training by role-playing and the purposeful utilization of relaxing activities was designed to improve patients' competence in dealing with stress (see Kallinke *et al.*, 1982). Relaxation training using breathing exercises completed the programme. Salt intake was to be influenced mainly by providing information, for which process the didactics of the health-belief-model (Becker *et al.*, 1979) was utilized. We continually encouraged the patients to take an active part in the coordination of the sessions, so that the groups finally had the character of self-help groups.

Patients met once a week for twelve sessions in the doctors' waiting room. Three booster sessions were added at monthly intervals. There were no more than 12 patients in each group. Although the doctor's assistant worked as a group leader, the doctors themselves were involved in the programme and at three times participated in the sessions in order to discuss health relevant topics. Group leaders received intensive training (a 40-hour course including trial therapy sessions), and during the therapy period were closely supervised by professional psychologists at weekly intervals.

In this study, a total of 15 general practices in a rural part of Lower Saxonia (West Germany) participated. The total sample of patients consisted of 261 obese essential hypertensives, all receiving antihypertensive medication. In each practice, the patients were assigned to either an experimental group or a control group matched for blood pressure values, body weight and age (readings after the initial interview as seen in Table 1).

While the experimental groups ($n = 155$) were given behavioural treatment, the control groups ($n = 106$) received intensified individual counselling by the doctor at 4-week intervals over a period of half a year. Blood pressure, body weight, and medication were recorded and discussed during these appointments.

Table 1. Initial values in experimental group (EG) and control group (CG) (t-test for independent samples).

		$\bar{x}$	s	n	t-test
Systolic BP	EG	153.6	18.9	155	NS
	CG	153.1	16.2	106	
Diastolic BP	EG	97.1	10.6	155	NS
	CG	97.6	9.7	106	
Body weight	EG	88.8	15.7	155	NS
	CG	86.2	12.7	104	
Body height	EG	165.8	8.6	155	NS
	CG	165.9	8.2	106	
Age	EG	50.1	10.6	155	NS
	CG	51.1	9.4	106	

Thus, we tested the hypothesis that group work is more effective in blood pressure treatment than individual counselling by the doctor.

Before treatment and half a year after treatment, we interviewed each patient concerning medication compliance, salt consumption, health behaviour (eating habits and bodily exercise), and health knowledge. For each variable an index was computed in such a way that high values indicate desired behaviour. After the interview, we recorded body weight and blood pressure under resting conditions.

Changes from first to second interview were analysed by a multivariate test, Hotelling T2. We observed the following results.

Experimental group: T2 = 229.91; $F = 44.26$; df = 5, 103; $p < 0.001$.
Control group: T2 = 9.43; $F = 1.77$; df = 5, 60; $0.20 > p > 0.10$.

This indicates that significant changes in the dependent variables occurred in the experimental group only.

Table 2 shows the changes in the dependent variables from first to second interview (t-test for dependent samples) in the experimental group. Body weight was reduced by 5.2 kg ($s = 5.0$) in the experimental group compared with 1.1 kg ($s = 3.8$) in the control group, which is a highly significant difference. Eighty-five percent of all patients who had undergone stress coping training were of the opinion that their stress coping in everyday life had improved on account of the training. Blood pressure towards the end of treatment was lowered by 14.4/7.4 mmHg in the experimental group and by 6.2/3.1 mmHg in the controls, which represents a significant difference between groups. For both groups, medication was re-evaluated by the doctor on the basis of blood pressure changes. In 34.2% of the experimental patients, medication was either discontinued or reduced, whereas only 17.8% of controls lowered medication. Since medication has an effect on blood pressure values, there were no further

Table 2. Experimental group: changes in the dependent variables from first to second interview.

Variable	1st M	Interview (S)	2nd M	Interview (S)	t-test for dependent samples t	df	p
Body weight (kg)	87.75	(16.61)	82.69	(17.72)	10.20	107	<0.001
Compliance	4.12	(1.19)	4.25	(1.16)	1.06	107	NS
Reduction of salt intake	3.75	(1.54)	4.88	(1.54)	8.54	107	<0.001
Health behaviour	2.22	(0.84)	2.93	(0.84)	8.54	107	<0.001
Health knowledge	13.18	(2.94)	14.10	(2.44)	3.48	107	<0.001

Hotelling $T^2 = 229.91$; $F = 44.26$; df = 5, 103; $p < 0.001$.

differences between the numbers of well-stabilized patients in experimental group and control group after the reduction of antihypertensive drugs (see Table 3). At this time the number of non-stabilized patients with hypertensive blood pressure values according to WHO-standards in both groups decreased significantly from 32 to 22% (χ^2 McNemar = 5.14; df = 1; $p < 0.05$). Thus, the specific effect of group treatment compared with intensified counselling mainly consisted in a greater reduction of weight and of antihypertensive medication. Counselling by itself also proved to have some effect.

On the whole, the results obtained using practice staff as group leaders were comparable to those obtained by professional psychologists. Again, group work was highly acceptable to doctors and patients. There were only 15% therapy drop-outs (missing three or more therapy sessions). Thus, we were encouraged

Table 3. Experimental and control group (second interview participants only): blood pressure classification according to WHO standards.

Classification	Exp. group	Control group	Total
First interview			
Normotensive	6 (4.7%)	4 (4.9%)	10 (4.8%)
Borderline	84 (65.1%)	49 (60.5%)	133 (63.3%)
Hypertensive	39 (30.2%)	28 (34.6%)	67 (31.9%)
	129 (100%)	81 (100%)	210 (100%)
Second interview			
Normotensive	19 (14.7%)	5 (6.4%)	24 (11.6%)
Borderline	82 (63.6%)	56 (71.8%)	138 (66.7%)
Hypertensive	28 (21.7%)	17 (21.8%)	45 (21.7%)
	129 (100%)	78 (100%)	207 (100%)

1st interview: $\chi^2 = 0.47$; df = 2; NS.
2nd interview: $\chi^2 = 3.39$; df = 2; NS.

Table 4. Changes in body weight and Broca-index between first and second interview.

	$\overline{X}$	s	diff.	n	t-test
Body weight (kg)					
1st Interview	88.5	14.3	5.5	430	22.21
2nd Interview	83.0	14.1			$p < 0.0001$
BROCA-Index					
1st Interview	137.9	21.6	9.8	430	8.75
2nd Interview	128.1	28.4			$p < 0.0001$

to test the practicability of group work in general practice on a nationwide basis.

STUDY III: GROUP WORK ON A NATIONWIDE BASIS

Group work according to the programme which we developed in our second study is now being practised in more than 200 general practices all over West Germany. In order to secure a high standard of quality, physicians only receive the therapy programme if they or their assistants have attended the 40-hour training course, which can be completed over two weekends.* Besides improving knowledge of the theoretical foundations of behaviour change, the objectives of the course are principally to learn about the practice of group work by means of role-playing and by trial therapy sessions. While doing their first course with patients, the group leaders are supervised by professional psychologists.

Although not all the physicians and the patients who utilize our patient programme are participating in our evaluation study, we can present the data of 430 obese essential hypertensives from 63 general practices who completed the course in 1985. Again, the patients were interviewed before the beginning of treatment and half a year after the termination of group work.

The data show that the mean age of the patients is 51.5 years ($s = 11.6$), and that there is a high proportion of women (83.0%).

Table 4 presents the reduction of weight and of Broca-index between first and second interview. The health behaviour of the patients once again has significantly improved ($p < 0.001$, Wilcoxon test). Patients reported more positive eating habits and more bodily exercise after intervention.

Medication was withdrawn or reduced in 35% of all patients. After these adjustments of medication, blood pressure was further lowered (see Table 5). Thus, according to the WHO classification, the number of patients with

---

*This strategy could only be realized with industrial support. In cooperation with Galenus Mannheim Company, whose financial and organizational resources were very helpful, we trained both practice staff and doctors in the use of our group programme. Group leaders were further supported by coworkers of the company who had previously received intensive training.

Table 5. Change in blood pressure between first and second interview.

	$\bar{X}$	s	diff.	n	t-test
Systolic BP					
1st Interview	151.2	19.9	7.8	426	8.36
2nd Interview	143.4	17.7			$p < 0.0001$
Diastolic BP					
1st Interview	91.6	10.8	4.2	426	8.19
2nd Interview	87.4	8.1			$p < 0.0001$

hypertensive blood pressure values was lowered from 33.9% before treatment to 10.9% about half a year after treatment.

A positive effect has also been demonstrated on health status. While only 32.4% of the patients rated their health as good or very good before group treatment, after treatment this number increased to 57.7% ($p < 0.001$; Wilcoxon test). The number of patients using additional salt during their meals decreased from 66.7% to 32.8% ($p < 0.001$; Wilcoxon test). Only 15% of the patients did not finish the programme and thus dropped out of treatment.

As the therapy programme has proved to be effective on a nationwide basis, we intend more and more to try and integrate group work into the daily routines of those general practitioners who are interested in additional ways of improving the care of hypertensive patients. Scientific research on the outcome will be continued.

REFERENCES

Basler, H.-D. and Schwoon, D. R. (1977). Verhaltenstherapie und zugrundeliegende Lerntheorie. In Bock, H. E., Gerok, W. and Hartmann, F. (Eds), *Klinik der Gegenwart*, vol. 11; Urban and Schwarzenberg, München, pp. 664–676.

Basler, H.-D., Brinkmeier, U., Haehn, K. D. and Mölders-Kober, R. (1982a). Psychological group treatment of essential hypertension in general practice. *British Journal of Clinical Psychology*, **21**, 295–302.

Basler, H.-D., Brinkmeier, U., Haehn, K. D. and Mölders-Kober, R. (1982b). Psychologische Gruppenverfahren — Behandlung der essentiellen Hypertonie in allgemeinärztlichen Praxen. *Münchener Medizinische Wochenschrift*, **124**, 560–564.

Basler, H.-D., Brinkmeier, U., Buser, K., Haehn, K. D., Mölders-Kober, R. (1985a). Essentielle Hypertonie — Gruppenbehandlung Adipöser in Allgemeinpraxen durch qualifizierte Laien. *Münchener Medizinische Wochenschift*, **127**, 550–555.

Basler, H.-D., Brinkmeier, U., Buser, K., Haehn, K. D., Mölders-Kober, R. (1985b). Adipositastherapie in der Allgemeinpraxis — Gruppenbehandlung versus Gesundheitsberatung. *Zeitschrift für Allgemeinmedizin*, **61**, 148–154.

Becker, M. H., Maiman, L. A., Kirscht, J. P., Haefner, D. P., Drachman, R. H. and Taylor, D. W. (1979). Patient perceptions and compliance: recent studies of the health belief model. In Haynes, R. B., Taylor, D. W. and Sackett, D. L. (Eds), *Compliance in Health Care*. Johns Hopkins University Press, Baltimore, pp. 94–132.

Beiman, I., Graham, L. E. and Ciminero, A. R. (1978). Setting generality of blood pressure reductions and the psychological treatment of reactive hypertension. *Journal of Behavioural Medicine*, 1, 445-453.

Benson, H., Shapiro, D., Tursky, B. and Schwartz, G. E. (1971). Decreased systolic blood pressure through operant conditioning techniques in patients with essential hypertension. *Science*, 173, 740-742.

Benson, H., Kotch, J. B. and Crassweller, K. D. (1977). The relaxation response: a bridge between psychiatry and medicine. *Medical Clinics of North America*, 61, 919-938.

Blackwell, B., Bloomfield, S., Gartside, P., Robinson, A., Hanneson, I., Magenheim, H., Nidick, S. and Zigler, R. (1976). Transcendental meditation in hypertension: individual patterns. *Lancet*, I, 223-226.

Blanchard, E. B., Miller, S. T., Abel, G. G., Haynes, M. R. and Wicker, R. (1979). Evaluation of biofeedback in the treatment of borderline hypertension. *Journal of Applied Behavioural Analysis*, 12, 99-109.

Brauer, A. P., Horlik, L., Nelson, E., Farquhar, J. W. and Agras, W. S. (1979). Relaxation therapy for essential hypertension: a veterans administration outpatient study. *Journal of Behavioural Medicine*, 2, 21-29.

BZgA (Bundeszentrale für gesundheitliche Aufklärung (1980). *Abnehmen* — aber mit Vernunft, Köln.

Carnahan, J. E. and Nugent, C. A. (1975). The effects of selfmonitoring by patients in the control of hypertension. *American Journal of Medical Science*, 269, 69-73.

Jacobson, E. (1938). *Progressive Relaxation*. University of Chicago Press, Chicago.

Kallinke, D., Kulick, B. and Heim, P. (1982). Behaviour analysis and treatment of essential hypertensives. *Journal of Psychosomatic Research*, 26, 541-549.

Levine, D. M., Green, L. W., Deeds, S. G., Chwalow, J., Russell, R. P. and Finlay, J. (1979). Health education for hypertensive patients. *Journal of the American Medical Association*, 241, 1700-1703.

Pudel, V. (1978). *Zur Psychogenese und Therapie der Adipositas*. Springer, Berlin.

Sackett, D. L., Gibson, E. S., Taylor, D. W., Haynes, R. B., Hackett, B. C., Roberts, R. S. and Johnson, A. L. (1975). Randomised clinical trial of strategies for improving medication compliance in primary hypertension. *Lancet*, 1, 1205-1207.

Wilson, G. T. (1980). Behavior modification and the treatment of obesity. In Stunkard, A. J. (Ed.), *Obesity*. Saunders, Philadelphia, pp. 325-344.

Behavioural Medicine in Cardiovascular Disorders
Edited by T. Elbert, W. Langosch, A. Steptoe and D. Vaitl
©1988 John Wiley & Sons Ltd

10

The Processes Underlying Long-term Blood Pressure Reductions in Essential Hypertensives Following Behavioural Therapy

A. Steptoe

Department of Psychology, St George's Hospital Medical School, University of London, UK

INTRODUCTION

A large number of studies have been published over the last 15 years, showing that the blood pressure (BP) of patients with essential hypertension can be lowered using behavioural techniques (Johnston, 1985; see also Chapters 7 and 8 by Walter *et al.* and Richter-Heinrich *et al.*). Relaxation and meditation alone or in combination with biofeedback have proven effective in comparison with attention–placebo conditions that control for expectancies and other non-specific effects (Bali, 1979; Irvine *et al.*, 1986). Although responses have primarily been evaluated in the clinic, reduced BP has also been recorded using ambulatory methods over the working day (Agras *et al.*, 1983). Follow-up studies have shown that lower BP is maintained 1 year after treatment in patients given behavioural therapy (Patel and North, 1975; Agras *et al.*, 1983). Patel *et al.* (1985) more recently reported a 4-year follow-up of a randomized controlled trial in which men and women aged 35–64 who were identified on screening as having two or more coronary risk factors (BP $\geqslant 140/90$ mmHg, plasma cholesterol $\geqslant 6.3$ mmol/l, and current smoking $\geqslant 10$ cigarettes per day) were assigned to relaxation-based behavioural modification or a control group. The significantly greater BP reductions observed at 8 weeks and 8 months were maintained at 4 years, and the data also suggested reduced coronary morbidity (indexed as treatment for ischaemic heart disease or suspected myocardial infarction) in the experimental group.

These data indicate that behavioural methods are effective in lowering the BP of many hypertensives. Nevertheless, there is considerable uncertainty about the mechanisms responsible. Various possibilities have been discussed in detail by Johnston (1986). The present chapter explores some factors of potential importance, including the relationship of relaxation practice to BP reduction, the use of relaxation as a coping skill in everyday life, and the changes in habitual activities that may accompany behavioural therapy. These issues will be illustrated by data collected at the 4-year follow-up of the controlled trial described by Patel et al. (1981, 1985).

RELAXATION PRACTICE AND
BLOOD PRESSURE REDUCTION

The first question is whether BP reductions depend on the amount of relaxation practice that hypertensives carry out. Relaxation practice usually involves sitting quietly at home, trying to duplicate the experiences of a therapy session, sometimes with the aid of tape-recorded instructions. Most treatment programmes encourage patients to practice once or twice a day. It is possible that BP reductions are directly related to adherence with this schedule, and that there is a 'dose–response' association between practice and therapeutic effect.

A number of studies have collected data concerning relaxation practice by self-report, and assessed the relationship with BP change. Charlesworth et al. (1984) compared a 10-week stress–management programme, based on autogenic training and cognitive behaviour modification, with a no-treatment control in 40 mild hypertensives. Systolic and diastolic BP reductions were significantly correlated with the number of reported practice sessions. A positive correlation was also observed by Wadden (1983). On the other hand, Crowther (1983) found no association between BP reduction and the number of home practice sessions. Irvine et al. (1986) reported a negative relationship between home practice and BP response, although it was difficult in this case to distinguish cause and effect. However, it should be pointed out that studies using relaxation and related methods for the treatment of anxiety have also shown inconsistent effects (Lewis et al., 1978; Zuroff and Schwarz, 1978).

The 4-year reassessment of participants in the study described by Patel and colleagues allowed this issue to be considered with respect to the long-term maintenance of BP reduction. Briefly, 192 men and women who fulfilled the coronary risk criteria detailed earlier, were assigned at random to behavioural treatment and control groups. Both groups were given health advice concerning smoking, diet, and hypertension. In addition, the treatment group underwent eight 1-hour sessions of breathing exercises, deep muscle relaxation, meditation, and stress management. They were instructed to practice for 15–20 min twice daily with the aid of a tape recording, and to try to relax during everyday activities. Mean BP in the treatment group fell from 146.5/87.9 to

139.4/85.2 mmHg at 4 years, compared with 144.1/88.3 to 145.7/92.4 mmHg in controls. Significantly greater effects were also seen in the subjects whose systolic and diastolic BP both fulfilled hypertensive criteria pre-treatment. The 43 treatment subjects in this category showed a reduction from 165.8/100.6 to 150.5/92.3 mmHg over this period, while the 36 controls changed from 160.3/98.3 to 157.6/99.4 mmHg.

A questionnaire concerning relaxation practice and other factors was completed by 81 (82%) treatment and 72 (77%) control subjects at 4-year follow-up. Surprisingly, only 14 (17%) of the treatment group reported that they continued regularly to practise relaxation. Although the average BP reduction in these individuals ($-10.9/-6.98$ mmHg) was somewhat greater than that in the remainder ($-6.28/-1.71$ mmHg), the difference was not significant. A division was then made among the people no longer relaxing, between those who had practised for a considerable period, of at least 2½ years (subgroup B, $n = 49$), and those who said that they had never practised, or had stopped more than 18 months ago (subgroup C, $n = 15$; 5 subjects failed to respond). For convenience, the subjects currently practising were designated subgroup A. There was a significant difference between the diastolic BP change in subgroups A and C (-6.98 vs $+4.17$ mmHg, $p = 0.017$), while the systolic effect approached significance (-10.9 vs $+2.20$ mmHg, $p < 0.1$). This lends some support to the notion that practice is related to BP response. However, similar BP reductions were found in subgroups A and B. Additionally, it was apparent that these effects were not independent of initial BP level. Subjects in subgroups A and B had higher BP on average before treatment than subgroup C. These effects are shown in Figure 1, where the relationship between initial BP and response in the different practice categories is apparent.

The data shown in Figure 1 should not be interpreted to imply that BP changes at 4 years represent regression to the mean or some other adaptation phenomenon. It should be noted that controls with high initial BP showed a change averaging $-2.7/+1.1$ mmHg over the comparable period. What the pattern does suggest is that the tendency to persist with relaxation training was related to the initial risk status of participants. It will be recalled that not all subjects were hypertensive when they began treatment, since some entered the trial on the basis of elevated cholesterol and cigarette smoking rather than high BP. It was subsequently found that 10 of the 14 subjects who continued to relax at 4 years were initially hypertensive, compared with only 5 of the 15 subjects in subgroup C. It is possible that hypertensives were more convinced by the rationale for relaxation and stress management than subjects who entered the trial with other risk factors, so engaged in the programme more enthusiastically.

An additional analysis was therefore conducted, comparing the hypertensive subjects in subgroups A and C. Numbers were small in these categories, so the results must be treated with caution. Nonetheless, the diastolic BP reduction in subgroup A was significantly greater than that in subgroup C (-11.1 vs

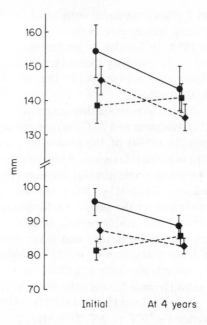

Figure 1. Relationship between BP pre-treatment and at 4 years' follow-up in groups varying in adherence to relaxation practice. Means ($\pm$ SEM) for systolic (top panel) and diastolic BP (bottom panel). ●——● Subgroup A: subjects continuing relaxation practice at 4 years; ◆----◆ subgroup B: subjects who relaxed regularly for at least 2½ years; ■ ---- ■ subgroup C, subjects who reported never relaxing, or who stopped within the first 2½ years.

+ 1.15 mmHg, $p = 0.039$), even though their initial BPs did not differ reliably. The results therefore give some support to the notion that relaxation practice correlates with BP reduction.

One possible explanation for the inconsistency in these data concerning relaxation practice is that reported practice levels are inaccurate. Subjects may bias their reports (perhaps to please the investigators), or forget the genuine pattern of practice. Technical developments in recent years have permitted the manufacture of special cassette recorders which unobtrusively monitor the number of times that relaxation tapes are played. Hoelsher et al. (1984) loaned these devices to volunteers with generalized anxiety disorder during treatment with progressive muscle relaxation. They found that, on average, patients overestimated relaxation practice by 126%. On self-report measures, 70% said they practised at least six times per week, but in terms of elapsed cassette playing time, only 25% fulfilled this criterion. Interestingly, the decreases in trait anxiety and neuroticism observed during the trial correlated significantly with objectively measured relaxation practice.

Two studies have also been conducted with hypertensives. Taylor *et al.* (1983) assessed use of a relaxation tape in 23 hypertensives. Again, patients overestimated practice time, although self-reported relaxation correlated highly with the objective measure ($r = 0.88$). However, neither self-report nor objective measures were related to BP responses. A different pattern emerged in the comparison of individual and group training in relaxation published by Hoelsher *et al.* (1986). In this case, both objective and subjectively defined relaxation practice correlated with systolic BP reduction ($r = 0.32$ and 0.39, respectively), but not with diastolic BP responses. Objective and self-report measures were themselves positively correlated.

These studies using timed audio-cassette playing indicate that although patients overestimate their practice levels, self-reports correlate across individuals with more objective measures. The relationship between these objective measures and BP response is not consistent. The studies have also been rather short (an 8-week treatment period in Taylor *et al.* (1983), and 4 weeks' treatment plus 6 weeks' follow-up in Hoelsher *et al.*, 1986), and it cannot be assumed that similar patterns will persist in the long term. Presumably over longer periods, investigators might wish to reduce patients' dependence on tape recordings.

The evidence relating relaxation practice with BP reduction does not present a clear cut picture at present. However, it can be concluded that some hypertensives show substantial BP reductions without apparently adhering to the relaxation schedule recommended by the therapist. Two possible explanations of this pattern might be considered. Firstly, less practice in relaxation may be needed than is generally advised. The level of one or two practice sessions daily is quite arbitrary, and a lower rate may produce similar BP responses. The second possibility is that it is not formal relaxation practice, but some other component of these treatment programmes that is the effective agent. This possibility is endorsed by the data presented in Figure 1, where subgroups A and B showed similar BP responses despite different levels of practice. The two additional elements that will be considered here are the use of relaxation as a coping skill, and the behavioural changes that might accompany relaxation-based treatment.

RELAXATION AS A COPING SKILL

Most behavioural treatments for essential hypertension emphasize the generalization of training into everyday life, and patients are encouraged to use the relaxation skills they have learnt when coping with stress at work and home. This use of relaxation as a coping skill may be more important than formal practice in generating and maintaining BP reductions. There are two ways in which relaxation might operate as a coping skill, and these need to be distinguished, since they have implications for the manner in which treatment programmes should be presented and focused.

Table 1. Use of relaxation as a coping skill and blood pressure change.

			Systolic			Diastolic		
		n	Mean initial	Mean change	SEM of change	Mean initial	Mean change	SEM of change
Do you ever 'tell' yourself to calm down and relax?	Often/ sometimes	73	145.39	−7.87	2.9	87.85	−2.91	1.8
	Never	8	153.23	+0.06	8.7	88.63	0.00	3.5

RELAXATION AND THE CONTROL OF STRESS RESPONSES

Hypertensives typically show large cardiovascular reactions when exposed to stressful environments, particularly those eliciting active behavioural responses (see Steptoe, 1984, 1986; Chapter 4, Wiedemann et al.). Relaxation may enable patients to control these pressor responses more effectively, and hence lower tonic BP levels. Certainly, many patients undergoing relaxation-based behavioural therapy report trying to use the treatment in this way. In the 4-year follow-up detailed earlier, 83% of subjects stated that they often or sometimes used relaxation in their daily lives, while 91% 'told' themselves to calm down and relax while under stress. A tendency towards greater BP reduction in those using these coping skills was also seen. Table 1 compares the initial BP and reduction over 4 years in subjects who did and did not report telling themselves to calm down under stress. Analysis using initial BP as a covariate showed a near-significant difference for systolic BP ($p = 0.082$).

However, it is far from established whether relaxation and other behavioural treatments do actually reduce cardiovascular reactivity to stress. This literature has recently been reviewed comprehensively by Jacob and Chesney (1986). The general pattern to emerge is that few studies have convincingly demonstrated that behavioural therapy reduces the cardiovascular reactions of hypertensive patients, although tonic BP level may be lowered. However, the mechanism has not been tested properly in many investigations. In particular, subjects have been tested in laboratory stress situations without being given instructions to try and use their relaxation coping skills, or an opportunity to prepare for the challenge. Many researchers appear to have assumed that lowered reactivity would emerge in some automatic way, without efforts on the part of patients. Studies that have given subjects instructions and time to prepare have shown reduced responses (e.g. Patel, 1975). It is also notable that in other settings (e.g. cancer chemotherapy, Lyles et al., 1982; experimental pain, Mills and Farrow, 1981), relaxation and related techniques have proven effective when explicitly used within the stressful situation. A clearer pattern may therefore emerge in future studies that are designed with these issues in mind.

RELAXATION AND COGNITIVE REAPPRAISAL

An alternative possibility is that relaxation modifies reactions not at the level of physiological responses, but through influencing the appraisal of the environment. Cognitive appraisal refers to the way in which people interpret the environment and stimuli that impinge upon them. The effects of altering appraisals on autonomic responses have been established in a number of experimental studies (e.g. Steptoe and Vögele, 1986). Behavioural therapies for hypertension either explicitly or implicitly encourage patients to identify stressful situations, and in some cases treatment has actually been directed towards modifying subjects' appraisals (e.g. Kallinke et al., 1982; Wadden, 1984). In other words, reactions may be reduced because patients no longer appraise their life situation in the same way, but perceive it as more benign or positive.

Unfortunately, there is little direct evidence concerning this process in the treatment of hypertension using relaxation-based programmes. However, the 4-year follow-up provided evidence at least consistent with this notion. Subjects in the treatment and control groups were asked whether the advice they had been given had affected their lives in general ways (apart from cardiovascular risk). The results indicated that more people in the treatment than control group reported that their lives had been improved. The effect was significant for many aspects, including relationships at work and at home, and enjoyment of life, as can be seen in Table 2. Of course, in this study it is difficult to tease out cause and effect, and reporting biases may also have been operating. Nevertheless, the results suggest that people's appraisal of their life situation may have been modified.

Table 2. General effects associated with behavioural therapy for coronary risk.

		Worse or no change (%)	Better (%)	p
Relationships at work	Treatment	72.9	27.1	0.01
	Control	90.8	9.2	
General health	Treatment	63.3	36.7	0.01
	Control	83.3	16.7	
Enjoyment of life	Treatment	64.6	35.4	0.04
	Control	80.6	19.4	
Personal and family relationships	Treatment	72.2	27.8	0.02
	Control	88.9	11.1	
General level of physical energy	Treatment	79.7	20.3	0.07
	Control	91.7	8.3	
Sexual life	Treatment	88.2	11.8	0.09
	Control	97.1	2.9	

BEHAVIOURAL THERAPY AND
CHANGES IN HABITUAL BEHAVIOUR

A final problem that should be considered is that relaxation-based behavioural therapy may not exert effects through relaxation training at all, but through alterations in chronic or habitual patterns of behaviour that themselves influence BP. As Johnston (1986) has pointed out, remarkably little is known about what patients actually do following behavioural treatment. There is a strong possibility that once patients have adopted the rationale for behavioural intervention — that BP, stress, and behaviour are intimately linked — they may adopt a 'healthier' lifestyle. This could include an increase in physical exercise and aerobic fitness that might itself have a hypotensive effect (Seals and Hagberg, 1984). Changes in alcohol intake might take place with concomitant BP responses (Potter and Beevers, 1984). It is also possible that subjects change their work practices, altering their commitment to work or the manner in which they carry it out. Theorell *et al.* (1985) have shown that people in 'high strain' occupations are especially vulnerable to hypertension, so alterations in work style might have a protective effect.

The involvement of these factors in behavioural treatment effects is speculative. However, it is important to draw attention to the fact that subtle variations in habits and behaviour may influence BP, and that such processes should be evaluated when studying the mechanisms underlying long-term BP reduction. The cognitive and behavioural components need to be assessed more rigorously in future investigations, in conjunction with measures of haemodynamic and endocrine parameters. A better understanding of the elements critical to success will assist in the identification of subjects most likely to benefit, and the development of more effective treatments.

REFERENCES

Agras, W. S., Southam, M. A. and Taylor, B. C. (1983). Long-term persistence of relaxation-induced blood pressure lowering during the working day. *Journal of Consulting and Clinical Psychology*, **51**, 792–794.

Bali, L. R. (1979). Long-term effect of relaxation on blood pressure and anxiety levels of essential hypertensive males: a controlled study. *Psychosomatic Medicine*, **41**, 637–646.

Charlesworth, E. A., Williams, B. J. and Baer, P. E. (1984). Stress management at the worksite for hypertension: compliance, cost-benefit, health care and hypertension-related variables. *Psychosomatic Medicine*, **46**, 387–397.

Crowther, J. H. (1983). Stress management training and relaxation imagery in the treatment of essential hypertension. *Journal of Behavioral Medicine*, **6**, 169–187.

Hoelsher, T. J., Lichstein, K. L. and Rosenthal, T. L. (1984). Objective versus subjective assessment of relaxation compliance among anxious individuals. *Behaviour Research and Therapy*, **22**, 187–193.

Hoelsher, T. J., Lichstein, K. L. and Rosenthal, T. L. (1986). Home relaxation practice in hypertension treatment: objective assessment and compliance induction. *Journal of Consulting and Clinical Psychology*, **54**, 217–221.

Irvine, M. J., Johnston, D. W., Jenner, D. A. and Marie, G. V. (1986). Relaxation and stress management in the treatment of essential hypertension. *Journal of Psychosomatic Research*, **30**, 437–450.

Jacob, R. G. and Chesney, M. A. (1986). Psychological and behavioral methods to reduce cardiovascular reactivity. In Matthews, K. A., Weiss, S. M., Detre, T., Dembroski, T. M., Falkner, B., Manuck, S. B. and Williams, R. B. (Eds), *Handbook of Stress, Reactivity and Cardiovascular Disease*. Wiley, New York, pp. 417–457.

Johnston, D. W. (1985). Psychological interventions in cardiovascular disease. *Journal of Psychosomatic Research*, **29**, 447–456.

Johnston, D. W. (1986). How does relaxation training reduce blood pressure in primary hypertension? In Dembroski, T. D., Schmidt, T. H. and Blümchen, C. (Eds), *Biobehavioral Factors in Coronary Heart Disease*. Karger, Basel, pp. 550–567.

Kallinke, D., Kulick, B. and Heim, P. (1982). Behaviour analysis and treatment of essential hypertensives. *Journal of Psychosomatic Research*, **26**, 541–550.

Lewis, C. E., Biglan, A. and Steinbock, E. (1978). Self-administered relaxation training and money deposits in the treatment of recurrent anxiety. *Journal of Consulting and Clinical Psychology*, **46**, 1274–1283.

Lyles, J. N., Burish, T. G., Krozely, M. G. and Oldham, R. K. (1982). Efficacy of relaxation training and guided imagery in reducing the aversiveness of cancer chemotherapy. *Journal of Consulting and Clinical Psychology*, **50**, 509–524.

Mills, W. W. and Farrow, J. T. (1981). The TM technique and acute experimental pain. *Psychosomatic Medicine*, **43**, 157–164.

Patel, C. (1975). Yoga and biofeedback in the management of 'stress' in hypertensive patients. *Clinical Science and Molecular Medicine*, **28** (suppl.), 171–174.

Patel, C. and North, W. R. S. (1975). Randomised controlled trial of yoga and biofeedback in the management of hypertension. *The Lancet*, **II**, 93–95.

Patel, C., Marmot, M. G. and Terry, D. J. (1981). Controlled trial of biofeedback-aided behavioural methods in reducing mild hypertension. *British Medical Journal*, **282**, 2005–2008.

Patel, C., Marmot, M. G., Terry, D. J., Carruthers, M., Hunt, B. and Patel, M. (1985). Trial of relaxation in reducing coronary risk: four years follow up. *British Medical Journal*, **290**, 1103–1106.

Potter, J. F. and Beevers, D. G. (1984). Pressor effect of alcohol in hypertension. *Lancet*, **I**, 119–122.

Seals, D. R. and Hagberg, J. N. (1984). The effect of exercise training on human hypertension: a review. *Medicine and Science in Sports and Exercise*, **16**, 207–215.

Steptoe, A. (1984). Psychophysiological processes in disease. In Steptoe, A. and Mathews, A. (Eds), *Health Care and Human Behaviour*. Academic Press, London, pp. 77–112.

Steptoe, A. (1986). Psychophysiological contributions to the understanding and management of essential hypertension. In Christie, M. J. and Mellett, P. G. (Eds), *The Psychosomatic Approach: Contemporary Practice of Whole-person Care*. Wiley, Chichester, pp. 171–189.

Steptoe, A. and Vögele, C. (1986). Are stress responses influenced by cognitive appraisal? An experimental comparison of coping strategies. *British Journal of Psychology*, **77**, 243–255.

Taylor, C. B., Agras, W. S., Schneider, J. A. and Allen, R. A. (1983). Adherence to instructions to practise relaxation exercises. *Journal of Consulting and Clinical Psychology*, **51**, 952–953.

Theorell, T., Knox, S., Svenssen, J. and Waller, D. (1985). Blood pressure variations during a working day at age 28 — effects of different types of work and blood pressure level at age 18. *Journal of Human Stress*, **11**, 36–41.

Wadden, T. A. (1983). Predicting treatment response to relaxation therapy for essential hypertension. *Journal of Nervous and Mental Disease*, **171**, 683–689.

Wadden, T. A. (1984). Relaxation therapy for essential hypertension: specific or non-specific effects? *Journal of Psychosomatic Research*, **28**, 53–62.

Zuroff, D. C. and Schwarz, J. C. (1978). Effects of transcendental meditation and muscle relaxation on trait anxiety, maladjustment, locus of control and drug use. *Journal of Consulting and Clinical Psychology*, **46**, 264–271.

Coronary Heart Diseases: Prevention and Rehabilitation

INTRODUCTION TO SECTION III

It is generally accepted that the genesis of coronary heart diseases such as angina pectoris and myocardial infarction is multifactorial, and it is estimated that conventional risk factors (hypercholesterolaemia, hypertriglyceridaemia, smoking, hypertension, diabetes, body fat, etc.) account for some 50% of disease events. For the remaining 50% it has been postulated that psychosocial characteristics are involved in the aetiology. In addition, it is possible that the probability of disease arising with standard risk factors is further increased by unfavourable psychosocial conditions. Emotionally intensive stressful events or the experience of psychosocial stress for a longer period favour the appearance of angina pectoris or myocardial infarction, provided that protective psychosocial conditions are absent. Among other items a low socioeconomic status, high psychosocial strain at work, life change events (mainly the experience of loss), type A behaviour, aggressive and hostile feelings and inhibition of emotional expression have been put forward as increasing risk, while hardiness and socio-emotional support have potentially risk-reducing characteristics. Symptoms of vital exhaustion and depressive feelings are regarded as prognostically significant for the clinical manifestation of coronary heart disease in subsequent months. It has further been suggested that these links are mediated through autonomic and endocrine reactions to challenging or threatening everyday situations, since these responses may favour the development of coronary sclerosis or the appearance of myocardial ischaemia.

In the biobehavioural approach, the traditional method of regarding standard risk factors, psychosocial risk factors and psychophysiological reactivity patterns is replaced by a holistic view. The problem of identifying individual characteristics relevant to coronary heart disease must be viewed in terms of identifying the closeness and stability of the interdependencies between diverse characteristics that potentially increase and decrease risk. The value of the biobehavioural perspective is evident in the contributions to this section. Three of the chapters are concerned with the management of biological and behavioural risk factors, while the remaining two chapters illustrate the role of psychosocial and psychophysiological parameters in predicting long-term outcome following infarction.

In Chapter 11, Scheuermann and coauthors demonstrate in a study of more than 9000 people without manifest coronary disease that it is possible to motivate blue collar and white collar workers equally to participate in a programme for the reduction of standard risk factors. Over the course of four years, the frequency of hypercholesterolaemia and smoking was reduced significantly in both groups. It would appear that local health programmes of this type may be useful for reducing the prevalence of standard risk factors, and may be effective with people from all social classes.

Roskies (Chapter 12) discusses the modification of a potentially important psychosocial risk factor: the type A coronary-prone behaviour pattern. In this controlled trial, people who participated in a 10-week cognitive-behavioural stress-coping programme showed significant reductions in type A behaviour assessed by structured interview. The programme is based on the hypothesis that type A individuals indiscriminately perceive many situations in their lives as challenges and respond to them with intensive psychophysiological stress reactions. The programme aims to reduce these high costs of coping by making type A persons into competent 'behavioural engineers', able to differentiate successfully between appropriate and inappropriate perceptions of challenge, and able to select coping strategies relevant to each situation.

The results of these two studies suggest that it is possible to reduce significantly the prevalence of coronary risk factors in healthy people. After infarction, it is necessary firstly to identify the conditions that lead to an unfavourable outcome or reduced future quality of life. When this has been done, attempts can be made to change these conditions with suitable intervention programmes.

In Chapter 13, Siegrist describes a treatment programme for post-infarction patients based on the hypothesis that behaviours characterized by continuous efforts in spite of the experience of distress increase risk for future morbidity. This behaviour may be particularly relevant within unfavourable occupational and social conditions. An intervention programme is described that is aimed at reducing the intensity, frequency and duration of this behaviour pattern. This promising approach is now being subjected to a systematic outcome evaluation.

Philip (Chapter 14) describes a study in which the prognostic significance of psychological assessments made in infarction patients shortly after discharge from intensive care is evaluated in terms of physical, psychological and social outcome at 4 and 12 months following discharge from hospital. It was found that the neurotic psychopathology identified in the 'Personal Disturbance' scale was the best predictor of social and psychological outcome, suggesting a practical method for identifying at an early stage those patients who require special attention.

Prognosis following infarction in younger patients is discussed in Chapter 15 by Langosch and co-workers. Their results focus on the relevance of psychological and psychophysiological data for an unfavourable course of disease over three to seven years. A lack of ability in handling strains, an inadequate estimation of ability to tolerate stress, pronounced achievement and competitive behaviour and increased psychological and autonomic activation when confronted with challenges are found in this study to be relevant to the long-term prognosis for young post-infarct patients.

Behavioural Medicine in Cardiovascular Disorders
Edited by T. Elbert, W. Langosch, A. Steptoe and D. Vaitl
©1988 John Wiley & Sons Ltd

11

The Role of Social Class in the Prevention of Cardiovascular Disorders

W. Scheuermann, W. Morgenstern, R. Scheidt, L. Buchholz
and E. Nüssel

Department of Clinical Social Medicine, University of Heidelberg

INTRODUCTION

The influence of social class on the development of coronary heart disease is well documented (Rose and Marmot, 1981; Liu and Cedres, 1982; Theorell, 1986). Prevention programmes should therefore try to take this influence into account, so that possible benefits are not restricted to a small proportion of the intervened population.

The Eberbach–Wiesloch Study (Nüssel, 1985), part of the WHO CCCCP-project (Comprehensive Cardiovascular Community Control Programme), is based on the assumption that health is decisively influenced by behaviour and environment and that the members of the community themselves are able to change these two factors and to establish a long-lasting health promotion.

Special emphasis is put on interpersonal interaction, whereas the use of mass media is restricted. An important basis of the model, which might, in sociological terms be called a 'bottom-up' approach of community prevention, is the setting up of a citizens' committee that plans and organizes all activities in close collaboration with the local physicians. The task of the physicians is to counsel the citizens to make sure that the activities comply with the ethical and scientific standards of medicine. The creativity and initiative of the population should not be restricted. All activities are voluntary and financially self-sustained. They comprise a very broad range of possibilities in all age groups and social classes: baby-swimming, bicycle competitions, blood pressure measurements in schools, factories, unions and clubs, discussions with artists, philosophers, theologists, to name only a few.

The main message is information and motivation; the final decision on what behaviour to adopt remains with the citizen. The aim of the intervention programme is a reduction of the main CHD-risk factors (hypercholesterolemia,

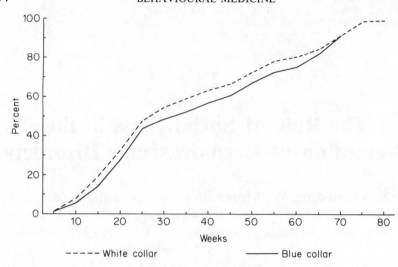

Figure 1. Time distribution of response to invitation 1976.

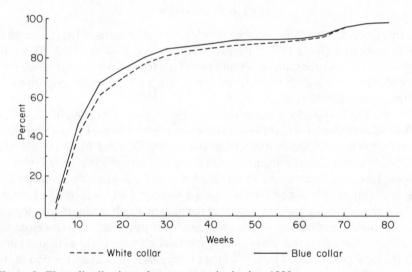

Figure 2. Time distribution of response to invitation 1980.

smoking, hypertension, and obesity), whose close relation to the prevalence of CHD has repeatedly been shown (Dawber *et al.*, 1957).

EVALUATION

In 1976, 9753 inhabitants of Eberbach and Wiesloch—two medium-sized towns near Heidelberg—aged 20–59 years, were physically examined in a screening investigation to establish the prevalence of the classical cardiovascular risk factors. This reflects a participation rate of 98%, which could only be achieved because the local physicians, authorities, and the citizens themselves supported the project on a broad scale.

Roughly 4 years later a similar participation rate was reached in a second monitoring of the same risk factors. To see whether there were differences depending on social level the screened population was divided into two groups: 'blue collar workers' and 'white collar workers', the first group in this case comprising the social classes IV and V, and the second the classes I, II, and III according to the social class definitions in England and Wales, which coincide approximately with corresponding social groups in Germany. This categorization permitted an overview concerning the four main variables: participation rate, hypercholesterolemia, percentage of smokers, and obese people. With such a sample size even small differences may prove to be statistically significant. As the whole project cannot be compared with a test under laboratory condition, we did not perform significance tests on our data. In these circumstances, statistics can be of secondary importance.

RESULTS

In 1976 during nearly the whole screening period, white collars came a little bit earlier to the screening than blue collars, whereas in the second screening the blue collar workers accepted the offer of the screening slightly more readily. The comparison between Figure 1 and Figure 2 also shows that in the second screening high participation rates were generally achieved faster.

Among blue collar workers in 1976 hypercholesterolemia, which was defined for values above 220 mg dl^{-1}, could be found slightly more often than among white collar workers, a difference that practically disappeared in 1980 (Table 1).

Table 1. Cholesterol (220 mg/dl +): (a) all, (b) males, (c) females.

	White collar	Blue collar
(a)		
1976	53.7%	56.8%
1980	46.7%	47.4%
Difference	− 7.0%	− 9.4%
(b)		
1976	57.5%	57.9%
1980	50.0%	50.5%
Difference	− 7.5%	− 7.4%
(c)		
1976	52.8%	55.0%
1980	43.7%	42.5%
Difference	− 9.1%	− 12.5%

Table 2. Smokers: (a) males, (b) females.

	White collar	Blue collar
(a)		
1976	40.9%	49.8%
1980	30.7%	41.7%
Difference	− 10.2%	− 8.1%
(b)		
1976	21.2%	19.9%
1980	17.9%	16.0%
Difference	− 3.3%	− 3.9%

The reduction of the prevalence was similar in both social groups in men, but was different in women, being pronounced in blue collar women.

There was also a considerable reduction in the percentage of smokers, with the biggest decrease in white collar men (Table 2). But here too the reduction in blue collar women was very slightly more marked than in white collar women.

A corresponding success could not be shown in regard to overweight, which was defined as a BROCA-index above 120 (Table 3). Whereas the percentage of overweight persons among the white collar population remained more or less unchanged, there was an increase of 3% in the lower social group. There were no remarkable sex differences.

DISCUSSION

It is generally believed that members of higher social classes adopt healthy lifestyles more readily than blue collar workers. Intervention programmes on a population-wide scale have to take such social differences into account.

The results presented in this paper generally do not show such a social bias. A screening for the main CHD-risk factors was accepted to nearly the same extent by both social classes examined here. A second screening showed that the response to the invitation among blue collar workers was slightly better than during the first screening. As the time-interval between invitation and examination might reflect the basic interest in one's own health, this result does not seem to implicate a negative response among the lower social classes in the Eberbach–Wiesloch study.

Table 3. Obesity (BROCA 120 +).

	White collar	Blue collar
1976	13.7%	16.9%
1980	14.6%	20.0%
Differences	+ 0.9%	+ 3.1%

This impression is enhanced by the trends in hypercholesterolemia and smoking. There seems to be no real difference between white and blue collar workers; hypercholesterolemia in women in the latter social group was actually slightly more reduced. This favourable result should not however disguise the fact that the percentage of smokers in blue collar men was still considerably higher.

The finding that there was no success in regard to overweight might in part be explained by the decrease in smokers. Further intervention activities in Eberbach and Wiesloch will take this feature especially into account.

We presume that this overall negligible bias due to social classes might be explained by the characteristics of the intervention model which gives the population the chance to influence intervention activities in a decisive manner. Whether this assumption is true requires a thorough evaluation of all the structures and processes in an urban community exposed to intervention.

In the framework of the German Cardiovascular Prevention Study (DHP = Deutsche Herz-Kreislauf-Präventionsstudie) we are trying to implement this 'Eberbach–Wiesloch strategy' in three further towns (Karlsruhe, Bruchsal, and Mosbach) in order to be able to evaluate these factors from the very beginning of the intervention programme. This was not possible to such an extent in the 'pioneer situation' of Eberbach and Wiesloch.

REFERENCES

Dawber, T. R., Moore, F. E. and Mann, G. V. (1957). Coronary heart disease in the Framingham Study. *American Journal of Public Health*, **47**, 4–24.

Liu, K. and Cedres, L. B. (1982). Relationship of education to major risk factors and death from CHD, CVD, and all causes. *Circulation*, **66**, 1308–1316.

Nüssel, E. (1985). Community-based prevention: The Eberbach–Wiesloch Study. In Hofmann, H. (Ed.), *Primary and Secondary Prevention of Coronary Heart Disease*. Springer, Berlin, Heidelberg, pp. 50–59.

Rose, G. and Marmot, M. G. (1981). Social class and coronary heart disease. *British Heart Journal*, **45**, 13–19.

Theorell, T. (1986). Untersuchungen zum Einfluß von Arbeitsplatzbelastungen und Beschäftigungssituationen auf das Kardiovaskuläre Risiko. In Halhuber, C. and Traenckner, K. (Eds), *Die koronare Herzkrankheit—eine Herausforderung an Gesellschaft und Politik*. Perimed, Erlangen, pp. 433–443.

Behavioural Medicine in Cardiovascular Disorders
Edited by T. Elbert, W. Langosch, A. Steptoe and D. Vaitl
©1988 John Wiley & Sons Ltd

12

A Stress Management Programme for Healthy Type As: The Montreal Type A Intervention Project

Ethel Roskies

Department of Psychology, University of Montreal, Canada

INTRODUCTION

This chapter will first summarize the methods and main findings of the Montreal Type A Intervention Project (Roskies *et al.*, 1986), and then describe in greater detail the stress management programme that proved to be the most effective of the three interventions tested. The opportunity offered in this chapter to focus on treatment content is particularly welcome, because it serves to correct the scant attention paid to the actual treatment process itself in most published reports of interventions for type As. It is appropriate, too, that this correction take place in a volume on behavioural medicine, because the problem is caused, in large part, by the attempt of behavioural researchers to follow reporting conventions established for pharmaceutical treatments, without allowing for the uniqueness of behavioural ones.

The biomedical research tradition requires that any report of a clinical trial must necessarily include information on treatment and outcome, of course, but also on sample selection and constitution, outcome measures employed and how they were used, and statistical analyses performed. Given the number of topics to be covered and the restrictions on article length in most journals, the researcher obviously must seek to condense wherever possible. For pharmaceutical researchers, the necessary economy can best be achieved by limiting description of the treatment; in most cases, sufficient information is conveyed simply by stating the name of the drug being tested and its dosage. Unfortunately, behavioural researchers, too, have tended to follow this practice of limiting treatment description, even though for behavioural treatments a label (e.g. relaxation training) is likely to conceal more than it reveals.

To cite examples specifically from type A research, two teams have recently reported success in modifying manifestations of the type A Behaviour Pattern (TABP), but published reports to date of the 'type A behavioural counseling' used by one (Friedman *et al.*, 1984) and the 'cognitive-behavioural stress management' used by the other (Roskies *et al.*, 1986) do not permit us to judge what is common to the two treatment approaches or how they differ. Even more confusing is the tendency to use the same label for what are quite obviously rather different treatments. Thus, Hart (1984), Jenni and Wollersheim (1979), Roskies (Roskies *et al.*, 1978, 1979; Roskies and Avard, 1982), and Suinn (Suinn, 1975; Suinn and Bloom, 1978) all claim to have used 'stress management' as a treatment for type As, but in one case it was considered a form of anxiety management while in another it was a form of anger control; in one study it was seen as a contrast to cognitive-behavioural treatment while in another it was seen as a part of it.

Behavioural treatments are obviously harder to describe than pharmaceutical ones because they are far less standardized in composition and administration. Thus, when dealing with a complex, multifaceted problem such as the TABP, the therapist rarely relies on a single intervention technique, but is likely to use a constellation of treatment strategies. Secondly, even when relatively well-known techniques are employed, their administration is inevitably modified by the complex interactions between therapist and client. But while the lack of precision in the description of behavioural treatments is understandable, nevertheless, it constitutes a serious handicap to progress in type A interventions; in the absence of detailed knowledge of what was done to whom under what conditions in a given programme, there is no basis for improving unsuccessful treatments or even replicating successful ones.

For behavioural treatments for type As to pass beyond the stage of alchemy, it is essential that they be presented in the same detail, and subject to the same careful scrutiny that is now reserved for measurement methods. By providing a detailed description of the assumptions and methods of the stress management treatment used by our research group, I hope to begin this long overdue and much needed process.

THE MONTREAL TYPE A INTERVENTION PROJECT

Purpose

The identification of the TABP as a major, independent risk factor for coronary heart disease (Review Panel on Coronary-Prone Behavior and Coronary Heart Disease, 1981) has given rise to a host of treatment efforts seeking to reduce coronary risk in type A individuals by modifying their behaviour. For type As who have already experienced a heart attack, the aim of treatment is to reduce the risk of reinfarction, while for the larger population of healthy type As (i.e. those without manifest signs of clinical heart disease), the goal is prevention. The treatments used for these purposes have varied from psychodynamic brief therapy, to jogging, to the various forms of stress management described above, but for healthy type As, at least, it was impossible to accept or reject any treatment, because of serious, methodological shortcomings in the studies testing them. Not only were samples extremely heterogeneous, making it difficult to determine who exactly was being treated for precisely what problem but, even more important, the criteria used to measure outcome were open to question. To track changes in incidence of coronary morbidity and mortality in apparently healthy, relatively young individuals would require unfeasibly large sample sizes and lengthy follow-up periods, but many of the measures that were used as substitutes bore no relationship either to heart disease or the TABP (see Roskies, 1982).

The Montreal Type A Intervention Project (MTAIP) was mounted in an effort to overcome some of the conceptual and methodological problems of previous intervention efforts with healthy type As. By careful selection of sample and outcome measures, and quality control of treatment delivery, it sought to provide a valid comparison of the efficacy of three short-term interventions (aerobic exercise, cognitive-behavioural stress management, and weight training) in reducing coronary risk within this population. The basic assumption was that the type As hypersensitivity and hyper-reactivity to everyday challenges and hassles constitutes a mechanism for coronary heart disease, with the corollary that any treatment resulting in a reduction of behavioural and physiological stress responses could also be considered to have reduced coronary risk.

Method

Sample

The sample for the study was composed of volunteers drawn from the population of male managers working at two large companies in the Montreal area. Potential participants were screened for (a) presence of type A, (b) presence of exaggerated cardiovascular and endocrine reactivity to a series of psychological stress tasks, and (c) absence of history or present signs of heart disease, hypertension or diabetes.

The sample for this study was carefully selected to ensure that treatment efficacy was tested in individuals exemplifying key characteristics of the target population: apparently healthy, employed at a level and in an environment in which type A behaviour is believed to flourish, and manifesting the distinguishing type A 'signs' of behavioural and physiological hyper-reactivity to stress. Managers constituted an appropriate group from which to select the sample because this is the occupational level at which type A behaviour is most prevalent and, apparently, also most harmful (Haynes *et al.*, 1980). The trial was limited to men because men and women differ significantly in their catecholamine stress responses (Frankenhaeuser, 1983) and, of the two sexes, it is men who are at considerably higher coronary risk. The restriction of recruitment to two companies was based on the belief that since the type A behaviour pattern represents an interaction between a predisposed individual and an eliciting environment (Friedman and Rosenman, 1974), it is important that participants in the clinical trial share as similar an environment as possible.

In all, 418 individuals began the selection process, but only 118 met all sample criteria and were enrolled in the programme. Of these, 107 fulfilled attendance and post-testing requirements and were included in the calculation of outcome, 33 in the aerobic exercise group and 37 each in the stress management and the weight training groups. The findings were limited to those receiving a complete dosage of treatment to ensure that each of the treatments was given the best possible conditions under which to manifest its efficacy.

Treatment

Individuals enrolled in the programme were stratified for age and level of physical fitness and then randomly assigned to one of the three treatments. Treatments were group-based, with 12–16 participants per group. The length of sessions (1 hour) and duration of treatment (10 weeks) were standard for all the treatments, but the number of required sessions per week varied according to the needs of the specific treatment approach. For stress management and weight training three weekly sessions were scheduled with attendance at two required, while for the aerobic programme four sessions were offered and three required. To be classified as completing treatment, individuals had to attend a minimum of 90% of the required sessions for their treatment group.

Both of the physical exercise programmes followed a similar format, beginning with a 10- to 15-minute warm-up period, and ending with a 10-minute cool-down period. The sole planned difference occurred in the middle section of the session when participants in the aerobic programme jogged, while those in weight training programme exercised on Nautilus equipment at intensities that generally exceeded the aerobic range, but for durations far shorter than those required to produce aerobic adaptations. Exercise prescriptions were individually tailored to participants' initial fitness level and then adjusted as necessary during the course of the programme.

To ensure once again that the treatments were tested under 'the best possible conditions', and to facilitate the adherence of healthy, busy men, a variety of strategies were used to maximize programme acceptability and minimize response costs. Group leaders were highly trained and experienced in working with a managerial population; participants were also furnished with written manuals explaining the content and rationale of the programme in which they were enrolled. The interventions were limited to the minimum period considered necessary to effect significant changes in aerobic fitness (10 weeks) and scheduled at the beginning of the workday (7.30 or 8 am). Treatment took place in settings close to the workplace and of high calibre; the two physical exercise groups met in private health clubs reserved for their exclusive use during programme hours. To minimize the possibility of dropout as a result of injury during physical exercise, participants in the aerobic treatment group were furnished with individually fitted jogging shoes, and arrangements were made with a Sports Medicine Unit for prompt treatment of pain or suspected injury.

A major hurdle for any group programme with busy managers is the need to deal with absences caused by business travel or other reasons. All the programmes made provision for this fact of life, the two exercise programmes by prescribing exercises that the participants could practice on their own, and the stress management programme by scheduling weekly make-up sessions for anticipated or past absences. With these provisions, an individual could miss up to 1 week of classes without apparent disruption of progress.

The validity of any clinical trial depends on the treatments being delivered as intended. Accordingly, we investigated participants' subjective evaluation of the treatment received, and verified whether the expected changes in aerobic fitness and muscle strength had occurred. Using a 7-point scale of 'worthwhileness', 82% of the sample (82% in the aerobic fitness group, 81% in the stress management group, and 83% in the weight training group) rated their treatment as 6 or 7 (i.e. very worthwhile). The physical changes observed were also those expected: joggers increased estimated maximal oxygen uptake and decreased basal heart rate significantly, but the other two groups did not. Conversely, and also as expected, the weight training group showed substantial increases on six of the seven strength determinations, the aerobic group improved on three determinations and the stress management group remained virtually unchanged. The positive results of these process measures, coupled with the attendance requirement that assured adequate programme exposure, led us to conclude that the treatments had been delivered as intended.

Outcome measures

The two criteria of treatment outcome were changes in behavioural and physiological reactivity to stress. Changes in behavioural reactivity were assessed by administering the Structured Interview (Rosenman, 1978) twice, before and after treatment. The Structured Interview (SI) is a 15- to 20-minute interview, in which predetermined questions about habits and daily activities are posed in a manner likely to evoke type A behaviours. Scoring is based on response style, rather than content. Using the Dembroski scoring protocol (Dembroski and MacDougall, 1983; Dembroski et al., 1978), individuals are scored on a 4-point scale for global type A behaviour, and on 5-point scales separately for speech loudness, explosiveness, and rapidity, response latency, competitiveness, and potential for hostility.

To circumvent rater bias, intentional or unintentional, the interviews were recorded and at the end of treatment were re-recorded in random order on new tapes, with all mention of time (pre-treatment vs post-treatment) or treatment group eliminated. Independent raters, who had no other connection with the project, then scored these tapes.

Physiological reactivity to stress was assessed during three laboratory sessions (selection, pre-treatment and post-treatment), but only the latter two scores were used to assess treatment efficacy. This strategy was used to circumvent the artificial cure that can be produced simply by habituation to the laboratory setting, with subsequent visits customarily yielding significantly lower reactivity scores compared to the first one (Lane, 1984).

Six comparable stress tasks served as stimuli (see Seraganian *et al.*, 1985) for a detailed description of the individual stress tasks and comparisons of their ability to evoke stress responses). Two tasks were presented at each session, and no individual received a given task more than once. Tasks were counterbalanced across groups for session administered, order of presentation, and time of day.

Initially, there were six dependent measures: systolic and diastolic blood pressure, heart rate, plasma epinephrine and norepinephrine, and cortisol. Unfortunately, three had to be discarded because measurement problems made it imprudent to utilize them for evaluation of treatment efficacy. For cortisol, less than a quarter of the sample showed a 25% increase above baseline during the course of the pre-treatment testing session, and even for those who did, there was no consistent pattern of elevation and recovery in response to the stress tasks. For the catecholamines, in contrast, the expected bell-shaped curve did occur, but large intra-assay variations (the same sample was split into two and each half was analysed separately) made us question the accuracy of the individual scores. Thus, the findings are based on changes in the three cardiovascular scores; individuals were assessed both for changes in intensity of response (percent increase above baseline) and duration (percent increase above baseline during a 4-minute recovery period following termination of the stressor).

Results

When the various treatments were compared in terms of their ability to modify behavioural reactivity, one treatment — cognitive-behavioural stress management — was clearly and consistently superior to the rest. It was significantly superior to the other two treatments both on global type A score and on five of the six components, showing reductions of 13–23% below pre-treatment values. In sharp contrast, the aerobic exercise group generally showed no change, while the weight training group was intermediate between the two others, with smaller and less consistent reductions of 0–12%; the differences between the two physical exercise groups, however, were not statistically significant. The credibility of these findings is enhanced by the fact that there were three groups per treatment, and the results were virtually identical in the different groups within each treatment.

For physiological stress responses, in contrast, none of the treatments could be said to achieve meaningful reductions. While there was a statistically significant drop pre- to post-treatment for the sample as a whole, there was no difference between treatments and, in any case, the reduction in reactivity was no greater than that attributable to habituation alone. In fact, when selection scores were juxtaposed against pre- and post-treatment ones, the greatest change occurred between selection and pre-treatment, a period in which no treatment had occurred. These results may reflect the inability of behavioural treatments in general to modify physiological hyper-reactivity, but they may also be the result of the inability of existing measures to accurately capture changes that do occur because of 'noise' in the measuring instruments and/or situations.

For the time being, therefore, we are left with the ability of this stress management programme to significantly reduce behavioural reactivity, as measured by the Structured Interview. This finding in itself is of considerable clinical interest, however, since Friedman has recently reported (Friedman et al., 1984) that in post-infarct patients, changes of this magnitude on the SI were associated with reduced recurrence and mortality. On this basis, the stress management programme requires and deserves further investigation.

STRESS MANAGEMENT FOR HEALTHY TYPE As

The basic belief guiding the construction of this intervention was that there is no all-purpose stress management programme that will serve as a universal panacea for all stress ills. Instead, when a therapist decides to apply stress management to a given condition, he or she is doing no more than making a choice of a general approach to treatment, one focusing on changing the way the person perceives and manages his or her transactions with the immediate environment. Still remaining to be accomplished before an actual treatment programme can be said to exist, is (a) detailed appraisal of the strengths and weaknesses of current coping patterns, (b) the delineation of specific goals for treatment, and (c) the selection of appropriate treatment methods for achieving these goals. Finally, and most important, the diagnosis and prescription must be couched in terms that are understandable by and acceptable to those for whom the treatment is destined.

Defining the problem

The sample for this study was considered to be at risk because of the presence of the TABP, but any treatment for this 'symptom' also had to take into account other, equally salient, sample characteristics: apparent health, substantial educational and occupational achievements, and lack of obvious distress as evidenced by the fact that project participants had not sought out treatment themselves. Thus, it would be patently ridiculous to view sample members as generally inadequate in managing their environment; on the contrary, based on their ability to fulfil valued social roles, these individuals were clearly above average in coping skills. Conversely, it would be equally unrealistic to define their coping problems as stemming from unusually stressful life circumstances; managerial jobs may be stressful to those who hold them, but they are less likely than blue collar jobs to be directly linked to physical and mental problems (Kasl, 1978), and still less so than total absence of work, i.e. unemployment (Fryer and Payne, 1986). In short, the TABP may be seen as a problem in coping but, paradoxically, the coping problems of this specific sample could not be ascribed either to an extraordinarily threatening environment, or to obvious deficiencies in managing the stresses they did encounter.

Nevertheless, coping competency can be evaluated not only according to the effectiveness with which a task is accomplished but also, and equally as important, by the cost of this effectiveness to the individual (Silber et al., 1961a, 1961b). In addition, the available evidence suggests that the type A may expend energy unnecessarily and/or ineffectively in coping with the inevitable hassles of daily life. Compared to less reactive individuals, type As are more likely both to evaluate even minor challenges or annoyances as stressful, and to react to these minor crises as intensely as to major ones. Participants in this programme had given concrete evidence of this hyper-reactivity by the fact that they had responded to mild stressors (the SI and the stress tasks in the laboratory) much more intensely than had some of their coworkers in the same company occupying similar positions. Furthermore, because of their insensitivity to bodily signs of fatigue and illness, type As are also more likely to proceed from one stressful situation to the next without allowing for rest and recuperation. Thus, instead of monitoring and controlling energy expenditures, the type A spends his or her abundant energy profligately, mobilizing resources indiscriminately to win a game of tennis, to solve a difficult and crucial work problem, or simply to fume at a too-slow elevator.

In this view of the TABP, the crucial coping defect lies not in the content of any single stress response, but in the indiscriminate mobilization and reaction to a variety of situations. The type A does not necessarily handle any specific stress episode badly, but it is the cumulative impact of perceiving too many situations as stressful and reacting too intensely and for too long that defines his or her increased vulnerability to CHD.

The goals of treatment

The aim of treatment for the healthy type A, therefore, is simply to reduce 'coping costs' by increasing the individual's *awareness* and *control* of stress perceptions and reactions. Healthy type As have demonstrated their ability to manage the environment, but the new challenge is to improve management of personal resources. Instead of responding indiscriminately and automatically to all the inevitable challenges and threats of daily living, the individual will ideally become both more *selective* in choosing his or her battles and more *skilled* in pursuing goals at minimum cost in personal upset and disturbed relations with others.

These goals cannot be achieved simply by presenting the individual with a pre-packaged coping formula, because there is no way to identify in advance all the situations in which hyper-reactivity is likely to occur, nor all the forms it is likely to take. Even within an apparently homogeneous group of healthy type A managers, life situations are too varied, possible stress responses too numerous, and individual differences too great, to rely on any single coping strategy (e.g. relaxation), or even a set combination of strategies. Instead, to effect any real and lasting change in habitual stress responses, the individual must learn to function independently as a behavioural engineer, capable both of discriminating between 'good' and 'bad' stress perceptions and responses in a given situation, and of devising and implementing coping strategies to meet the needs of that situation. To achieve this flexibility of response, there are four component skills to be mastered.

1. Increased *awareness* of the many levels — physiological, behavioural, emotional, and cognitive — and of the many situations in which dysfunctional responses are occurring.
2. *Acquisition* of multiple new coping strategies — via learning of new coping techniques and mobilization of existing ones — for evaluating and responding to potential stressors.
3. Ability to *evaluate* the effect of different coping strategies on mental and physical well-being.
4. Repeated *practice* of new coping patterns in an ever-widening variety of situations until these new patterns themselves become habitual.

This conceptualization of coping deficiencies, and the consequent goals of treatment, are likely to be acceptable to healthy type As for a number of reasons. First, this model is as much a recognition of health as a diagnosis of illness; rather than labelling existing coping strategies as 'bad' and seeking to eradicate them, it acknowledges the high level of coping competency already achieved by sample members and strives to build on this foundation. This recognition of existing functioning adequacy is an essential prerequisite to any attempt at intervention with this population who, quite rightly, will resist being cast in a sick role that is incongruent both with their values and their own perceptions of themselves. In fact, it is only these individuals' past record in successfully meeting difficulty challenges that makes it possible to envisage a short-term intervention for behaviours that are so deeply ingrained and amply reinforced!

A second advantage of this model is that it does not threaten cherished goals, but simply seeks to improve the methods used to reach these goals. Stress management for healthy type As is not an attempt to reconstruct the individual in the image of the 'healthy personality', or even to refashion him according to the tastes and preferences of the therapist. For instance, one would not seek to change a lifestyle based on serial sexual conquests into one committed to monogamy, or to advocate quiet walks in the woods to a devotee of gambling at Las Vegas. Instead, the scope of treatment is limited to showing individuals how to use resources more efficiently in pursuing existing goals and commitments.

The third major advantage of this model is that it leads to an intervention focused on active acquisition of new skills, rather than one stressing rest and inactivity. Given the barrage of publicity that the TABP and its negative consequences has received in recent years, it would indeed be the unusual type A who was not somewhat aware of and uneasy about his stress reactions. However, many Type As are caught in the dilemma of seeing no acceptable alternative to what they are currently doing; they are continuously advised to 'take it easy', but life in the rocking chair is not particularly appealing to these active people. The model presented here does not require the type A to become less active but, instead, emphasizes active pursuit of a new challenge, that of self-management.

The learning process

The programme presented here is designed for twenty sessions. The MTAIP scheduled 2-hourly sessions per week, with a third session available for individuals to make up an anticipated or past absence. Initially, the two session a week rhythm was adopted to make frequency comparable to the other treatments, but it proved to have considerable clinical utility in permitting more frequent opportunity to recognize and deal with learning problems, thus helping to prevent participants from becoming discouraged and dropping out.

The programme contains a number of coping techniques, such as training in relaxation, problem solving and communication skills (see Table 1), but is not primarily technique oriented. Effective coping, in my view, depends on more than the possession of a multitude of coping techniques; one must also know when and how to use them. And it is precisely in this area that the coping deficiencies of the type A are most evident; many sample members, for instance, may have already followed workshops on communication skills, but would not think of applying these skills to a marital conflict. The goal, therefore, is not only to teach new techniques but also to facilitate the effective use of existing ones.

Table 1. Programme structure.

Modules	Skills taught
1. Introduction	General overview
2. Relax Learning to control physical stress responses	Self-monitoring of physical and emotional tension signs. Progressive muscular relaxation (Bernstein and Borkovec, 1973; Goldfried, 1977)
3. Control yourself Learning to control behavioural stress responses	Self-monitoring of behavioural signs of tension. Incompatible behaviours, delay, communication skills (Stuart, 1974)
4. Think productively Learning to control cognitive stress responses	Self-monitoring of self-talk. Cognitive restructuring (Beck, 1976; Goldfried, 1977; Meichenbaum, 1985)
5. Be prepared Learning to anticipate and plan for predictable stress situations	Identification of recurrent stress triggers; stress inoculation training (Meichenbaum, 1985)
6. Cool it Learning emergency braking in unpredictable stress situations	Identification of signs of heightened tension; application of physical, behavioural, and cognitive controls. Anger-control (Novaco, 1975)
7. Building stress resistance Learning to plan for rest and recuperation	Identification of pleasurable activities. Problem-solving (D'Zurilla and Nezu, 1982; Goldfried and Davison, 1976)
8. Protect your investment Stress management as a lifelong investment	Relapse prevention (Marlatt and Gordon, 1985)

As in the learning of any complex skill, the acquisition of coping skills can be facilitated by dividing the matter to be learned into a series of graded steps. Thus, this programme is divided into eight modules (see Table 1). The first serves as a general programme introduction, while the next three are devoted to basic skill building, teaching the individual to monitor and modulate physical, behavioural, and cognitive responses to stress. The next two modules build on these basic skills by teaching participants how to combine them and apply them, first, to anticipating and planning for predictable stress triggers (i.e. trouble shooting) and, second, to regaining control when suddenly confronted by unpredictable and unexpected stress emergencies. The seventh module extends the scope of self-management to the realm of pleasures; the aim here is to teach the individual how to attain needed rest and recuperation by planning for them. The eighth and final module focuses on relapse prevention, awareness of possible reversions to old habits, and methods for managing these lapses.

For impatient type As, however, the step method can be difficult to accept unless they can clearly see the relationship between what they are doing today and their ultimate goals. The challenge then is to divide the matter into small enough steps to be manageable, but also to provide a map of the entire path so that the relevance of each part to the whole is clearly visible. To guide individuals through the programme, a written manual is provided to participants made up of eight road maps or 'rationales' (Roskies, 1987a,b). The first rationale constitutes a general introduction to and overview of the programme, defining the problem(s) to be treated, listing the goals of treatment, and summarizing programme content and methods. The remaining seven rationales serve as introductions to specific modules, defining what is to be learned in that module and why, and the steps involved in learning it. During the course of the programme this written manual helps the participant place the present task in the context both of past learning and future goals. After the programme, the manual can be used as a refresher course.

After the general introduction, the same basic sequence is used in the remaining seven modules: problem identification, learning of remedial techniques, application to a specific situation and evaluation of effects, generalization to other situations. To use the module on modification of behavioural stress responses as an example, the person first learns to monitor behavioural signs of tension (e.g. shouting, interrupting, grimacing, gulping of food, aggressive driving, etc.), and to identify the negative consequences of uncontrolled displays of tense behaviour (e.g. churning stomach, angry secretary, etc.). The next step is to select targets for change and identify existing coping techniques, or learn new ones, that could be used to change the behaviour. For instance, a person who wanted to reduce the barking quality of his voice on the telephone at work, could engage both in incompatible behaviours (pausing to relax before making a call or answering one, speaking slowly, listening carefully to the other person) and delay (10-second time out when he perceives that he is barking). After deciding which techniques to use, where and when (e.g. tomorrow morning at the office, every time I answer the phone), he would engage in a trial practice, monitoring both his success in using the techniques, and the effect of any changes in voice quality on feelings about himself, relationship to the person with whom he is speaking, content of telephone call, etc. Once the basic process of modifying a specific behaviour in a specific situation was familiar, he would gradually extend the range and complexity of target behaviours, developing, implementing, and evaluating coping strategies as needed. The same learning sequence from initial awareness to final generalization is repeated in each of the other modules.

A noteworthy departure in this programme from usual cognitive-behavioural procedures is the blending of the assessment and treatment phases; instead of completing an exhaustive inventory of the type A's coping problems before beginning intervention, the procedure used here is to alternate problem identification with remedial action, proceeding from module to module. This sequence was adopted to solve a common conundrum faced by therapists working with type As: to change behaviour the individual must become aware of what is dysfunctional in his current actions, but most type As are unaware of what they are actually experiencing and doing in stress situations and, even more important, unwilling to become aware of dysfunctional stress responses because they are convinced that there is nothing that can be done about it. Here we seek to build confidence in the therapeutic process by beginning with minimal disclosure (e.g. record keeping of variations in physical tension) and immediately instituting effective remedial action (e.g. relaxation training). As type As become increasingly confident of their ability to change dysfunctional responses, they also become more willing to recognize their existence.

A second distinctive characteristic of this programme is the emphasis on behavioural assignments or 'homework'. Each session has its accompanying homework assignment (see Roskies, 1987a,b, for facsimiles of the homework sheets) and, in fact, therapist–client meetings are designed mainly as a preparation for and as follow-up to the *in vivo* practices provided by the homework assignments. This focus on behavioural assignments reflects my belief that coping skills, like any other skill, can only be learned with repeated practice and corrective feedback. One does not learn to play tennis or speak French without multiple trial and error sessions, and the same principle holds true for relaxation or problem-solving. Furthermore, it is important that these skills be practised under the conditions and in the environment in which they are to be used; learning to cope better with daily hassles is best done while one is actually experiencing them.

Convincing time pressured type As to add still another demand to an overburdened day is far from an easy task, but a number of techniques have enabled me to reach a compliance rate of 75–90% with the homework assignments. One important aid to adherence is the physical format in which these homework assignments are presented. Each is a finished product, numbered, titled, and pre-packaged, indicating that behavioural assignments are not simply afterthoughts, but occupy a central role in the programme. Furthermore, the task to be done is clearly described; the title page of each assignment indicates the topic, what is to be done, and for what purpose. Of even greater value in making the assignment understandable, is the example sheet that is included in each one; here, participants can see concretely how a completed assignment might look. Finally, to minimize response costs, participants are furnished with prepared response sheets requiring only a minimum of writing on their parts (Roskies, 1987b).

A second major aid to adherence is the emphasis placed on the review of homework assignments during sessions. At least half of each session is devoted to reviewing the homework assignment of the previous session, and participants are encouraged to read directly from their homework sheets, rather than responding in broad, general terms. To further emphasize the importance of homework, most of the time and attention, particularly in early sessions, is focused on those who have done the assignment. Managers who are also type As are likely to be very sensitive to group expectations, and to conform to a norm of compliance if it is established early and firmly enough.

CONCLUSIONS

The stress management programme described in this chapter is not intended as the final word on treatment of healthy type As. However, it is the treatment for this population with the strongest empirical support to date and, to the best of my knowledge, it is the only treatment described in sufficient detail to permit replication by others. By laying bare what we did and why we did it, I hope to stimulate other researchers in the area to describe their treatments in sufficient detail to permit synthesis of the common elements and empirical testing of the differences. Only in this way can we correct our mistakes and build on our strengths.

Acknowledgements

The research reported here was financed by Health and Welfare, Canada. Co-principal investigators for the MTAIP were Peter Seraganian, Robert Oseasohn, and James A. Hanley. Dr Lorraine Poitras was my co-therapist for the stress management programme.

REFERENCES

Beck, A. T. (1976). *Cognitive Therapy And The Emotional Disorders*. International Universities Press, New York.

Bernstein, D. A. and Borkovec, T. D. (1973). *Progressive Relaxation Training: A Manual For The Helping Professions*. Research Press, Champaign, Illinois.

Dembroski, T. M. and MacDougall, J. M. (1983). Behavioral and psychophysiological perspectives on coronary-prone behavior. In Dembroski, T. M., Schmidt, T. G. and Blümchen, G. (Eds), *Biobehavioral Bases of Coronary Heart Disease*. Karger, Basel, pp. 106–129.

Dembroski, T. M., MacDougall, J. M., Shields, J. L., Pettito, J. and Lushene, R. (1978). Components of the Type A coronary-prone behavior pattern and cardiovascular responses to psychomotor challenge. *Journal of Behavioral Medicine*, **1**, 159–176.

D'Zurilla, T. and Nezu, A. (1982). Social problem-solving in adults. In Kendall, D. (Ed.), *Advances in Cognitive-Behavior Research and Therapy*, vol. 1. Academic Press, New York, pp. 202–274.

Frankenhaeuser, M. (1983). The Sympathetic-adrenal and pituitary-adrenal response to challenge: Comparison between the sexes. In Dembroski, T. M., Schmidt, T. G. and Blümchen, G. (Eds), *Biobehavioral Bases of Coronary Heart Disease*. Karger, Basel, pp. 91–105.

Friedman, M. and Rosenman, R. H. (1974). *Type A Behavior and Your Heart*. Knopf, New York.

Friedman, M., Thoresen, C. E., Gill, J. J., Powell, L., Ulmer, D., Thompson, L., Price, V. A., Rabin, D. D., Breall, W. S., Dixon, T., Levy, R. A. and Bourg, E. (1984). Alteration of Type A behavior and reduction in cardiac recurrence in post-myocardial infarction patients. *American Journal*, **108**, 237–248.

Fryer, D. and Payne, R. (1986). Being Unemployed: A review of the literature on the psychological experience of unemployment. In Cooper, C. L. and Robertson, I. T. (Eds), *International Review of Industrial and Organizational Psychology 1986*. Wiley, Chichester, pp. 235–278.

Goldfried, M. R. (1977). The use of relaxation and cognitive relabeling as coping skills. In Stuart, R. (Ed.), *Behavioral Self-Management: Strategies, Techniques and Outcomes*. Brunner/Mazel, New York, pp. 82–116.

Goldfried, M. R. and Davison, G. (1976). *Clinical Behavior Therapy*, Holt, Rinehart and Winston, New York.

Hart, K. E. (1984). Anxiety management training and anger control for Type A individuals. *Journal of Behavior Therapy and Experimental Psychiatry*, **15**, 1–7.

Haynes, S. G., Feinleib, M. and Kannel, W. B. (1980). The relationship of psychosocial factors to coronary heart disease of the Framingham Study. III. Eight-year incidence of coronary heart disease. *American Journal of Epidemiology*, **111**, 37–58.

Jenni, M. A. and Wollersheim, J. P. (1979). Cognitive Therapy, Stress Management Training and the Type A Behavior Pattern. *Cognitive Therapy and Research*, **3**, 61–73.

Kasl, S. V. (1978). Epidemiological contributions to the study of work stress. In Cooper, C. L. and Payne, R. (Eds), *Stress at Work*. Wiley, New York, pp. 3–48.

Lane, J. D. (1984). Reliability of cardiovascular responses to psychological stress. *SPR Abstracts*, **21**, 586.

Marlatt, G. A. and Gordon, J. R. (Eds) (1985). *Relapse prevention: maintenance strategies in the treatment of addictive behaviors*. Guilford Press, New York.

Meichenbaum, D. (1985). *Stress Inoculation Training*. Pergamon, New York.

Novaco, R. (1975). *Anger Control: The Development and Evaluation of an Experimental Treatment*. D. C. Heath, Lexington, Massachusetts.

Review Panel on Coronary-Prone Behavior and Coronary Heart Disease (1981). Coronary-prone behavior and coronary heart disease: A critical review. *Circulation*, **63**, 1199–1215.

Rosenman, R. H. (1978). The Interview Method of Assessment of the Coronary-Prone Behavior Pattern. In Dembroski, T. M., Weiss, S. M., Shields, J., Haynes, S. G. and Feinleib, M. (Eds), *Coronary-Prone Behavior*. Springer-Verlag, New York, pp. 55–70.

Roskies, E. (1982). Type A intervention: finding the disease to fit the cures. In Surwit, R., Williams, R. B., Steptoe, A. and Biersner, R. (Eds), *Behavioral Treatment of Disease*. Plenum Press, New York, pp. 71–86.

Roskies, E. (1987a). *Stress Management for the Healthy Type A: Theory and Practice*. Guilford Press, New York.

Roskies, E. (1987b). *Stress Management for the Healthy Type A: A Skills Training Program*. Guilford Press, New York.

Roskies, E. and Avard, J. (1982). Teaching healthy managers to control their coronary-prone (Type A) behavior. In Blankstein, K. R. and Polivy, J. (Eds), *Self-Control and Self-Modification of Emotional Behavior: Advances in the Study of Communication and Affect*. Plenum Press, New York, pp. 161–183.

Roskies, E., Kearney, H., Spevack, M., Surkis, A., Cohen, C. and Gilman, S. (1979). Generalizability and durability of treatment effects in an intervention program for coronary-prone Type A Managers. *Journal of Behavioral Medicine*, **2**, 195–207.

Roskies, E., Spevack, M., Surkis, A., Cohen, C. and Gilman, S. (1978). Changing the coronary-prone Type A behavior pattern in a non-clinical population. *Journal of Behavioral Medicine*, **1**, 201–216.

Roskies, E., Seraganian, P., Oseasohn, R., Hanley, J. A., Collu, R., Martin, N. and Smilga, C. (1986). The Montreal Type A intervention project: major findings. *Health Psychology*, **5**, 45–69.

Seraganian, P., Hanley, J. A., Hollander, B., Roskies, E., Smilga, C., Martin, N., Collu, R. C. and Oseasohn, R. (1985). Psychophysiological reactivity: issues in quantification and reliability. *Journal of Psychosomatic Research*, **25**, 393–405.

Silber, E., Coelho, G. V., Murphy, E. B., Hamburg, D. A., Pearlin, L. I. and Rosenberg, E. B. (1961a). Competent adolescents coping with college decision. *Archives of General Psychiatry*, **5**, 517–527.

Silber, E., Hamburg, D. A., Coelho, G. V., Murray, E. B., Rosenberg, E. B. and Pearlin, L. I. (1961b). Adaptive Behavior in Competent Adolescents. *Archives of General Psychiatry*, **5**, 354–365.

Stuart, R. B. (1974). Communication skills. Paper presented at the annual meeting of the Association des specialistes en modification du comportement. Moncton, New Brunswick, Canada, June.

Suinn, R. M. (1975). The Cardiac Stress Management Program for Type A Patients. *Cardiac Rehabilitation*, **5**, 13–15.

Suinn, R. M. and Bloom, L. J. (1978). Anxiety Management Training for Pattern A Behavior, *Journal of Behavioral Medicine*, **1**, 25–35.

Behavioural Medicine in Cardiovascular Disorders
Edited by T. Elbert, W. Langosch, A. Steptoe and D. Vaitl
©1988 John Wiley & Sons Ltd

13

Effort and Distress in Coronary Patients: How to Modify

Karin Siegrist
*Herz-Kreislauf-Klinik, Bad Berleburg and Department of Medical Sociology,
Medical School, University of Marburg*

INTRODUCTION

But I am not type A, Freya said, when we were
all sitting in the sauna. I'm not in high
need for control as some of our patients are.
Some are unable to express their emotions. They
do not attach anything to themselves or themselves to anything, except for success. — Of course
you are type A, I replied, and of course you are
attached to people and things.

One common misunderstanding about type A behavior pattern (TABP) is the
'naturalistic' one: the construct is taken as a fair reproduction of a person's
behavior with photographical accuracy. Most of the literature on TABP is
favorable to this type of error. I would like to present some arguments in favor
of a very cautious use of the TABP concept. A construct is a construct
and remains a construct, although certain individuals might look like its
personification. What is interesting about TABP and the motivation thought
to be underlying—an exaggerated need for control—is its potential for
provoking effort with distress (E&D). Competitiveness, overcommitment to
work, and perfectionism are thought to be coronary prone under certain
circumstances only: when they elicit a reaction of E&D in the organism as a
whole. It is this E&D reaction that behavior modification aims at, not the
behavior pattern *per se*. The reaction has some determinants other than TABP,
namely a social one (not to mention biological factors) and it is only when they
interact that there is cardiovascular risk.

As an introduction I would like to present some recent discussions of E&D as a coronary risk factor and pay particular attention to the role of TABP within social risk constellations. The second part gives an overview and discussion of behavior modification trials in patients and individuals at risk. My own somewhat eclectic approach to reduce E&D in coronary patients is developed in the third part. Finally I shall briefly outline an evaluation of that programme which is under way.

RECENT EVIDENCE RELATING EFFORT WITH DISTRESS AND CORONARY RISK

One can describe 'stress' in a way Karl Marx once described capitalism: stress is extremely productive and efficient, it leads to formidable physiologic changes. Often adaptation is the endpoint of the stress process. Stress provides the energy necessary for emotional behavior (Meerson, 1984), which is an expensive search for the optimal adaptive response. But capitalism did not offer the same chances of growth to everybody and not everybody could adapt to the changes it implied. The stress process does not end up with better coping abilities for all. Some get into circles of overactivation not followed by adequate phases of regeneration. In this case 'effort with distress' (cf. Frankenhaeuser, 1980; see also Siegrist, 1987, whose 'active distress' is closely related to E&D) is experienced. This means on the behavioral level: strong efforts to cope with high demands are associated with anger and, when success is doubtful, with frustration and perception of lack of control. The activation of two stress axes typically parallels this pattern of emotions and behavior: the sympathico-adrenal-medullary and the pituitary-adrenocortical, the first being particularly associated with the components of effort and anger, the second being related to feelings of frustration and helplessness. If sustained activation of both stress axes occurs again and again, effort with distress appears to be a risk factor of cardiovascular disease. A considerable amount of epidemiologic, clinical, and experimental evidence concerning its relevance in etiology has been accumulated (Beamish et al., 1985; Schmidt et al., 1986).

Some psychosocial risk factors and how they might work

The best single social predictor of cardiovascular disease (CVD) is social status. Low status has evolved as a risk factor for cardiovascular complications in different societies in the past decades (Marmot, 1982). It has been demonstrated that the class-related risk is only to a minor degree explained by health-related behaviors like smoking, overeating or poor compliance with medical regimen. There is, however, growing evidence for an accumulation of job strains and status insecurity in the lower classes, whereas the positive side of options and rewards is only poorly developed.

The best single psychological predictor of CVD risk has been TABP. But some recent prospective studies have failed to replicate earlier findings (Shekelle *et al.*, 1986), although others did (Haynes *et al.*, 1983; Siegrist, 1987). When does TABP exert its explanatory power, when does it not? In the Framingham study the behavior pattern did explain cardiovascular morbidity especially when somatic or social risk factors were present at the same time. In a longitudinal study on industrial workers in the FRG TABP was found to be associated with hypertension and hypercholesterolemia only in the subgroup of workers in low positions doing their job under conditions of low job security, high quantitative demands and low rewards. For those who were better off strong commitment to the job and perfectionism did not affect cardiovascular risk.

Different indicators of E&D have been found to be associated with CVD and its risk factors. Experimental studies indicate that the mechanisms underlying this association might be described in terms of hyper-responsiveness to environmental stressors. If we leave out central nervous information processing and behavior for a while in order to focus on endocrine and physiological reactions we find an impressive body of evidence for the role of hyper-reactivity. Catecholamines and cortisol, both important endpoints of the formerly described stress-axes — if chronically over-reacting — seem to be a factor in elevating blood pressure (Henry *et al.*, 1977). The impact of frequent over-reactions of this kind on the functioning of physiological buffer mechanisms has been investigated. A lot of studies have been carried out to ascertain the predictive value of blood pressure (BP) and heart rate (HR) reactions to challenge for future hypertension. The results thus far are not quite consistent, but there is some evidence for hyper-reactivity being predictive of elevated BP levels in the future. Unfortunately, there are as yet very few studies that measure BP reactions in the individual's specifically challenging environment. Hyper-reactivity in the work setting provides us with a more realistic picture of what is going on in everyday life than clinical casual or experimentally induced BP elevations.

Several researchers have tried to differentiate reaction patterns that are supposed to be predictive of different disease outcomes. A reaction pattern characterized by strong HR and systolic BP reactions seems more predictive of hypertension, whereas a pattern characterized by a marked rise of diastolic BP may be relevant for the development of CVD (for a discussion, see Sime *et al.*, 1980).

If we assume that differences in neuroendocrine and physiological reactivity cannot be ascribed to genetic factors only, we come back to higher nervous information processing. If subjects exhibit marked differences in physiological reactivity this may be because of equally marked differences in dealing with environmental stressors. Pronounced anger and anxiety reactions in situations of high demand are discussed as relevant psychological variables (Manuck *et al.*, 1985). A more complex way of perception and of coping with external challenges in conceived under the label TABP. Rosenman, one of the founding fathers in this research tradition, recently described it as a 'particular action–emotion complex that is exhibited by an individual who is engaged in a relatively *chronic* and excessive struggle to obtain [all] . . . in the shortest period of time or against the opposite efforts of others' (Rosenman, 1986).

From the very beginning the construct TABP has included sociological as well as psychological aspects. Classical trait psychology has failed to grasp the heart of the matter. Type A is more precisely described by what people do than by their personality traits. Chronic engagement in 'excessive struggle', as Rosenman stated, may be called behavioral hyper-reactivity. Instruments to measure TABP concentrate on that aspect. The hypothesis, however, that behavioral hyper-responsiveness must be paralleled by endocrine and physiological hyper-reactivity has not been consistently confirmed. There seems to be a good deal of confusion concerning the coronary prone potential of TABP, if we look at the following quotation: '. . . a necessary, but insufficient condition of producing specific aspects of Type A is a general, perhaps heritable hyper-responsivity to environmental challenge . . .' (Matthews and Rakaczky, 1986).

In view of the fact that the conditions under which TABP is detrimental to cardiovascular health are still controversial, the issue of ecological validity should be reconsidered. It is only as part of a psychosocial risk constellation that TABP is stressful and has an impact on cardiovascular health: this is the basic assumption in favor of which I would like to put forward some arguments. E&D modification—this would be the second assumption—can find a more solid foundation, if the underlying risk constellations are explored instead of focusing on the role of TABP as a partly inherited temperament.

Effort with distress producing constellations: theoretical considerations, a model and some empirical evidence

Recent investigations into the biochemical processes involved in the stress reaction provided insights into its molecular basis (Beamish *et al.*, 1985). What can the behavioral sciences tell us about psychosocial risk constellations eliciting the stress reaction, particularly the E&D pattern? It is taken for granted that the rising incidence of CVD seen in our century is associated with the fundamental social changes referred to as urbanization and industrialization. If we compare Western culture and society to Japan it becomes apparent that industrialization is compatible with different lifestyles. Ours is shaped by the rapid pace of life typical of an achievement society. Everybody, the common ideology suggests, has got a chance to lead his or her life in accordance with the value of achievement. Moreover, eagerness to compete and commitment to work will be recognized and rewarded regardless of a person's current social characteristics. TABP is the behavior pattern favored by achievement society. It seems paradoxical to call it a risk factor, if it leads one to be in harmony with the values of one's society. There is another paradox: TABP is more common among higher status groups whereas CVD incidence is higher among lower status groups. To make sense of these findings we may ask sociology and social psychology for some help. Twenty years ago the American sociologist Merton (1968) analyzed achievement ideology as a very unrealistic description of the social system. He showed different forms of deviant behavior to be caused by the gap between the ideology of equally distributed chances on the one hand and real social inequality and its impact on an individual's biography on the other.

In the meantime considerable research on class-related self-conceptions, social orientations, and lifestyles has been done. Kohn (Kohn and Schooler, 1983) has developed a general model of social stratification, job conditions, and multiple dimensions of personality and behavior. The results of various empirical studies including longitudinal investigations, support the hypothesis that stratification-related conditions of life have an impact on the psychological functioning and behavior of individuals. The job condition found to be most strongly related to class was substantive complexity of work. Men and women in higher positions with complex and self-directed work tend to believe that the society in which they live and their own capacities make a self-directed orientation efficacious. They feel personally responsible for what they do, feelings of self-worth are pronounced, as is trustfulness towards other people. Men and women in lower positions who experience low complexity of work, often feel closely supervised and suffer from job insecurity. They are typically working under greater external time pressure, and it is more likely that they are held responsible for things outside their control. They exhibit lower levels of self-confidence, higher levels of anxiety than their luckier counterparts, consider self-direction impossible and are not very trustful towards others. Would not TABP seem a very expensive coping strategy under these circumstances?

At this point it is necessary to underline the relativity of place in hierarchy. As our society offers a complex and multidimensional stratification system, a negative effect of status on psychological functioning is to be expected not only when we compare white collar to blue collar positions, but also, when we make comparisons within middle class white collar strata. The one who perceives his or her job as less complex, less interesting, and more oppressive than the job of some colleague, may be called 'relatively deprived'.

If relative social status is related to self-concepts, competence (verbal and other) and to expectancy towards other people, it is a factor in identity formation. Identity means that individuals can relate with what others think about them even if their views are quite heterogeneous to what they themselves consider to be their selves. It implies further that individuals can relate what they did yesterday to what they do today and are able to make plans for tomorrow. The normally unquestioned ground of identity lies in reliable functioning of the organism.

These briefly outlined concepts from the social sciences should be of some help to build up a model of psychosocial risk constellations. Sustained activation in the sense of E&D is to be expected if status, identity, and current behavior pattern are not in harmony over a longer period of time. If status or relative position in social hierarchy offers little chances to develop one's capacities, little opportunities to control the world around and very limited opportunities to get strong commitment to work rewarded, then TABP is a very expensive coping style and E&D are to be expected. Identity is permanently threatened under these circumstances, because the 'looking-glass self', i.e., self as reflected by significant others differs markedly from what the individual considers his or her self to be and even more markedly from the anticipated self that his or her sustained drive to achieve aims at. Type As' chronic and excessive struggle 'against the opposing efforts of others', is also a struggle against their place in hierarchy.

It has been stated that the type A never gives up despite the intensity and duration of the struggle (Rosenman, 1986). This persistence would be surprising, if there was not a strong motivation basis of TABP. As Siegrist has pointed out (Siegrist et al., 1980) a pronounced need for control over the social world around can lead to the 'Sisyphus syndrome' (see also Glass, 1977). Explained by a learning-generalization model or in psychodynamic terms as a compensation for insufficient attachment relations in early life, high need for control in adult life is associated with unrealistic appraisal of demands and opportunities, of one's coping potential, and the social roles one can aspire to. The changes in TABP in the course of individual biographies over time have been referred to as 'coping career' (Siegrist, 1987). In the beginning of this career 'vigor', i.e. work commitment (hard driving) and perfectionism are the dominant dimensions of TAB with increasing external demands or threat together with the effects of aging (decrease of coping potential), the more negative aspects like impatience, irritability, latent hostility, and inability to withdraw and relax become increasingly important.

This is not the place to go into further detail on the conceptual level, nor is it possible to present empirical evidence in an extensive manner. Nonetheless, based on epidemiologic data, I would like to demonstrate that 'coping career' might be a useful concept. Second, I will try to show that TABP as a way of coping with environmental stimuli — perceived as threats to an individual's need for control — is harmful to cardiovascular health only if it is part of a psychosocial risk constellation. Preliminary evidence is drawn from a prospective study on 416 male blue collar workers, aged 25–55 years (mean = 40.8 + 9.6), initially free from manifest CVD, who were followed over 3 years (final sample $n = 310$). The study was done to find out if levels in the risk factors hypertension and hypercholesterolemia could be ascribed to levels of external demands and threats in interaction with TABP. In order to validate the concept of 'coping career', the assumption was tested that the later stage of the career should be related to severe sleep disorders as signs of adaptive breakdown. It could be shown that in fact those workers who woke up frequently during the night or stayed awake in the early morning scored high on 'immersion', encompassing the aspects of impatience, irritability, latent hostility, and inability to withdraw from work obligations. External demands which, together with high need for control, provoked E&D, were found to be above average in the group with disturbed sleep. On the other hand, a relationship between severe sleep disorders and coronary events has been established in prospective studies (for an overview and for the study presented here, see Siegrist, 1987). Siegrist and coworkers wondered whether lack of deep and undisturbed regeneration at night would not be predictive of manifestations of CVD. On the basis of very small numbers they found sleep disturbances lasting for 4 weeks to be associated with a higher risk of acute myocardial infarction (AMI) in the two subsequent years.

Need for control in control-limiting social contexts was considered. Does it produce cumulative experience of E&D so that a relationship with BP or low density lipoprotein (LDL) can be observed? The researchers defined as 'control-limiting' the context of the low status unskilled worker as compared to the less oppressive context of the skilled worker. The unfavorable job context with its poor opportunity and reward structure makes high need for control a particularly unrealistic coping pattern. Therefore a closer relationship between TABP and indicators of cardiovascular risk in the unskilled than in the group of the skilled workers is expected. It could be demonstrated by linear structural equation models that this assumption is correct. Comparing the groups who did not differ in mean BP, there was a marked effect of 'vigor' on BP levels in the unskilled group. When a similar model was computed to explain LDL, the results were basically the same. The risk factors smoking and overweight together with age explained relatively little in the less privileged but had all their usual explanatory power in the more privileged group.

We do not know as yet how far these results can be generalized to different populations. Will the model outlined above be valuable in white collar populations, where control-limiting and oppressive working conditions may be less obvious so that the notion of 'relative deprivation' becomes more important? It is the working hypothesis of the chapter presented here that the model can be applied to different social groups.

Effort with distress in coronary patients

Given the above evidence for the role of a risk constellation associated with E&D in the etiology of CVD, the next question that seems relevant for behavior modification in post-MI patients is whether the specific interactions of TABP with external situations relate to the course of the disease once a coronary event has taken place.

Over recent years, epidemiologic and experimental studies have in fact demonstrated detrimental effects of natural and laboratory stressors on the cardiovascular system. A retrospective case control study on 380 patients with early MI (age 30–55) and on 190 healthy controls matched for age and occupational position established a relationship between psychosocial factors and a premature AMI (Siegrist et al., 1980). Findings of a follow-up study on 75% of the patients about 18 months after disease onset support the notion of a 'coping career': Patients who experienced high demands and oppressive working conditions scored higher on 'need for control' (particularly on dimensions of 'immersion') at follow-up than at the first interview during cardiac rehabilitation some weeks after disease onset. In the meantime 13 patients had died from a coronary event. To find out whether an extreme psychosocial risk constellation (chronic work stress and stressful life events and pronounced TABP before AMI) would predict mortality, we compared proportions of high risk persons within the group of the deceased to respective proportions within the surviving patients and within the healthy controls. If we attach the factor 1 to the healthy controls, there is a 1:4.3:7.2 relation of controls:survivors:deceased. The model presented is a simple additive one. Because of small numbers interaction effects of TABP and social context could not be tested. Unfortunately the interaction of cardiovascular parameters relevant to the course of disease could not be analyzed.

More convincing from the cardiologic point of view is a recent study on the impact of psychosocial stress and social isolation on mortality after MI (Ruberman et al., 1984). A total of 2300 male survivors of MI were interviewed. Independent of traditional risk factors, cardiac function, and cardiac vulnerability after MI the authors found a strong effect of psychosocial stress and social isolation on mortality for cardiac causes after 3 years. TABP was not predictive in this context. As interactions between oppressive social situation and TABP had not been hypothesized, they were not tested. We do not know as yet whether a respective risk constellation might be equally predictive of mortality.

Experimental studies tell us about the mechanisms whereby natural stressors might affect the course of the disease. Different kinds of laboratory stimuli like mental arithmetic or the Stroop–colour–word interference test are supposed to be adequate substitutes for natural stressors. Stressors which elicit efforts at active coping have produced marked physiologic reactions and hemodynamic alterations in post-MI patients. Under specific circumstances, the reactions were accompanied by signs of regional myocardial ischemia (Deanfield et al., 1984). Tavazzi et al. (1984) provoked lung edema in 2 MI patients out of 48, who had never experienced this complication before. Several authors have documented life-threatening cardiac arrhythmia triggered by strong emotional reactions to social stressors (Lown, 1984). Two classes of determinants of cardiovascular reactions must be considered: severity of the disease and intensity of the stress reaction. Both are relevant to the issue of E&D modification.

TRIALS OF BEHAVIOR MODIFICATION
IN CORONARY PATIENTS AND IN PERSONS AT RISK

What is the logic of behavior modification in individuals with CVD and in individuals at risk of developing the disease? Following the above line of argument one would expect assessment of psychosocial stress factors as the first step in intervention, in order to select those persons who suffer from recurrent experience of E&D. Unfortunately, many studies done in this area do not clearly define in behavioral terms who should undergo behavior modification.

Perhaps the most impressive work in this field has been carried out by Patel *et al.* (1985). On screening they identified about 200 men and women who had at least two of the following risk factors: hypertension ($\geqslant 140/90$ mmHg), elevated levels of plasma cholesterol ($\geqslant 243.6$ mg 100 ml^{-1}), and current cigarette smoking habit ($\geqslant 10$ cigarettes day^{-1}). After random allocation either to a behavior modification or control group, an 8-week treatment phase started. The group sessions comprised relaxation techniques and meditation, desensitization towards everyday stressors, and cognitive restructuring. Effects of treatment on risk factors were assessed at the end of the program, after 8 months, and after 4 years. Compared to the control group, short-term and medium-range effects on all parameters were found. Concerning BP levels, a long-term effect could even be demonstrated. Screening for cardiovascular morbidity after 4 years brought further evidence for the role of behavioral factors. In the treatment group the incidence of CVD was significantly lower than in the control group. The same holds true for mortality due to MI. Of course it would be interesting to know who profits most from stress management and relaxation in terms of psychosocial risk.

Another approach that has been quite successful is TABP modification in healthy type As as well as in post-MI patients exhibiting the behavior pattern. Two important questions have been answered positively:

1. Is behavior modification possible in a substantial amount of type A persons?
2. Is there an impact of lowered TABP on cardiovascular health or its risk factors (e.g. plasma cholesterol level) (Gill *et al.*, 1985; Friedman *et al.*, 1984).

Finally a type of intervention should be noted in which disease onset is the criterion for including an individual into the program of behavioral therapy. The underlying assumption is that MI is a very stressful life event for everybody to whom it might occur. Life events, particularly loss events, are known to require a great deal of adaptation energy. Therapy consists in continuous support given to the patient. Coping with disease and coping with stressful situations — maybe perceived as even more stressful in the post-MI situation — is thought to be enhanced via stress management in groups (Rahe *et al.*, 1979) or via regular exchange with a health professional (Frasure-Smith and Prince, 1985). Different researchers have been successful, as it seems, in reducing psychological indicators of distress, like anxiety and depression, and in reducing morbidity (Rahe *et al.*, 1979) or mortality (Frasure-Smith and Prince, 1985).

Certainly such results are encouraging for everybody working in the field. But some shortcomings should be mentioned: Intervention on the basis of a coronary event considered stressful for everybody seems not very specific. The same holds true for intervention on the basis of the assumption that sustained activation in the sense of E&D is a risk factor for the total population in modern western society. In the other type of therapeutic approach it is the coping pattern only that is defined as a stress factor, whereas the social context with its demands and rewards, its opportunities and threats, is totally left out.

Seemingly, there has been a lack of sociologically informed approaches.

EFFORT AND DISTRESS MODIFICATION:
A PROGRAM FOR CORONARY PATIENTS

The setting in which the therapeutic team is on the look out for candidates to be enrolled into the E&D modification program is a cardiac rehabilitation clinic. The majority of the patients—members of the middle and upper middle classes—have recently been hospitalized for AMI and/or coronary bypass surgery. They spend 4 to 6 weeks in the rehabilitation center. The purpose of rehabilitation is manifold: diagnostic procedures are conducted and effectiveness of therapies is evaluated. Patients improve their physical stress tolerance by doing regular exercise. In addition to more common medical procedures a lot of the clinic's activities are concerned with the psychological and social consequences of being ill. Health education and different kinds of relaxation techniques are supposed to be helpful for those who have to adapt to life with a chronic disease. Psychological counselling and psychotherapy are available to those patients who present abnormal emotional reactions to physical illness.

Patient selection

It is not known how best to select the most appropriate treatment for any individual patient. There are desirable and there are realistic modes of patient referral. As a consequence of the theoretical reflections on TABP a standardized pre-treatment interview, including measures of social context and indicators of subjective distress, would have to be carried out with all the patients who seem to be under stress and/or seem to be type A. This is the only way of obtaining sufficient information for identifying patients at high risk in psychosocial terms. On the other hand, it is impossible to screen dozens of patients per week thoroughly for an E&D producing risk constellation. The dominant referral source for E&D modification candidates is the physician. Physicians have to learn that their wards contain patients who have experienced severe E&D in the past and who are at high risk if they continue their old lifestyle which may have been an expensive way of adaptation to their social context. Doctors are required to become particularly attentive to indicators of subjective distress like sustained feelings of anger or helplessness or severe sleep disturbances. To ascertain that such disorders go back to the situation prior to MI/surgery, i.e. are not secondary to medical illness, a short retrospective questionnaire has been developed by the author. It is handed out to each patient at arrival so that the doctor gets some help to structure the initial interview as far as psychosocial factors are concerned. Further criteria for patient selection are indicators of behavioral and/or physiologic hyper-reactivity to stressors which are part of the clinic's everyday life, such as waiting for a diagnostic procedure or having to perform a physical exercise test. In some cases a psychomental stress-test has been carried out (Stroop–colour–word–conflict task).

Finally self-referral is an important source for E&D modification candidates. If patients consider themselves as being in need of behavior modification, commitment to the group tends to be high.

There are also more implicit criteria for selection. They are summed up in the following description of the typical participant. It is a man in his late forties, whose pronounced TABP makes him work at least 12 hours per day. The first time in his life he realized that he felt very bad was at the intensive care unit immediately after MI. Apparently he has reached a good position in social hierarchy but there are some aspects of his social context that seem threatening to him. He does not suffer from a general lack of coping skills nor is he emotionally disturbed. The lack of fit between his exaggerated need for control and certain control-limiting features of his context is interwoven with his biography: there are as many biographies as there are individuals.

Potential goals of E&D modification

At the end of the program the patients should have available some tools that facilitate coping with their relevant stressors. They should be able to act as their own change agents in the near future when they return to their everyday activities. The tools are:

1. Familiarity with a method of relaxation (Benson's relaxation Response), its roots, its purpose, and the technique.
2. Enhanced ability to recognize symptoms of an E&D reaction.
3. A more reflective relationship to one's TABP together with an enhanced ability to withdraw so that irritability, hostility, and sustained activation become less common.
4. Ability to locate TABP-related norms within the development of industrial society.
5. Ability to analyze one's own particular version of TABP in biographical terms.

6. Enhanced understanding of one's social context with its potential demands and rewards, its opportunities and threats.
7. Ability to detect ideas and beliefs which are out of keeping with one's real social circumstances.
8. Ability to deal with anticipated processes of stigmatization that might occur at the work place or at home where the patient might be labelled 'chronically ill'.
9. Awareness of factors in the environment and in the organism that provoke anxiety and depression.

Taken together: the E&D reaction should be reduced in intensity, duration, and frequency and, at the same time, returning to normal should be facilitated.

In so far as these goals are attained, positive effects on the risk factors hypertension, hypercholesterolemia, and smoking may occur. A reduction of cardiovascular morbidity and mortality is hypothesized.

The program of E&D modification

The setting is a comfortable and quiet room with a blackboard. The therapist makes the patients, 8 to 10 participants, form a circle with their chairs. During a short pre-treatment interview they have been told that we will meet twice a week and that there will be six group sessions, each 90 minutes, with some information given by the therapist at the beginning, almost an hour of group discussion in the middle, and preparation for relaxation and relaxation practice at the end.

Relevant concepts from sociology and psychology are outlined in the beginning of each session. The therapist presents basic ideas about organism-environment exchange and the importance of cognitive and emotional processes for adaptation to potential stressors. Selective information on neuronal control of bodily function should provide some insight into the role of stress as an etiologic factor. At the same time, it offers a view of the individual's chances of enhancing cardiovascular health by using more adaptive coping strategies.

Several homework sheets are handed out over the course of the program so that 'lessons' can be repeated and attempts be made to personalize the more general information. Three sheets are particularly important: (1) The Need For Control Homework Sheet, (2) the Reactivity To Acute Stress Sheet, and (3) the In-And-Out-Of-Circles-Of E&D Sheet.

1. *The Need for Control Homework Sheet* enumerates the six dimensions of the above described version of TABP (Siegrist, 1987):
'Immer- 1. Need for approval, coping with success and failure
sion'   2. Competitiveness, independence and latent hostility
         3. Work commitment, hard driving
         4. Perfectionism, need for making plans } 'Vigor'
'Immer- 5. Time urgency, impatience and irritability
sion'   6. Inability to withdraw from work obligations.

The participants are asked to answer several questions concerning their own coping styles. First they have to think about the relationship between TABP and social norms and values. The question of which dimension is relevant to them has to be answered second. Has there been unrealistic appraisal of social context or of the person's capacities to deal with external demands in the past? Did the unrealistic appraisal, in turn, lead to experiences of subjective distress? The next step is to make a decision as to whether the relevant behaviors are to be changed in the future. This decision includes a reflection on the possibility of change in one's particular environment.

Other questions deal with the impact of CVD on performance of social roles. What does it mean to have a chronic disease in middle adulthood? Is it perceived as a form of deviance? The experience of threat to the body which often implies a threat to identity—could it be coped with? And, finally, does this experience of being ill pose the most severe problems to individuals with a strong need for control?

The Need For Control Sheet is discussed in the third and fourth session, when basic information on E&D has been given and the participants know about each other's risk constellations. The therapist points out the importance of making concrete plans of TABP modification, because otherwise everyday routines will prove difficult to change. Doubts about anticipated reactions from significant others: colleagues, superiors, family, friends, are exchanged in the group. This leads to the issue of how to advertize behavior change, and to whom. It is quite helpful if for one of the group, disease onset lies somewhere in the past, so that behavior modification has been tried already. If modification has been successful the others are encouraged. On the other hand the efforts behind become apparent.

2. *The Reactivity To Acute Stress Sheet* is discussed during the fifth session and deals with patients' cognitive, emotional, behavioral, and physiologic reactions to Stroop–colour–word–interference test (for a description, see Siegrist *et al.*, 1987). Usually at least one of the group members has been enrolled in a follow-up study on the course of CVD in relation to psychosocial risk factors and as hypothetically influenced by the E&D modification program.

The Sheet presents a more didactic version of the interview used in the study concerning the person's interpretation of the test. Do the candidates relate to it their everyday stressors? What were the individuals' thoughts and feelings before the test began, during the test, and during the 3-minute resting period afterwards? Did strong negative feelings affect performance? If there has been marked physiologic arousal, has it been perceived? What about the attribution of causality, when at the end of the test the candidate makes more and more mistakes, almost inevitably? Around these questions, each group member is asked to name typical strategies to cope with similar situations of acute stress. The discussion of strategies should help to clarify the distinction between 'effort' in the sense of phasic activation without marked negative feelings and E&D

as a more sustained activation associated with anger, tenseness, irritation, and helplessness.

It is interesting to note that patients enrolled in the study and participating in the program often apply Benson's Relaxation Response during the resting period after the test. They have not been told to do so before. Having practised the relaxation technique twice under therapeutic control, they were able to apply it as a coping strategy in an entirely new kind of stressful situation.

3. *The In-And-Out-Of-Circles-Of E&D Sheet* tries to sum up what has been learnt before. It is handed out at the end of the fifth session. Participants are supposed to study it in detail on their own in order to be prepared for the last session. E&D is presented as a result of different classes of determinants. First industrial achievement society has to be taken into account as a, maybe, necessary, but insufficient condition of producing E&D. Then social context is to be considered. What about status and what about emotional bonds? Does place in society as far as it is defined by status and bonds seem to be relatively stable or does it seem to be threatened? In case of threat even minor stressors may lead to E&D. Is there a strong need for control? How are the two related: perception of place as more or less safe and secure and a more or less pronounced need for control? Are the respective perceptions realistic? The sheet suggests that there is a relationship between a chronic risk constellation defined by TABP and place, and E&D reactions occurring in particular situations of demand. Subjects are asked to analyze their thoughts, feelings, symptoms, and behaviors exhibited in recurrent situations of challenge that ended up subjective distress in the past. How to withdraw when the E&D reaction has already begun? Finally they are invited to reflect upon aspects of their biographies. What is the *status quo* like in terms of age, severity of disease, importance of work role, importance of family and friends, and leisure activities?

When these questions have been discussed we come back to each member's personal goals. We tell each other how we will try to make life less stressful. Then we lean back, close our eyes, and practise relaxation together.

EFFORT WITH DISTRESS MODIFICATION IN CORONARY PATIENTS—IS IT EFFECTIVE?

The goals of the program have been described in some detail. After 2 years of experience with groups of coronary patients a study on goal attainment has been started. Included are male survivors of first MI, age ≤ 55 years, who have not undergone cardiac surgery. They are randomly allocated either to the E&D modification group (together with patients that are not enrolled in the study) or to the control group. Both groups participate in the general program the clinic offers (see above (3)). Thus control group members also become familiar with basic ideas about psychosocial stress.

The effectiveness of the E&D modification program is measured in the following ways:

1. Extensive documentation of cardiovascular functioning and of risk factors provides us with valuable control information.
2. E&D modification implies that there has been E&D in the etiology of the disease. By means of a structured interview and a TABP questionnaire at the beginning of the stay in the rehabilitation clinic we try to find out if this is the case. In addition we ask for attitudes towards behavior modification and concrete plans to change aspects of the patient's situation. Emotions of anxiety and depression secondary to MI are explored.
3. To specify E&D as a risk factor a Stroop test is applied, where several measures of BP and HR are taken and ECG is recorded. A short structured interview tries to improve the ecologic validity of the test.
4. The first assessment of effectiveness takes place at the end of the rehabilitation period. The following measures are taken again: TABP, attitudes towards behavior modification and concrete plans to change the situation at home, and, finally, negative emotions secondary to MI.
5. Measures of BP, plasma lipoproteins and other risk factors are taken; we do not, however, consider them to be valuable criteria of effectiveness at present. Therapeutic approaches like diet and pharmacological methods are supposed to have a strong and immediate impact on coronary risk factors. It seems difficult to control for their effects.
6. At an 18-month follow-up the above enumerated measures are to be taken again (With a slight modification: Instead of asking for concrete plans, we will ask for change that has been realized). In addition, clinical assessments of cardiac status, an exercise stress-test and the Stroop test will be repeated. Cause of death will be explored in those patients who did not survive.
7. On the basis of the data set outlined above it should be possible to test the following hypotheses:

(a) Patients who experienced E&D before MI profit more from the modification program than those who did not experience E&D.
(b) This holds true not only in terms of coronary prone behavior (TABP, changes in social roles) and emotions (anxiety, depression), but also of levels of BP, LDL, and stress tolerance.
(c) As intervening variables, general willingness to change aspects of lifestyle and outcome expectancy towards E&D modification are to be taken into account.
(d) Important control variables are age, cardiac functioning, risk factors, and complications as measured during the stay in the rehabilitation clinic.

In order to test our hypotheses properly we intend to include about 200 patients in our study.

REFERENCES

Beamish, E. E., Singal, P. K. and Dhalla, N. S. (Eds) (1985). *Stress and Heart Disease*. Martinus Nijhoff, Boston, Dordrecht, Lancaster.

Deanfield, J. E., Shea, M., Ribiero, P., de Landesheere, Ch., Wilson, R., Horlock, P. and Selwyn, A. (1984). Transient ST-segment depression as a marker of myocardial ischaemia during daily life. *American Journal of Cardiology*, **54**, 1195-1200.

Fischer, C. S. (1973). On urban alienation and anomie. *American Sociological Review*, **38**, 311-326.

Frankenhaeuser, M. (1980). Psychobiological aspects of life stress. In Levine, S. and Ursin, H. (Eds), *Coping and Health*, Plenum Press, New York.

Frasure-Smith, N. and Prince, R. (1985). The ischemic heart disease life stress monitoring program: impact on mortality. *Psychosomatic Medicine*, **47**, 431-445.

Friedman, M., Thoresen, C. E., Gill, J. J., Powell, L. H., Ulmer, D., Thompson, L., Price, V. A., Rabin, D. D., Breall, W. S., Dixon, T., Levy, R., Bourg, E. (1984). Alteration of type A behavior and reduction in cardiac recurrences in postmyocardial infarction patients. *American Heart Journal*, **108**, 237.

Glass, D. C. (1977). *Behavior Patterns, Stress and Coronary Disease*, Erlbaum, Hillsdale.

Gill, J. J., Price, V., Friedman, M., Thoresen, C. E., Powell, L. H., Ulmer, D., Brown, B. (1985). Reduction in type A behavior in healthy middle-aged American military officers. *American Heart Journal*, **110**, 503-514.

Haynes, S. G., Feinleib, M., Eaker, D. (1983). Type A behavior and the 10 year incidence of coronary heart disease in the Framingham study. In Rosenman, R. H. (Ed.), *Psychosomatic Risk Factors and Coronary Heart Disease*. Huber, Bern.

Henry, J. P., Stephens, P. M. (1977). *Stress, Health, and the Social Environment. A Sociobiologic Approach to Medicine*. Springer, New York, Heidelberg, Berlin.

Kohn, M. L. and Schooler, C. (1983). *Work and Personality: An Inquiry into the Impact of Social Stratification*. Ablex Publishing Corporation, Norwood, NJ.

Lown, B. (1984). Cardiovascular collapse and sudden cardiac death. In Braunwald, E. (Ed.), *Heart Disease. A Textbook of Cardiovascular Medicine*. Saunders, Philadelphia, London.

Manuck, S. B., Proietti, J. M., Rader, S.-J., Polefrone, J. M. (1985). Hypertension, affect, and cardiovascular response to cognitive challenge. *Psychosomatic Medicine*, **47**, 189-200.

Marmot, M. (1982). Socio-economic and cultural factors in ischaemic heart disease. *Advances of Cardiology*, **29**, 68-76.

Matthews, S. K. and Rakaczky, C. J. (1986). Familial aspects of type A behavior pattern and physiologic reactivity to stress. In Schmidt, T. H., Dembroski, T. M. and Blümchen, G. (Eds), *Biological and Psychological Factors in Cardiovascular Disease*. Springer, Berlin.

Meerson, F. (1984). *Adaptation, Stress and Prophylaxis*. Springer, Berlin.

Merton, R. (1968). *Social Theory and Social Structure*. The Free Press, New York.

Patel, Ch., Marmot, M. G., Terry, D. J., Carruthers, M., Hunt, B., Patel, M. (1985). Trial of relaxation in reducing coronary risk: four year follow-up. *British Medical Journal*, **290**, 1103-1106.

Rahe, R., Ward, H. W. and Hayes, V. (1979). Brief group therapy in myocardial infarction rehabilitation: three to four-year follow-up of a controlled trial. *Psychosomatic Medicine*, **41**, 229-242.

Rosenman, R. H. (1986). Current and past history of type A behavior pattern. In Schmidt, T. H., Dembroski, T. M. and Blümchen, G. (Eds), *Biological and Psychological Factors in Cardiovascular Disease*. Springer, Berlin.

Ruberman, W., Weinblatt, E., Goldberg, J., Chaudhary, B. S. (1984). Psychosocial influences on mortality after myocardial infarction. *The New England Journal of Medicine*, **30**, 552–559.

Schmidt, T. H., Dembroski, T. M., Blümchen, G. (Eds), (1986). *Biological and Psychological Factors in Cardiovascular Disease*, Springer, Berlin.

Shekelle, R. B., Hulley, S. B., Neaton, J. D., Billings, J., Borhani, N. O., Gerace, T. A., Jacobs, D., Lasser, N., Mittlemark, M. and Stamler, J. (1986). Type A behavior and risk of coronary heart disease in the Multiple Risk Factor Intervention Trial. In Schmidt, T. H., Dembroski, T. M., Blümchen, G. (Eds), *Biological and Psychological Factors in Cardiovascular Disease*. Springer, Berlin.

Siegrist, J. (1987). Impaired quality of life as a risk factor in cardiovascular disease. *Journal of Chronic Disease*, **40**, 571–578.

Siegrist, J., Dittmann, K., Rittner, K. and Weber, I. (1980). *Soziale Belastungen und Herzinfarkt*. Enke, Stuttgart.

Siegrist, J., Matschinger, H., Klein, D. and Grünewald, R. (1987). Pressure response and heart rate reaction in a blue collar population at cardiovascular risk. *Journal of Hypertension*, **4**, Suppl. **6**, 260–262.

Sime, W. E., Buell, J. C., Eliot, R. S. (1980). Cardiovascular responses to emotional stress (quiz interview) in post-myocardial infarction patients and matched control subjects. *Journal of Human Stress*, **6**, 39–46.

Tavazzi, L., Mazzuero, G., Giordano, A., Zotti, A. M. and Berlotti, G. (1984). Hemodyamic characterization of different mental stress tests. In L'Abbate, A. (Ed.), *Breakdown in Human Adaptation to 'Stress'*, vol. II, part 4. Martinus Nijhoff Publishers, Boston.

Behavioural Medicine in Cardiovascular Disorders
Edited by T. Elbert, W. Langosch, A. Steptoe and D. Vaitl
©1988 John Wiley & Sons Ltd

14

Psychological Predictors of Outcome after Myocardial Infarction

Royal Edinburgh Hospital, Edinburgh

INTRODUCTION

Coronary heart disease is a major ailment throughout Europe and North America. Some individuals suffer only mild symptoms which are inconvenient but only moderately restrictive, others endure years of incapacitating pain which can intrude into all aspects of their lives. Frequently the first indication of coronary heart disease is a myocardial infarction; for many patients this is also the last indicator since about one-quarter of patients suffering a first infarction die within a few hours. The short-term outcome of myocardial infarction is best measured by physical parameters, in particular by mortality. Patients who have survived an attack and leave hospital alive have had a good short-term outcome. However, for the great majority of patients it is the extent to which they adjust to the physical, emotional, and social implications, real and perceived, of having had a heart attack that is the gauge of long-term outcome.

It is difficult to think of any single measure of long-term outcome after a myocardial infarction. Death is clearly an unsatisfactory outcome, yet so also is being alive but severely restricted and handicapped by residual effects of the acute episode. Continuing organic morbidity, the other traditional measure is also insufficient as a measure of outcome. In recent years it has become increasingly common to talk about 'psychosocial outcome' or 'quality of life', reflecting an awareness that outcome must be measured in psychological and social as well as organic terms. The most commonly used psychosocial indicators are return to work, social activities, domestic harmony, and individual emotional state. As yet there is no generally accepted structured measure of any of these indicators. It can only be hoped that the present diversity of assessment will provide the basis for an agreed index of outcome which is tolerant of differences in culture and professional bias. Interest in psychosocial aspects of outcome developed in parallel with the move toward early mobilization of the post-infarction patient and the belief that planned exercise enhanced general well-being as well as restoring physical function. Since treatment, whether acute or rehabilitative, is intimately linked with outcome, it is not surprising that rehabilitation of patients who survive an acute myocardial infarction is defined as covering every aspect of the patient, 'including his physiological, clinical, psychological, and social problems' (WHO, 1969). The consensus of expert opinion is that not all patients require specialist rehabilitation, a good outcome for the majority of patients can be attained using local resources coordinated by the primary care physician (International Society and Federation of Cardiology, 1983). Thus in any series of post-infarction patients there will be a continuum of rehabilitative need from very little, for example, simple guidance on exercise, cessation of smoking and the like, to the maximum represented by regular attendance at a specialist clinic and contact with a wide range of specialist staff.

If only a limited number of patients require specialized rehabilitation how should those at risk be identified? Many studies have demonstrated that while psychosocial outcome is not well predicted by physical state prior to leaving hospital, such outcome is influenced by pre-discharge emotional state. The term 'emotional upset' is a rather global concept which has been measured in a wide variety of ways including direct examination of patients by a psychiatrist, the analysis of nursing reports and casenotes, as well as patient self-report using interviews, questionnaires, and formal psychological tests. In some respects this diversity of measurement has been beneficial since it demonstrates that the relationship between emotional state in the ward and subsequent outcome is not specific to any particular measure or any particular definition of outcome. When we move beyond simply demonstrating a relationship between upset and outcome and try to make predictions about which individual patients are most likely to have poor outcomes, then diversity of measurement frustrates attempts to draw together the findings of different researchers. The choice of which psychological dimensions to use is heavily influenced by the theoretical standpoint of the researcher; behaviourists, trait theorists, and social psychologists will favour the use of measures and constructs which can be accommodated within their particular theory. Although there is apparently no limit to the number of 'personality' tests created by psychologists, the imposition of the simplest rules of psychometrics and of test evaluation allows the more idiosyncratic of these to be eliminated and permits us to subsume most tests under a much smaller set of replicable psychological dimensions. Within general psychology anxiety and extraversion are two such replicable dimensions. While emotional upset can be considered from the framework of general psychology and considered as part of the normal range of reacting or behaving, it can equally be viewed from a psychopathological perspective. Methods based on this perspective, whether interviews, ratings or self-report scales, are concerned with the identification of morbid mental states. Some of these can be considered to be exaggerated forms of normal moods or characteristics, others occur extremely rarely in the population at large and yet others can be seen as qualitatively distinct from normal experience. Measures derived from general psychology have a more or less gaussian distribution of scores. Psychopathological scales, on the other hand, are almost always J-shaped in distribution when applied to the population at large, they are almost always categorical or classificatory in purpose and cutting points are determined by clinical criteria. Some dimensions, such as anxiety, can be construed from both a normal and psychopathological perspective so that any assessment of 'emotional upset' requires both kinds of measures to be used. Failure to do so leads to apparently contradictory findings in the literature and erroneous conclusions about the treatment and rehabilitative needs of patients who have suffered a myocardial infarction.

METHODS

My colleagues and I have reported on various aspects of the emotional state of infarction patients in the Coronary Care Unit, in the hospital ward, and at outpatient follow-up (Cay et al., 1972; Dellipiani et al., 1976; Philip et al., 1979). Some comments made by Johnston in his review of psychological interventions in cardiovascular disease (Johnston, 1985) caused me to look again at our information on a large cohort of patients who had been followed up, without intervention, over a 12-month period. In his review Johnston concluded that psychological interventions in post-infarction patients had very modest effects. Echoing the WHO report cited earlier in this chapter he indicated that such intervention should not be given routinely to all patients but only to those who clearly required help. His assertion that '. . . it is almost certainly very difficult to identify, at an early stage, those patients who will require assistance . . .' was challenging. It seemed worthwhile to look again at the data to see if Johnston's assertion could be refuted.

The group studied comprised 203 men who had survived an acute attack of myocardial infarction or ischaemia long enough to be admitted to the Coronary Care Unit of the Royal Infirmary of Edinburgh. They formed a consecutive series of such admissions, with the exception of those who died in the intensive care unit. The group and the physical, psychological, and social information gathered on them has been described in detail elsewhere (Cay et al., 1973) and will be repeated here only when necessary.

The main part of the psychological information was gathered by means of interview and questionnaire between 8 and 10 days after transfer from Coronary Care Unit to a general medical ward. Earlier contacts were kept brief so as to maintain the cooperation of both patients and staff. Patients were invited to attend follow-up clinics at 4 months and 12 months after discharge from hospital.

This chapter will focus on the extent to which physical diagnosis and four measures of emotional state predicted selected outcome variables. Almost all patients admitted to Coronary Care Units are presumed to have suffered a heart attack and a definitive diagnosis of myocardial infarction is made in about two-thirds of such patients. In the present group 131 of the 203 patients had a definite diagnosis of myocardial infarction. Most of the remaining patients were diagnosed as having had an attack of myocardial ischaemia. Both diagnostic groups had similar experiences from the onset of their 'attack' to transfer from intensive care to a general hospital ward and their outcome in psychosocial terms was similar.

Two of the measures of emotional state were based on an interview conducted by a psychiatrist. *Antecedent stress* was deemed to be present when there was clear evidence at interview of an increase in tension or anxiety before the acute attack which precipitated treatment. Where patients claimed to have suffered from tension or anxiety for most of their lives, antecedent stress was recorded as 'not present'. A formulation of *psychiatric disorder* was based on the psychiatrist's evaluation of present mental state and history. It also incorporated an assessment of each patient's personality and social history.

The remaining measures were developed within the framework of formal theories of personality, those of Cattell (1973) and Foulds (1965, 1976). The measures are objective, standardized instruments for which there is available a substantial body of information relating to normal subjects and to patients with physical or mental illness. Cattell has produced a family of anxiety scales which are at the trait end of the trait-state continuum and are firmly based in general psychology. Because our study involved repeated assessments we used the Eight-Parallel Form Anxiety Battery (Scheier and Cattell, 1960) to make frequent assessments of anxiety with minimum repetition of individual items. The battery was also attractive in its attempt to combine the convenience of pencil and paper assessment with benefits of disguised 'objective' subtests tapping different aspects of anxiety. Accordingly the measure of *general anxiety* reported here was Form C of the Battery completed after 7 days in the ward.

Foulds' theory of personality is concerned with the interplay between normal and abnormal psychological processes. Emphasis is placed on the close links between personal maturity and integrity and the ease with which an individual can establish and maintain close interpersonal relationships with one or more others. Threats to the integrity of the individual's identity of self are signalled by signs and symptoms of anxiety, depression and other pathological features. These signs and symptoms also signal a diminished capacity to maintain relationships with others which, in turn, leads to an impairment of everyday functioning. The *Personal Disturbance* scale (Foulds and Hope, 1968) comprises 20 items covering a wide range of neurotic psychopathology. In the standardization sample no normal scored over 4 so that all scores of 5 and above are taken to denote personal disturbance. Although there is a loss of richness by doing so, it is possible to use the Personal Disturbance scale independent of its theoretical background. Used in this way it should be considered simply as a psychologically rather than psychiatrically based means of identifying individuals manifesting a significant degree of psychological disturbance.

Table 1. Correlations between physical diagnosis and emotional upset in the ward.

	1	2	3	4	5
Physical diagnosis (1)	—	0.020	0.072	− 0.140	0.110
Antecedent stress (2)		—	0.384[†]	0.106	0.134
Psychiatric disorder (3)			—	0.161	0.166*
General anxiety (4)				—	0.300[†]
Personal disturbance (5)					—

*$P<0.05$; [†]$P<0.001$.

Table 2. Breakdown of group according to physical diagnosis and measures of emotional upset.

Physical diagnosis	Myocardial infarction 131 (65%) Other diagnosis 72 (35%)
Antecedent stress	Absent 82 (43%) Present 110 (57%) No information on 11 cases
Psychiatric disorder	Absent 68 (34%) Present 131 (66%) No information on 4 cases
General anxiety	145 patients tested; mean 4.83; SD 2.04 No useable tests on 58 cases
Personal disturbance	Absent 106 (64%) Present 61 (36%) No information on 36 cases

RESULTS

Table 1 shows how physical diagnosis and the four measures of emotional upset are correlated. There is no association between physical diagnosis and any measure of emotional upset. The presence of antecedent stress and being diagnosed as having psychiatric disorder are significantly correlated as are having a high general anxiety score and being classed as being personally disturbed. These correlations, although statistically significant are small in terms of common variance in the measures and this is even more true of the just-significant correlation between the psychiatrist's formulation of disorder and the self-report of personal disturbance. The four measures are, therefore, sufficiently independent to warrant each being examined as a potential predictor of later outcome.

Table 2 shows the composition of the group in terms of physical diagnosis and the various measures of emotional upset. Patients recovering from a heart attack are easily tired and have limited powers of concentration. This constrains psychological measurement, especially where it involves structured tests or assessments. In all, 12 patients died in hospital and others had to be returned

Table 3. Physical and social outcome of the group at 4- and 12-month follow-up.

	4 months Number	(%)	12 months Number	(%)
Physical outcome				
Dead at follow-up	11 of 189	(6%)	24 of 190	(13%)
no information	2		1	
Readmitted to hospital	36 of 179	(20%)	65 of 165	(39%)
no information	1		2	
Current angina	78 of 162	(48%)	76 of 158	(48%)
no information	18		9	
Current breathlessness	99 of 162	(61%)	94 of 158	(60%)
no information	18		9	
Current ischaemia	17 of 162	(10%)	25 of 158	(16%)
no information	18		9	
Social outcome				
Return to work				
(a) As active as before	57	(42%)	59	(45%)
(b) Less active	37	(27%)	41	(31%)
(c) Retired since myocardial infarction	4	(3%)	9	(7%)
(d) Unemployed since myocardial infarction	37	(27%)	22	(17%)
no information	10		4	
Reduced income	36 of 165	(23%)	No data	
no information	15			
Poor financial state	73 of 165	(44%)	No data	
no information	15			
Reduced social activity	58 of 165	(37%)	49 of 162	(30%)
no information	15		5	

Table 4. Psychological outcome of the group at 4- and 12-month follow up.

	4 months Number	(%)	12 months Number	(%)
Personal disturbance	45 of 136	(33%)	No data	
no information	44			
Psychiatric disorder	92 of 156	(59%)	90 of 160	(56%)
no information	24		7	
Reported problems				
(a) Physical activity	58 of 156	(37%)	73 of 160	(46%)
no information	24		7	
(b) At work	45 of 128	(35%)	44 of 131	(34%)
no information	20		6	
(c) Financial difficulty	39 of 156	(25%)	32 of 160	(20%)
no information	24		7	
(d) Domestic problems	34 of 156	(22%)	21 of 160	(13%)
no information	24		7	

to the Coronary Care Unit for further intensive care. Physical diagnosis can be made without the active participation of the patient and a psychiatric formulation can be made in the course of flexible interviewing which can be spread over a number of sessions according to the state of the patient. It should not be surprising, therefore, to note that in Table 2 the most formal assessments had the lowest completion rates. The other main feature of this table is the disparity between the proportion deemed to have psychiatric disorder and the numbers classed as personally disturbed. The disparity is largely due to the different cutting points used by the two measures. The majority (74%) of patients classed as personally disturbed are also deemed to be psychiatrically disordered, whereas a minority (43%) of the psychiatrically disordered are classes as personally disturbed.

Tables 3 and 4 show the overall picture for each outcome measure at 4- and 12-month follow-up. Patients were followed up at 4 months and again at 12 months following discharge from hospital when physical and psychosocial state were separately examined by a physician and a psychiatrist. *Physical outcome* was measured by mortality, being readmitted to hospital and the presence of angina, breathlessness and ischaemic attacks. *Social outcome* was assessed through return to work, assessment of loss of income, financial state and the extent to which social activities had been reduced as a consequence of infarction. *Psychological outcome* was measured by the Personal Disturbance scale, assessment of psychiatric disorder, and by the patients' report of difficulties or problems regarding physical activity, work, finance or domestic matters. The figures presented for mortality and readmission to hospital at 4 and 12 months follow-up are cumulative; all other figures are cross-sectional and relate to state at the time of follow-up examination.

Table 3 shows that 6% of those discharged alive from hospital were dead within 4 months and this figure increased to 13% by the time of 12 months follow-up. The overall incidence of mortality in Scots of this age group is slightly more than 1% in any given year; patients who survive the acute phase of myocardial infarction or severe ischaemia are over ten times more likely to die in the following year than the average citizen of comparable age. However, it must not be forgotten that the majority survive, albeit with a high incidence of continuing morbidity as assessed by re-admission to hospital or by the presence of angina, breathlessness or ischaemia. Two-thirds of the patients who were working prior to the acute episode of illness had returned to work by the time of the 4-month follow-up; most were working as actively as before but a significant minority had reduced their work load or had changed to less active jobs. This state of affairs had not changed materially at 12 months. Loss of work or reduced earning capacity was reflected in about one-quarter of the patients being assessed as having less income at the first follow-up. Despite sickness benefits almost one-half of the group were considered to be in a marginal or poor financial state. Lastly, about one-third of all patients were considered to have had their social lives curtailed as a result of having had a heart attack and the passage of time did not improve this restriction to any great extent.

A similar degree of temporal stability characterizes the indices of psychological outcome presented in Table 4. The proportion of personal disturbance at 4 months and psychiatric disorder at both follow-up dates is not greatly different from that assessed in the ward; on both measures the bulk of patients assessed as distressed in the ward continued to be seen as distressed at follow-up with relatively few patients either improving or deteriorating.

More than one-third of patients reported problems at work or in overall physical activity, with complaints in the latter area being even more frequent at 12 months. At 4 months, financial difficulties were reported by 1 patient in every 4, while domestic or family problems were almost as common. By 12 months these were reduced, although only for domestic problems was the reduction great enough to warrant notice.

Taken together, Tables 3 and 4 indicate that survivors of an acute coronary episode continue to have a high mortality rate and a large incidence of physical morbidity which does not reduce with the passage of time. In the absence of specific rehabilitation or other therapeutic intervention the high levels of emotional upset displayed in hospital continue unabated in the months following discharge. This composite picture is the backcloth against which is pursued the search for measures which predict physical, psychological and social outcome.

Final physical diagnosis was of minimal value in predicting the outcome listed in Tables 3 and 4, only presence of angina at 4 months being related to diagnosis ($\chi^2 = 5.93$, df $= 1$, $P < 0.01$) in that more patients with a diagnosed infarction (56%) had angina compared with other patients (35%). Physical outcome at follow-up was not predicted by any of the four emotional measures so that attention can be focused on the extent to which these measures predicted social and psychological outcome. Two general points need to be made about Tables 5 and 7; the figures are whole number percentages which facilitate comparisons both between and within tables, while the chi-square values have been calculated using raw figures. For statistical analysis the 'retired' and 'unemployed' categories of return to work were combined.

Antecedent stress was a poor predictor of social and psychological outcome with significant associations being limited to psychiatric disorder and patient's report of domestic difficulties, both at 4-month follow-up only. The presence of psychiatric symptoms at interview in the ward did not predict any aspect of social outcome at 4- or 12-month follow-up either, but did anticipate reports of physical and domestic difficulties at 4 months as well as work difficulties at 1 year. Table 5 indicates the close link between psychiatric disorder in the ward and at follow-up.

Personal disturbance assessed in the ward predicted all the psychological outcome measures at 4 months as well as financial state from the social measures. Table 6 also shows that being personally disturbed in the ward was related to

Table 5. Psychiatric disorder and social outcome at 4 and 12 months.

	4-month follow-up		12-month follow-up	
	Symptoms present %	Absent %	Symptoms present %	Absent %
Return to work				
As active as before	37	52 $\chi^2 = 3.15$	38	57 $\chi^2 = 5.19$
Less active	31	22 df = 2, NS	33	28 df = 2, NS
Retired since myo-	3	2	8	4
cardial infarction				
Unemployed	29	24	20	11
Income				
No change	74	84 $\chi^2 = 1.68$	No data	
Reduced	26	16 df = 1, NS	No data	
Financial state				
Satisfactory	50	67 $\chi^2 = 3.67$	No data	
Poor	50	33 df = 1, NS	No data	
Social activity				
No change	60	67 $\chi^2 = 0.40$	65	77 $\chi^2 = 1.95$
Reduce	40	33 df = 1, NS	35	23 df = 1, NS

work status 1 year later but not to such status at 4 months. At the later follow-up those patients who had been disturbed in the ward were more likely to be unemployed; a similar but non-significant $(0.10 > p < 0.05)$ association between psychiatric disorder in the ward and work status at 1 year was seen. Table 7 shows that predictive value of the Personal Disturbance scale extends to the prediction of financial difficulties at 12 months.

Tables 5 and 7 show very clearly that while the assessment of psychiatric disorder and measurement of personal disturbance overlap in content and purpose they do not predict one another to an equal extent. Being personally disturbed in the ward entails a higher probability of being disturbed at 4 months and also showing psychiatric symptoms at both follow-up assessments. Being psychiatrically disordered in the ward did not predict personal disturbance at follow-up. General anxiety measured in the ward carried no predictive implications for outcome at 4 or 12 months with the exception of psychiatric disorder at the earlier follow-up.

It can be concluded from these findings that the Personal Disturbance scale is the best predictor of psychological and social outcome among the four measures of emotional upset. Prediction is stronger for outcomes which are reflections of mental state and patient's perceptions of situations and, not surprisingly, is stronger for 4-month rather than 12-month outcome.

Within psychology it is common to express the relationship between variables, including predictive relationships, in terms of common variance. Within medicine different methods and conventions have been developed to assess the adequacy of predictive or screening tests. Sensitivity and specificity taken together give

Table 6. Personal disturbance and social outcome at 4 and 12 months.

| | 4-month follow-up | | 12-month follow-up | |
| | Disturbance | | Disturbance | |
	present %	Absent %	present %	Absent %
Return to work				
As active as before	40	48 $\chi^2 = 0.80$	29	52 $\chi^2 = 11.54$
Less active	28	27 df = 2, NS	31	29 df = 2, $p < 0.005$
Retired since myocardial infarction	0	4	9	7
Unemployed	33	22	31	12
Income				
No change	74	83 $\chi^2 = 1.24$	No data	
Reduced	26	17 df = 1, NS	No data	
Financial state				
Satisfactory	40	71 $\chi^2 = 12.16$	No data	
Poor	60	29 df = 1, $p < 0.001$		
Social activity				
No change	52	66 $\chi^2 = 2.09$	64	76 $\chi^2 = 1.85$
Reduced	48	34 df = 1, NS	36	24 df = 1, NS

Table 7. Personal disturbance and psychological outcome at 4 and 12 months.

| | 4-month follow-up | | 12-month follow-up | |
| | Disturbance | | Disturbance | |
	present %	Absent %	present %	Absent %
Personal disturbance				
Normal	38	85 $\chi^2 = 25.42$	No data	
Disturbed	62	15 df = 1, $p < 0.001$	No data	
Psychiatric disorder				
No symptoms	20	57 $\chi^2 = 15.98$	32	54 $\chi^2 = 5.42$
Symptoms present	80	43 df = 1, $p < 0.001$	68	46 df = 1, $p < 0.05$
Physical difficulties				
No problems	48	76 $\chi^2 = 10.11$	51	60 $\chi^2 = 0.64$
Problems reported	52	24 df = 1, $p < 0.001$	49	40 df = 1, NS
Work difficulties				
No problems	49	77 $\chi^2 = 7.69$	56	76 $\chi^2 = 3.65$
Problems reported	51	23 df = 1, $p < 0.01$	44	24 df = 1, NS
Financial difficulties				
No problems	65	86 $\chi^2 = 7.72$	70	86 $\chi^2 = 3.92$
Problems reported	35	14 df = 1, $p < 0.01$	30	14 df = 1, $p < 0.05$
Domestic difficulties				
No problems	62	85 $\chi^2 = 8.07$	89	86 $\chi^2 = 0.10$
Problems reported	38	15 df = 1, $p < 0.005$	11	14 df = 1, NS

Table 8. Personal disturbance and the prediction of financial state.

| | | Personal disturbance | | |
		Not PD	PD +	
Financial state	Satisfactory	65	21	86
	Poor	27	32	59
		92	53	145

$\phi = 0.30$	Sensitivity	54%
Variance in common = 0.09%	Specificity	76%
	Misclassification	34%

an overall correct classification percentage for the predictive measure under scrutiny. Misclassification comprises the combined percentage of false positives and false negatives identified by the test under scrutiny relative to the total number of individuals in the sample. Misclassification can be corrected by allowing for the known or estimated incidence of cases in the population from which the sample was drawn. Where the known incidence of a condition is low the adequacy of a screening test depends greatly on its sensitivity; where the incidence is high then predictive adequacy depends on specificity.

Table 8 shows the relationship between being personally disturbed in the ward and being seen to be in a poor financial state at 4-month follow-up. The phi (ϕ) correlation between the variables is 0.30 and the variance in common is 9%. The sensitivity of the Personal Disturbance scale in predicting financial state at follow-up is 54% (32 cases out of 59), the specificity 76% (65 cases out of 86) and the overall misclassification rate is 34% (27 + 21 cases out of 145). Very similar rates of sensitivity, specificity, and overall misclassification are obtained for the Personal Disturbance scale as a predictor of perceived difficulties in physical exertion, work, finance and in the home. Knowing a patient's standing on Personal Disturbance in the ward helps to determine whether he will report problems or difficulties in these areas at follow-up. If, for instance, it was planned to include advice on financial budgeting or eligibility for social benefits as part of aftercare, it would be useful to be able to predict which patients would be most in need of such a service and also those for whom such a service would be superfluous. In the absence of any other information, allocation to such an aftercare service on the basis of Personal Disturbance would be accurately carried out for two-thirds of the patients considered.

Because the Personal Disturbance scale is higher on specificity than on sensitivity its predictive strength lies mainly in its ability to minimize the number of false positives. Johnston (1985) has concluded that the effects of psychological interventions in survivors' myocardial infarction are modest. One reason for such a conclusion is the lack of adequate selection of patients requiring such intervention. If patients have not been selected or have been selected using a measure which yields a high proportion of false positives, individuals who do not require intervention and hence will show no 'improvement' at the end of the intervention, then any beneficial effects on true positives will be swamped by the lack of effect on the false positives. Contrary to Johnston's conclusion, it is possible to identify patients who are likely to need assistance. Further, it is possible to identify such patients using simple but psychometrically sound measures which could be administered by suitable trained non-psychologist health care staff.

REFERENCES

Cattell, R. B. (1973). *Personality and Mood by Questionnaire.* Jossey-Bass, San Francisco.

Cay, E. L., Vetter, N. J., Philip, A. E. and Dugard, P. (1972). Psychological reactions to a coronary care unit. *Journal of Psychosomatic Research*, **16**, 437–447.

Cay, E. L., Vetter, N. J., Philip, A. E. and Dugard, P. (1973). Return to work after a heart attack. *Journal of Psychosomatic Research*, **17**, 231–243.

Dellipiani, A. W., Cay, E. L., Philip, A. E., Vetter, N. J., Colling, W. A., Donaldson, R. J. and McCormack, P. (1976). Anxiety after a heart attack. *British Heart Journal*, **38**, 752–757.

Foulds, G. A. (1965). *Personality and Personal Illness.* Tavistock, London.

Foulds, G. A. (1976). *The Hierarchical Nature of Personal Illness.* Academic Press, London.

Foulds, G. A. and Hope, K. (1968). *Manual of the Symptom Sign Inventory.* University of London Press, London.

International Society and Federation of Cardiology (1983). *Myocardial Infarction, How to Prevent, How to Rehabilitate.* International Society of Cardiology, Zürich, Switzerland.

Johnston, D. W. (1985). Psychological interventions in cardiovascular disease. *Journal of Psychosomatic Research*, **29**, 447–456.

Philip, A. E., Cay, E. L., Vetter, N. J. and Stuckey, N. A. (1979). Personal traits and the physical, psychiatric and social state of patients one year after a myocardial infarction. *International Journal of Rehabilitation Research*, **2**, 479–487.

Scheier, I. H. and Cattell, R. B. (1960). *Handbook for the I.P.A.T. 8 — Parallel-Form Anxiety Battery.* I.P.A.T., Champaign, Illinois.

World Health Organisation (1969). *The Rehabilitation of patients with Cardiovascular Disease.* World Health Organisation, Copenhagen.

Behavioural Medicine in Cardiovascular Disorders
Edited by T. Elbert, W. Langosch, A. Steptoe and D. Vaitl
©1988 John Wiley & Sons Ltd

15

Psychosocial Predictors of Cardiac Health after Myocardial Infarction at a Young Age

W. Langosch, H. Borcherding, G. Brodner and K. Wybitul
Benedikt Kreutz Rehabilitationszentrum, Südring 15, 7812 Bad Krozingen

INTRODUCTION

It is estimated that about 4% of all myocardial infarctions occur in men under the age of 40 years old (Lamm, 1981). Based upon the data of the Register Study Heidelberg, this would mean that each year about 3000 men in the Federal Republic of Germany, aged under 40, will suffer their first myocardial infarction (Nüssel *et al.*, 1981). In the Federal Republic of Germany, myocardial infarction is the fifth most frequent cause of death for men in the age group 25–45 years (Federal Office of Statistics, 1985). The total number of men dying of a myocardial infarction, represents 2.6% of those affected below the age of 45 years.

It has been shown that 61%–75% of men in this age group have a survival rate of 1–5 years (Nüssel *et al.*, 1981); for patients who have survived the pre-hospital phase between 68%–80% showed a 10 year rate of survival (Georgiou *et al.*, 1978, Gertler *et al.*, 1964). The long-term mortality of younger patients compares slightly more favourably than with older patients (Bergstrand *et al.*, 1981, Gertler *et al.*, 1964); but when taking the population group corresponding in age as a reference group, then the relative risk of mortality of the younger post-infarction patients is about 10 times as high (Gohlke, 1984).

In the determination of long-term prognosis, the extent of coronary atherosclerosis, the degree of the left ventricular dysfunction and the frequency of ventricular arrhythmias are considered (Gohlke, 1984). Over a period of 16 years 35.3% of the patients suffered a re-infarction (Roth *et al.*, 1967). During an observation period of 13 years 27.5% survived the re-infarction (Gertler *et al.*, 1964) while 46.1% of the patients reported angina pectoris symptoms during this time (Gertler *et al.*, 1964).

In summary, it can be stated that after surviving a myocardial infarction at a young age the relative mortality risk is clearly increased during subsequent years. The most frequent cause of death being sudden death from heart disease or a re-infarction. Angina-pectoris symptoms, dyspnoe, and re-infarction are the most frequent non-deadly complications.

As prognosis relevant for the appearance of serious cardiac complications, the risk factors to be considered are nicotine abuse, hyper-cholesterolemia, hyper-triglyceridemia, hypertension, and diabetes mellitus (Georgiou *et al.*, 1978; Gohlke *et al.*, 1980), although their significance is not undisputed (Bergstrand *et al.*, 1982). However, Epstein and Wilhelmsen (1982) suggest that even in the case of an insufficient connection between risk factor and the risk of getting ill again, the avoidance of a risk factor may contribute to a slowing down of the process of disease, and thus, to a comparatively better prognosis.

Possible psychological risk factors for the appearance of serious cardiac complications (re-infarction, cardiac death) after myocardial infarction, may include extraordinary stress and social isolation (Ruberman *et al.*, 1984), type-A modes of behaviour according to self-judgement (Jenkins *et al.*, 1976), a comparatively higher emotional stability and a lesser developed feeling of weakness (Nirkko *et al.*, 1982), an increased depressiveness (Bruhn *et al.*, 1969) and an increased dominance as well as a dissimulation of the limitations due to the disease (Brodner *et al.*, 1985) are discussed. Psychophysiological considerations emphasizing the importance of a synergistic activation of the sympatho-adrenomedullary axis and of the hypophysis-suprarenal gland cortex axis for the development and the further course of the coronary disease and its clinical manifestations (Langosch 1988; Siegrist and Matschinger, 1985) are discussed in addition to coronary associated psychophysiological parameters.

The general hypothesis is that the appearance of serious cardiac complications (cardiac death, re-infarction, worsened cardiac status) is dependent, firstly, on cardiological findings (number of significantly stenotic coronary arteries, degree of left-ventricular dysfunction, significant ventricular arrhythmias), secondly, on the presence of standard risk factors, thirdly, on the presence of psychosocial risk factors, and fourthly on the activation of coronary associated physiological parameters under psychological stress.

METHODOLOGY

Patients

The original sample was composed of 252 male patients having suffered and survived an ascertained transmural myocardial infarction before 40 years of age. Cardiological, psychological, psychophysiological, and job-related examinations were carried out within the first 12 months after their myocardial infarction for 187 patients, and for the remaining 65 patients 48 months after their first infarction. The average age of the first group at the time of examination was 36.6 years, and of the second group 39.7 years. An in-patient re-examination was carried out for 152 of these patients during 1984 and 1986 although this was not due to a worsening of clinical symptoms in any of the patients re-examined. The follow-up examination took place 3 years ($n = 45$), 5 years ($n = 53$) and 7 years ($n = 21$) after the initial in-patient examination for the first group, and 4 years ($n = 62$) and 6 years ($n = 28$) after the initial in-patient examination for the second group.

After excluding patients who had died in the meantime ($n = 19$), and 21 patients who had to undergo heart surgery, 212 patients were available for a re-examination. Within the group of 60 patients ($= 20\%$) who had refused to participate in the control examination, some basic medical, job-related, and social data were obtained from 51 patients ($= 85\%$) by means of a telephone inquiry. A subsequent check proved that the participants and the non-participants questioned by telephone were not significantly different to the number of patients who had suffered a re-infarction, to the number of patients for whom another stay in hospital had become necessary because of their heart disease, to the number of patients who had participated in the meantime in a health cure, and to their marital status. However, significantly more patients of the non-participant group were unemployed, and there were some differences in the affiliation to an occupational group: among the non-participants the self-employed were comparatively over-represented and the executives under-represented.

Examinations

In the initial in-patient examination patients were examined cardiologically, psychologically, psychophysiologically, and job-related. The cardiological data also comprised findings of invasive testing (coronary angiography, ventriculography, floating catheterization) and non-invasive testing (electrocardiogram at rest, exercise-ECG, Holter-monitoring and X-ray of the thorax). Standard risk factors were partially acquired by means of case history data (e.g. abuse of nicotine), partially by means of corresponding tests determined on admission, and before leaving hospital (cholesterol-, triglyceride-, uric acid data, blood pressure, overweight according to Broca, and diabetes mellitus).

The psychological data were obtained via written responses to PSM (Langosch et al., 1980), a questionnaire measuring habits, FPI-A (Fahrenberg et al., 1978), SES (Hampel, 1977), and interviews (standardized type-A interview, and behaviour analysis for infarction patients).

The psychophysiological examination comprised the standardized presentation of six rest and five stress conditions (intensive concentrated demands under noise, self-controlled time pressure, stringent given time pressure, and emotional stress through cognitive analysis of current and future problems). ECG, electrodermal activity, and respiration rate were continuously monitored, and blood pressure was taken semi-automatically after each phase of stress and rest. Self-response measures of feelings during the different stressful phases were also obtained from standard rating scales, in addition to performance scores in each task. The selection of the different psychophysiological variables and their compliance to difference index-values was carried out according to consideration of content, and derivation from the activation theory, of the proven association between cardiologic findings and defined statistic distribution criteria (a detailed description of the methodology of examination and evaluation is found in Langosch et al., 1983).

Job-related stress and demand factors were obtained through interviews. However, only those factors that were validated by direct observations of the patient at work or of conditions where the patient would return to work after infarction were included in the final analyses. The data pool to be analysed comprised 21 cardiological variables, 10 statements of standard risk factors, 67 psychological variables, 70 psychophysiological factors, and 26 job-related factors.

Group divisions

Group divisions were carried out according to the following three criteria:

1. survival re-infarction during the observation time;
2. appearance of serious cardiac complications (re-infarction and cardiac death) during the observation period;
3. changes in the cardiac status from the initial to the re-examination according to cardiological experts (improved, unchanged, worsened cardiac status in re-examination).

Considering the relatively small number of patients with survival re-infarction, it was decided not to compare this group with the remaining patients, but to compare it with a further group which may be regarded as similar in initial cardiological findings. Therefore, for the 19 patients who had suffered a re-infarction, a further 19 patients were found who were cardiologically comparable to the initial examination in the following factors: Number of significantly ($> 50\%$) stenotic coronary arteries ($\chi^2 = 0.30$, df = 3, $p = 0.95$), angina pectoris symptoms according to the NYHA-classification ($\chi^2 = 1.70$, df = 3, $p = 0.64$), dysrhythmia in Holter-monitoring ($\chi^2 = 5$, 97, df = 5, $p = 0.31$), working tolerance according to ergometric strain when lying ($t = 0.21$, df = 36, $p = 0.76$), maximum heart rate volume ($t = 0$, 33, df = 35, $p = 0.74$), number of dys- or acinetic segments of the left ventricle ($t = 0.46$, df = 36, $p = 0.65$), and extent of the left ventricular malfunction ($\chi^2 = 0.64$, df = 2, $p = 0.73$). These two groups were then compared on the basis of the remaining factors in the initial examination, by means of a logistical regression analysis. Thus, an attempt was made to predict the criterion 're-infarction'. Data from patients who later underwent heart surgery or who died were not included in the regression analysis.

The patient group with serious cardiac complications was comprised of 19 patients with survival re-infarction, and 11 further patients who died of cardiac problems. This group of 30 patients was compared with the remaining patients ($n = 201$) on the basis of initial examinations. As patients who further underwent heart surgery were not considered in both groups, two patients from the total of 13 who died from cardiac problems, were also excluded. Job-related data were not included in this group comparison as it could not be clarified for the deceased how far the job-related factors, determined in the initial examination, applied to the time when work was resumed until death. A prognosis was then made for the appearance of serious cardiac complications by means of the logistical regression analysis technique, where the selection of the predictors orientated on the results of the preceeding group comparison.

After re-examination, 40 patients were judged unchanged, and 56 patients as worsened by comparison to the initial examination. Based on the initial data, first, an attempt was made to show differences between these three groups with different developments in the cardiac status, and secondly to predict by means of logistical regression analysis whether the cardiac status will worsen or whether it will remain unchanged in the future. The patient group with an improved cardiac status was excluded from the logistical regression analysis, as a binary coded variable was acceptable as a criterion, and because it was expected that the group of patients with unchanged cardiac status would contrast more clearly with the two remaining groups on the basis of achievement behaviour. It was assumed that pronounced achievement-oriented behaviour may be judged as prognostically unfavourable only in connection with a worse cardiac original status, e.g. a pronounced coronary sclerosis or a strong malfunction of the left ventricle. However, in the presence of good initial cardiological findings, e.g. no vascular disease or a low number of dys- or akinetic segments, comparable achievement-oriented behaviour within the observation period of 1 to 7 years will have few unfavourable effects upon the cardiac status. Therefore, the group of patients with stable cardiac status should demonstrate a comparatively lesser development of achievement-oriented behaviour compared to the group of patients with worsened cardiac status.

Considering the sample size it was decided that the number of predictors in the logistical regression analysis should not exceed six. It was also decided that, independent of the results of the respective group comparisons, each predictor group should contain at least one standard risk factor and one cardiological finding. Apart from this, the selection of the variables for the regression analysis should be carried out by taking into consideration the significance level and the respective sample size, as the logistical regression analysis can only be carried out with patients who have a complete data set. For each logistical regression analysis, a summary table reports the results of two statistical tests and the corresponding values. The statistical test χ^2 (Chi^2) tests the hypothesis that the term entered (removed) at that step significantly improves prediction. A small p-value indicates a significant improvement at that step. The goodness-of-fit χ^2 tests the hypothesis that the model at that step fits the data adequately. A small p-value means that the predicted values do not fit the data. For the various statistical analyses conducted the following tests were applied: when comparing the groups χ^2-test, t-test, one-way analysis of variance. Significance level was set at $p < 0.10$ to enable recognition of statistical tendencies, and as a result of the small sample size. The BMDP-library version 1987, was used to conduct these analyses.

RESULTS

Comparison of patients with versus without survival re-infarction at initial examination (groups parallelized according to cardiological findings)

The results show that at the initial examination the groups are almost parallel in nature and differ only in three cardiological factors; the non-re-infarction group shows a slightly higher pulmonary capillary pressure at rest. It is also noticeable that both groups differ neither in standard risk factors nor in job-related stress and demands.

The re-infarction patients were more often annoyed and aggressive; they felt less efficient, complained of more heart symptoms, judged themselves at the beginning of the psychophysiological examination as more tense, and made more mistakes under concentrative demands and noise. After emotional stress they showed a clear rise in systolic blood pressure, and during the first 2 minutes of the type-A interview they showed a marked rise in the maximum heart frequency.

The predictors variables heart symptoms, job efficiency, number of mistakes under concentrative demands, and rise of the systolic blood pressure after emotional stress were chosen for the logistical regression analysis. The number of significantly stenotic coronary arteries and the continuation of nicotine consumption after an infarction were also considered as further predictors. It was refrained from including the type-A variables in the regression analysis because of the low number of subjects to whom this procedure had been applied.

The six variables yield a significant prognosis of the criterion 're-infarction'. The best predictor was the increased number of mistakes during intensive concentrative demands under noise, followed by smoking after the infarction, and an increased rise of systolic blood pressure after emotional stress. It is surprising that the extent of the coronary sclerosis has proved to be a variable with little significance for the prognosis.

Table 1. Patients with vs without re-infarction (groups parallelized according to medical findings).

	$\overline{X}_R$ ($n = 19$)	S_R	$\overline{X}_{NR}$ ($n = 19$)	S_{NR}	t	p	df
Extra job	0.17 $n = 6$	0.41	1.25 $n = 8$	1.49	1.96	0.08	8.4
Max. ST-segment depression (EC)	0.04 $n = 19$	0.09	0.00 $n = 19$	0.00	2.18	0.04	18
Pulmonary capillary pressure in rest (FC)	8.00 $n = 19$	2.65	10.21 $n = 19$	4.29	-1.91	0.07	30
Systolic blood pressure, max. value (FC)	195.00	21.02	177.37	33.10	1.96	0.06	30.5
Aggressiveness potential (type-A interview)	4.00 $n = 5$	0.71	3.29 $n = 7$	0.49	2.08	0.06	10
Anger (type-A interview)	2.60 $n = 5$	0.89	1.71 $n = 7$	0.49	2.22	0.05	10
Job efficiency	3.29 $n = 17$	1.16	4.07 $n = 15$	0.88	-2.10	0.04	30
Heart symptoms (PSM-1, z-value)	0.34 $n = 18$	1.04	-0.34 $n = 18$	0.81	2.17	0.04	34
Openness (FPI-9)	9.42 $n = 12$	2.75	7.43 $n = 14$	2.85	1.88	0.07	24
Systolic blood pressure, diff: speech-rest (PPE, z-value)	0.44 $n = 13$	0.97	-0.32 $n = 15$	0.82	2.27	0.03	26
Heart frequency — max. diff: type-A final rest	0.20 $n = 5$	10.64	10.00 $n = 7$	3.51	-2.31	0.04	10
Number of mistakes under concentrative demands	3.62 $n = 13$	1.45	2.43 $n = 15$	1.16	2.36	0.03	25
Tense: basic rest (PPE)	3.77 $n = 13$	0.73	3.13 $n = 15$	1.19	1.73	0.10	23.6

R: patients with re-infarction, NR: patients without re-infarction, FC: floating catheter, PPE: psychophysiological examination.

Table 2. Logistic regression analysis prognosis of re-infarction (re-infarction $n = 9$), remaining ($n = 129$).

Predictors	Improvement of prediction χ^2	p	Goodness of fit χ^2	p
0.			65.28	1.00
1. Number of mistakes under concentrative demands (PPE)	3.53	0.06	61.76	1.00
2. Smoking	2.40	0.12	59.35	1.00
3. Systolic blood pressure diff: speech-rest (PPE)	2.06	0.15	57.29	1.00
4. Heart symptoms (PSM-1)	1.11	0.29	56.18	1.00
5. Job efficiency	0.15	0.70	56.03	1.00
6. Number of significantly stenotic coronary arteries	0.03	0.86	56.00	1.00

*Patients operated on or dead have not been considered.

Comparison of patients with serious
cardiac complications with the remaining patients

Patients who suffered subsequent serious cardiac complications showed during the initial examination only a smaller maximum heart minute volume and a tendency to a lower cardiac index.

They report that they are less composed, unable to recover quickly, sleep less, are more worried about their health, and make more mistakes during concentrative demands under noise; and yet they judge their efficiency better by comparison to the remaining patients. Again it is noticeable that the standard risk factors do not permit a separation of both groups. This further indicates that candidates for serious cardiac complications hardly differ from the remaining patients in cardiological findings.

The following variables were chosen for the logistical regression analysis: bad recuperation ability, subjective ability to take stress, and number of mistakes under intensive concentrative demands. Smoking was listed as a standard risk factor, and the number of significantly stenotic coronary arteries as well as the cardiac-index (maximum heart-rate volume under stress per m^2 body surface), which is an indicator for the dysfunction of the left ventricle, were used as cardiological findings.

Table 3. Patients who died and patients with re-infarction vs remaining patients without heart operation*.

	X_C $(n=30)$	S_C	X_{NC} $(n=201)$	S_{NC}	t	p	df
Cardiac index	7.70 $n=27$	1.80	8.26 $n=184$	1.64	−1.64	0.10	209
Max. heart stroke volume (FC)	14.50 $n=27$	3.46	15.94 $n=185$	3.34	−2.15	0.03	210
Bad recuperation on weekend (z-value)	0.37 $n=26$	0.98	−0.06 $n=178$	0.97	2.14	0.04	202
Sleep hours/night	6.83 $n=26$	1.49	7.30 $n=181$	1.02	−2.06	0.04	205
Body-referred worries (PSM-4)	20.00 $n=27$	4.82	17.79 $n=176$	6.20	2.09	0.04	40.5
Subjective ability to take stress (PSM-14)	25.62 $n=26$	4.59	23.08 $n=197$	5.62	2.20	0.03	197
Calmness (FPI-6)	5.16 $n=19$	2.01	6.09 $n=141$	2.18	−1.76	0.08	158
Number of mistakes under concentrative demands (PPE)	3.28 $n=18$	1.45	2.57 $n=159$	1.39	2.05	0.04	175

*In this comparison the job-related findings of the initial examination have not been considered as for the later deceased the validity of statements in case of resuming work could not be secured.
C: patients with serious cardiac complications (cardiac death, re-infarction), NC: patients without serious cardiac complications.

Table 4. Logistic regression analysis: prognosis of cardiac complications* (complications $(n = 12)$, remaining $(n = 13)$).

Predictors	Improvement of prediction χ^2	p	Goodness of fit χ^2	p
0.			79.05	1.00
1. Subjective ability to take stress (PSM-14)	3.96	0.05	75.09	1.00
2. Bad recuperation on weekends	6.51	0.01	68.58	1.00
3. Number of mistakes under concentrative demands (PPE)	1.71	0.19	66.86	1.00
4. Cardiac index	1.49	0.22	65.38	1.00
5. Number of significantly stenotic coronary arteries	0.84	0.36	64.54	1.00
6. Smoking	0.56	0.46	64.00	1.00

*Operated patients have not been considered.

The logistical analysis has lead to a good adaptation of the realistic distribution of the criterion; the best predictors are a limited ability to recuperate and the subjective impression of being able to cope easily with stress. Smoking, the number of significantly stenotic coronary arteries, and the cardiac index prove, on the other hand, to be less significant for the prognosis of serious cardiac complications.

Changes in cardiac status from initial in-patient to re-examination

The cardiac status from clinical results of the re-examination conducted for all patients by the same cardiologist, were compared with findings from the initial examination. Patients judged as having a worsened status, in comparison with patients regarded as unchanged, have a more pronounced coronary sclerosis, are more frequently overweight, state more frequently that they wish to change their habits, behave more competitively in their job, are more achievement motivated, had a higher heart frequency during the psychophysiological examination, feel more tense during this measure, and showed fewer delayed correct reactions under more stringent given time pressure.

Compared with patients whose cardiac status has improved, those whose cardiac status has worsened have a more pronounced coronary sclerosis, a larger number of dys- or acinetic segments, a higher working tolerance, a lower pulmonary capillary pressure under stress and were more frequently overweight. They smoked more rarely in the last year preceding the initial examination, thought themselves less efficient, subjected to increased time pressure, and were more depressive. They showed a lower breathing volume and a higher heart frequency during the psychophysiological examination. They also experienced less frequent overlapping of work in their job. The variables achievement

Table 5. Changes in cardiac status from the initial in-patient to the re-examination.

	$\bar{X}_i$ (n=48)	S_i	$\bar{X}_u$ (n=40)	S_u	$\bar{X}_w$ (n=56)	S_w	F	p	df
Kaltenbach-Score	15.02*	10.13	15.03*	9.07	22.04*,*	13.97	5.71	0.00	2/127
Number of affected segments	2.93 n=43	1.12	3.51 n=37	1.47	3.48 n=50	1.47	2.46	0.09	2/127
Working tolerance (Watt, FC)	108.13**,* n=46	25.42	127.85** n=39	32.88	125.38* n=53	28.38	6.24	0.00	2/135
AP-free working, tolerance (Watt, FC)	100.39**,* n=46	34.35	125.59** n=39	34.55	119.55* n=53	34.34	6.46	0.00	2/135
PCP—rest value (FC)	10.35 n=46	4.43	8.36 n=39	3.16	9.25 n=53	4.25	2.60	0.07	2/135
PCP—max. value (FC)	19.63* n=46	9.56	15.74 n=39	8.70	15.17* n=53	7.03	3.90	0.02	2/135
Systolic blood pressure, max. value (FC)	184.35* n=46	30.60	199.74* n=39	31.20	191.37 n=51	24.88	3.02	0.05	2/133
Smoking behavior (last 12 months)	79.5% n=44		52.6% n=38		53.8% n=52		5.65 χ^2	0.00	4
Overweight (Broca >10%)	14.6% n=48		25% n=40		35.7% n=56		6.06 χ^2	0.05	2
Job overlappings	1.31* n=29	1.14	0.73* n=22	1.03	0.78 n=18	0.81	2.51	0.09	2/66

Variable	i: $\bar{X}$	n	SD	u: $\bar{X}$	n	SD	w: $\bar{X}$	n	SD	F	p	df
Latency time (type-A interview)	4.21	n=28	1.07	3.17	n=12	1.80	3.89	n=9	1.17	2.74	0.07	2/46
Job efficiency (self-rating)	4.05	n=44	0.78	3.82	n=38	1.01	3.53	n=49	1.45	2.42	0.09	2/128
Habits changed	3.46*	n=44	1.19	2.80*,***	n=39	0.98	3.71***	n=52	1.04	8.37	0.00	2/132
Job competition (PSM-11)	18.60	n=44	5.73	16.19*	n=38	5.40	19.83*	n=43	6.05	4.16	0.02	2/122
Haste/impatience (PSM-12)	16.64	n=44	4.70	18.11	n=38	4.68	18.74	n=50	4.10	2.67	0.07	2/129
Achievement motivation (PSM-15)	36.61	n=43	8.22	35.72***	n=36	5.27	39.38***	n=48	7.23	3.12	0.05	2/124
Depressiveness (FPI-3)	3.56	n=34	3.13	4.70	n=30	3.43	5.12	n=41	3.09	2.30	0.10	2/102
Number of delayed reactions under stringent given time pressure (PPE)	0.03	n=42	0.99	0.28	n=28	0.69	−.20	n=45	0.91	2.52	0.08	2/112
Psychic activation: (PPE, z-value)	0.58	n=41	0.46	0.41	n=27	0.30	0.65	n=45	0.45	2.55	0.08	2/110
Heart frequency-$\bar{X}$, habitual value (PPE)	79.95	n=43	12.13	78.86	n=27	8.87	84.65	n=45	8.86	3.53	0.03	2/112
Breathing volume-$\bar{X}$, habitual value (PPE)	90.43***	n=40	46.68	79.59	n=27	54.99	54.17***	n=44	34.87	7.23	0.00	2/108

i: Improved cardiac status at in-patient re-examination; u: unchanged cardiac status at in-patient re-examination; w: worsened cardiac status at in-patient re-examination.

Level of significance according to Bonferroni tests: $*p<0.05$, $**p<0.01$, $***p<0.001$.

Table 6. Logistic regression analysis: Prognosis of changes in cardiac status* (unchanged $(n = 18)$, worsened $(n = 25)$).

Predictors	Improvement of prediction χ^2	p	Goodness of fit χ^2	p
0.			60.57	0.05
1. Kaltenbach-Score	7.37	0.01	53.21	0.14
2. Achievement motivation (PSM-15)	8.08	0.00	45.13	0.34
3. Number of delayed correct reactions under stringent given time pressure (PPG)	3.09	0.08	42.04	0.43
4. Smoking	1.41	0.24	40.63	0.44
5. Depressiveness (FPI-3)	1.22	0.27	39.41	0.45
6. Heart frequency, habitual value (PPE)	0.06	0.81	39.35	0.41

*Operated and deceased patients have not been considered.

motivation, depressiveness, heart frequency during the psychophysiological examination, number of delayed correct reactions under high time pressure, Kaltenbach-score as an index for the extent of the coronary sclerosis, and smoking, were enlisted as predictors into the logistical regression analysis.

With a satisfactory adaptation to the distribution of the criterion, the extent of achievement motivation and the degree of severity of the coronary sclerosis proved to be the best predictors. The other variables hardly contributed to the prognosis whether the cardiac status was stable or would worsen in future.

DISCUSSION

An important common finding from the various mean value comparisons and logistical regression analyses is that psychosocial and psychophysiological findings are significant for all three criteria (survival re-infarction, serious cardiac complications, future changes in cardiac status), even with the appropriate consideration of cardiac findings and standard risk factors. For the long-term future of younger post-infarction patients it is clearly necessary to determine a complex risk constellation composed of psychosocial, psychophysiological, and cardiac findings in addition to standard risk factors.

Biobehavioral characteristics of patients prone to develop cardiac complications

Candidates for the appearance of a re-infarction are marked by an increased aggressiveness potential, cardiac problems, and less effective behaviour under stressful making conditions, as well as more pronounced reactivity of systolic blood pressure after emotional stress. As aggressiveness is regarded as an essential component of type-A behaviour (Friedman, 1979), the significance of anger and aggressiveness for the re-infarction found in this study, corresponds with the findings of Jenkins *et al.* (1976) and the result of Friedman *et al.* (1986). When taking the increased number of mistakes under stressful conditions and the increased rise of systolic blood pressure after emotional stress as indications of a less effective handling of psychic stressors, a reduction in self-reported job efficiency can be understood as a symptom of excessive demands. Indeed, considering that smoking has proved to be a prognostically significant risk factor for a re-infarction, this results in the following constellation of risk factors for a re-infarction. Endangered patients are those who feel excessive demands are placed upon them and are more aggressive, who do not stop smoking and dispose of little effective forms of coping with psychological stressors, and who react with an increase in systolic blood pressure when confronted with psychic stress. The prognostic significance of symptoms of vital exhaustion which can already be determined for the occurrence of the myocardial infarction (Appels *et al.*, 1986) seem, therefore, to be also valid for the re-infarction.

It may be concluded that patients with increased aggressiveness and symptoms of exhaustion, who continue smoking, and who demonstrate increased systolic blood pressure reactivity as a result of ineffective stress coping strategies, are subject to an increased risk of myocardial infarction. The assumption that only one subgroup of aggressive patients with symptoms of exhaustion have an increased physiological reactivity accords with the opinion of Dembroski and McDougall (1983) that of the type-A persons only a minority shows an increased cardiovascular reactivity.

The illustrated psychosocial and psychophysiological risk constellation is largely independent of cardiac findings, for, on the one hand, they have been successfully controlled through parallelizing the groups, and, on the other, it can be seen from the logistical regression analysis that the extent of the coronary sclerosis is contributing comparatively little to the prognosis of re-infarction, although it is known from other studies that the stenotic degree is an important determinant for the progression of the coronary sclerosis (Roskamm *et al.*, 1983).

When comparing patients who have suffered a re-infarction or who have died as a result of cardiac problems with the remaining patients, it is again striking that cardiac findings hardly enable a differentiation between these two groups. Neither the extent of the coronary sclerosis nor the number of dys- or acinetic segments, or the degree of left-ventricular malfunction determined by means of a ventriculography, permit a separation of these two groups. Only the cardiac index and the maximum heart minute volume differentiate between the groups, with patients with serious complications showing more favourable results.

The determined standard risk factors also yield no differentiation between the two groups and have, therefore, no clear significance for prognostic purposes. This opinion is supported by the logistical regression analysis in which the number of narrowed vessels, cardiac index, and smoking are confirmed as variables of little relevance.

As a result of the psychological findings patients may be identified by symptoms of excessive stress (reduced ability to recuperate, little sleep), heightened body-referred worries, increased irritability, as well as little effectiveness in handling psychosocial stress, and also by an increased cardiac ability to endure stress according to self-judgement. This suggests that in spite of comparable working tolerances these patients judge their ability to cope with stress more easily. There is apparently a contradiction within the endangered patient between the subjective judgement of their cardiac ability to cope with stress and the general efficiency perceived by them. This indicates that such patients do not think their symptoms of excessive stress relevant for their cardiac status. The alternative assumption of an extensive denial or dissimulation of cardiac symptoms is most unlikely as they mention no fewer heart symptoms.

The patients at risk, in spite of the presence of symptoms of excessive stress and in spite of being generally worried about their health, are convinced that cardiacally they can cope with stress by comparison to the rest of the patients. These patients at risk apparently make no contingency between the two facts 'cardiac ability to cope with stress' and 'presence of symptoms of excessive stress', so that it must be assumed that they will be more worried about their general state of health in the future when symptoms of excessive stress appear, yet without worrying about their cardiac status. These patients behave as if they had a sound heart and feel generally excessively stressed because of an inefficiency in coping with psychosocial stress. Apparently, they have avoided the necessary analysis of their changed life situation as a result of the disease by trivializing the effects of the disease on their behaviour and the unfavourable effects of chronic excessive stress on the further duration of the disease. This interpretation aligns with the pronounced feeling of weakness described by Nirkko et al. (1982) as well as with the dissimulation of limitations due to the disease with patients who suffer further serious cardiac complications (Brodner et al., 1985). It is, however, unsatisfactory, that no physiological parameter could be identified which may be understood as a link between this psychological constellation and the manifestation of survival re-infarction or cardiac death. This refers to the necessity of supplementing the psychophysiological measurement by further recordings, and in particular biochemical, parameters.

It has been seen that patients with re-infarction and patients with serious cardiac complications show a reduced effective coping of psychosocial stress and the presence of symptoms of excessive stress. Such stress related problems are indicative of serious cardiac complications. However, they pertain more closely to total or vital exhaustion. Further cardiac findings and standard risk factors both proved to be of less prognostic relevance for younger post-infarction patients. This similarity of findings is not surprising, however, as the re-infarction patients are included in both criteria groups.

Patients whose cardiac status has worsened are, by comparison to those showing a stable cardiac status, mainly identified by a more pronounced coronary sclerosis, a more pronounced achievement and competitively-oriented behaviour, an increased psychological and partly physiological activation during psychosocial stress, and by a tendency to feelings of insufficiency. This constellation is mainly characterizing patients who show compensatory achievement behaviour, that is for those whom chronic achievement behaviour is the preferred strategy for coping with their fear of loss of self-esteem (Langosch, 1988).

The negative effects of chronic compensatory achievement behaviour upon the cardiovascular system can also be derived from the neurophysiological theory of anxiety by Gray (1982). The anxiety of losing one's self-esteem, the constant anticipation of not being successful, of failure, criticism, etc., results in a hyperactivation of the behavioural inhibition system, which leads in turn, because of a gradual exhaustion of the noradregenic input in the hypothalamus, finally to helplessness, to feelings of insufficiency, and to a stimulation of the hypophysis-suprarenal gland system. Pronounced compensatory achievement behaviour, which may be defined as a constant active avoidance behaviour, and coping with anticipated punishment stimulation, is associated with a hyper-activation of the sympatho-adrenomedullary axis. Thus, a synergistic activation of the two stress axes results from the synergistic hyperactivation of these two emotional systems. Results of animal experiments by Kaplan *et al.* (1985) support the assumption that a synergistic activation of the two stress axes may be significant for the progression of the coronary sclerosis. Kaplan *et al.* found that after a repeated confrontation with unstable social situations the dominant animals showed more pronounced morphological changes in the coronary arteries.

In the logistical regression analysis, high achievement motivation proved to be the best individual predictor, followed by the Kaltenbach Score as an indicator for the degree of severity of coronary sclerosis. Since Roskamm *et al.* (1983) demonstrated that after an observation period of an average of 3.5 years, progression of coronary sclerosis is mainly found in patients who already had a multilocular vascular affection when initially examined. It may be hypothesised that the predicted progression of the coronary sclerosis is additionally accelerated by the constant synergistic activation of the two stress axes, as it has been postulated in the presence of compensatory achievement behaviour. A surprising finding is that the percentage of smokers was found to be highest in the group of patients whose cardiac status was rated as improved at re-examination. When considering that these patients have a less severe degree of coronary atherosclerosis, this result indicates that smoking is an important risk factor for myocardial infarction at a young age, even when the degree of coronary atherosclerosis may be low (Gohlke *et al.*, 1981). However, smoking does not appear to be a significant predictor for the direction of changes in the cardiac status post-infarction demonstrated by the results of the logistical regression analysis. A worsening of the cardiac status would then result for those younger post-infarction patients who show signs of compensatory achievement-oriented behaviour and who have a pronounced coronary sclerosis according to the findings of this study. This must be qualified by indicating that in the psychophysiological examination indications were found for pronounced psychosocial activation and an increase in physiological activation; the synergistic activation of the two stress axes could not be proven, however, as biochemical characteristics were not recorded.

Implications for patient management

If for the occurrence of re-infarction, serious cardiac complications and for a worsening of the cardiac status psychosocial factors are essential, the question of possible psychotherapeutic intervention arises. Such therapy may help to delay or prevent the occurrence of these unfavourable cardiac developments.

The risk of re-infarction may be reduced at an early stage by improving the ability of patients to cope with psychosocial stress by means of stress-coping training (cf. Langosch et al., 1982). By reducing the level of aggressive behaviour through anger-management programmes (Novaco, 1975, 1976), and by reducing the increased reactivity of systolic blood pressure by relaxation techniques (Patel, 1986) risk of myocardial re-infarction should diminish. In addition the risk of serious cardiac complications may also be maintained at a low level by improving the discrimination between symptoms of excessive stress, and by re-attributing these symptoms as warning signals for overstressing the cardiovascular system, and finally by recognizing and accepting necessary psychological adaptations to the limitations of efficiency as a result of myocardial infarction.

The risk for a worsening of the cardiac status may also be reduced through stress-coping techniques, and by improving the discrimination between self-overstressing and self-punishing cognitions, and in addition by establishing a helpful personal dialogue to replace the self-overstressing and self-punishing instructions with self-encouraging and problem-oriented cognitions. It becomes clear that for younger post-infarction patients great importance must be attached to a comprehensive stress-coping training if there is to be a reduction in the risk of unfavourable cardiac conditions and developments.

It must be stated that these findings may only be transferred with limitations to older post-infarction patients as Roskamm et al. (1982) state that younger and older myocardial infarction patients have only a limited comparability. Finally, as a result of the small sample size of the individual groups it is necessary to conduct further prospective studies to validate these findings.

Acknowledgement

This research was supported by a grant from the Federal Ministry of Research and Technology, number 070631915. Responsibility for the contents of this publication lies with the authors.

REFERENCES

Appels, A., Mulder, P., van't Hof, M., Jenkins, C. D., van Houtem, J. and Tau, F. (1986). The predictive power of the A/B typology in Holland: results of a 9.5-year follow-up study. In Schmidt, T. H., Dembróski, T. M. and Blümchen, G. (Eds), *Biological and Psychological Factors in Cardiovascular Disease*. Springer, Berlin, pp. 56–62.

Bergstrand, R., Vedin, A., Wilhelmsson, C. and Wilhelmsson, L. (1981). Myocardial infarction among men below age 40 in Göteborg. In Roskamm, H. (Ed.), *Myocardial Infarction at Young Age*. Springer, Berlin, pp. 23–28.

Brodner, G., Langosch, W. and Borcherding, H. (1985). Psychologische Veränderungen einige Jahre nach Herzinfarkt. In Langosch, W. (Ed.), *Psychische Bewältigung der chronischen Herzerkrankung*. Springer, Berlin, pp. 240–257.

Bruhn, J. G., Chandler, B. and Wolf, S. (1969). A psychological study of survivors and nonsurvivors of myocardial infarction. *Psychosomatic Medicine*, **31**, 8–19.

Dembroski, T. M. and MacDougall, J. M. (1983). Behavioral and psychophysiological perspectives on coronary prone behavior. In Dembroski, T. M., Schmidt, T. H. and Blümchen, G. (Eds), *Biobehavioral Bases of Coronary Heart Disease*. Karger, Basel, pp. 106–129.

Epstein, F. H. and Wilhelmsen, L. (1982). Do the standard risk factors alter their role after the first myocardial infarction? In Mathes, P. and Halhuber, H. J. (Eds), *Controversies in Cardiac Rehabilitation*. Springer, Berlin, pp. 18–20.

Fahrenberg, J., Selg, H. and Hampel, R. (1978). *Das Freiburger Persönlichkeitsinventar FPI*, Hogrefe, Göttingen.

Federal Office of Statistic (1985). *Statistisches Jahrbuch 1985 für die Bundesrepublick Deutschland*. Kohlhammer, Stuttgart, Mainz.

Friedman, M. (1979). The modification of Type A behavior in post-infarctions. *American Heart Journal*, **97**, 551–560.

Friedman, M., Thoresen, C. E., Gill, J. J., Ulmer, D., Powell, L. H., Price, V. A., Brown, B., Thompson, L., Rabin, D. D., Breall, W. S., Bourg, E., Levy, R. and Nixon, T. (1986). Alternation of type A behavior and its effect on cardiac recurrences in post myocardial infarction patients: summary results of the recurrent coronary prevention project. *American Heart Journal*, **112**, 653–661.

Georgiou, V., Athanassiades, D., Hadjigeorge, C., Kaurouklis, C. and Agoustakis, D. (1978). Die Langzeitprognose der koronaren Herzerkrankungen bei jungen hospitalisierten Patienten. *Herz/Kreislauf*, **10**, 279–283.

Gertler, M. M., White, P. D., Simon, R. and Gottsch, L. G. (1964). Long term follow up of young coronary patients. *American Journal of Medical Sciences*, 145–154.

Gohlke, H. (1984). Herzinfarkt im jungen Erwachsenenalter. In Roskamm, H. (Ed.), *Koronarerkrankungen: Handbuch der inneren Medizin*, vol. IX/3. Springer, Berlin, pp. 785–803.

Gohlke, H., Stürzenhofecker, P., Thilo, A., Droste, C., Görnandt, L. and Roskamm, H. (1981). Coronary angiographic findings and risk factors in postinfarction patients under the age of 40. In Roskamm, H. (Ed.), *Myocardial Infarction at Young Age*. Springer, Berlin, pp. 61–77.

Gray, J. A. (1982). *Neuropsychology of Anxiety*. Oxford University Press, Oxford.

Hampel, R. (1977). Adjektiv—Skalen zur Einschätzung der Stimmung (SES). *Diagnostica*, **2**, 43-60.

Jenkins, C. D., Zyzanski, S. J. and Rosenman, R. H. (1976). Risk of new myocardial infarction in middle aged men with manifest coronary heart disease. *Circulation*, **53**, 342-347.

Kaplan, J. R., Manuck, S. B., Clarkson, T. B. and Prichard, R. W. (1985). Animal models of behavioral influences on atherogenesis. In Katkin, E. S. and Manuck, S. B. (Eds), *Advances in Behavioral Medicine*, vol. 1. JAI press, Greenwich, Connecticut, pp. 115-163.

Lamm, G. (1981). The epidemiology of acute myocardial infarction at young age. In Roskamm, H. (Ed.), *Myocardial Infarction at Young Age*. Springer, Berlin, pp. 5-12.

Langosch, W. (1988). Umfassende Behandlung des Postinfarktpatienten durch den Hausarzt: Welche psychosozialen Aspekte sind von besonderer Relevanz? In Halhuber, M. J. (Ed.), *Umfassende Herzinfarkt—Nachsorge in Klinik und Praxis*. Hans Huber, Bern, in press.

Langosch, W., Brodner, G. and Foerster, F. (1983). Psychophysiological testing of postinfarction patients. A study determining the cardiological importance of psychophysiological variables. In Dembroski, T. M., Schmidt, T. H. and Blümchen, G. (Eds), *Biobehavioral Bases of Coronary Heart Disease*. Karger, Basel, pp. 197-227.

Langosch, W., Seer, P., Brodner, G., Kallinke, D., Kulick, B. and Heim, P. (1982). Behavior therapy with coronary heart disease patients: results of a comparative study. *Journal of Psychosomatic Research*, **26**, 475-484.

Langosch, W., Prokoph, J. H. and Brodner, G. (1980). Der psychologische Screeningbogen für Patienten mit Myokardinfarkt (PSM) bei verschiedenen kardiologischen Diagnosegruppen. In Fassbender, C. F. and Mahler, E. (Eds), *Der Herzinfarkt als psychosomatische Erkrankung in der Rehabilitation*. Boehringer, Mannheim, pp. 89-123.

Nirkko, O., Lauroma, M., Siltanen, P., Tuominen, H. and Vanhala, K. (1982). Psychological risk factors related to coronary heart disease. Prospective studies among policemen in Helsinki. *Acta Medica Scandinavica* (suppl), **660**, 137-146.

Novaco, R. W. (1975). *Anger Control: the Development and Evaluation of an Experimental Treatment*. D. C. Heath, Lexington, M.A.

Novaco, R. W. (1976). Treatment of chronic anger through cognitive and relaxation controls. *Journal of Consulting and Clinical Psychology*, **44**, 681.

Nüssel, E., Buchholz, L. and Scheidt, R. (1981). Myocardial infarction in young men in the Heidelberg Register Area. In Roskamm, H. (Ed.), *Myocardial Infarction at Young Age*. Springer, Berlin, pp. 13-16.

Patel, C. (1986). Prevention paradox in coronary heart disease. In Schmidt, T. H., Dembroski, T. M. and Blümchen, G. (Eds), *Biological and Psychological Factors in Cardiovascular Disease*. Springer, Berlin, pp. 553-549.

Roskamm, H., Gohlke, H., Stürzenhofecker, P., Droste, C., Thomas, H., Samek, L., Schnellbacher, K. and Betz, P. (1983). Der Herzinfarkt im jugendlichen Alter (unter 40 Jahren): Koronarmorphologie, Risikofaktoren, Langzeitprognose der Erkrankung und Progression der Koronargefäßsklerose. *Zeitschrift für Kardiologie*, **72**, 1-11.

Roth, O., Berki, A. and Wolff, G. D. (1967). Long range observations in fifty-three young patients with myocardial infarction. *American Journal of Cardiology*, **19**, 331-338.

Ruberman, E., Weinblatt, E., Goldberg, J. D. and Chaudhary, B. S. (1984). Psychosocial influences on mortality after myocardial infarction. *New England Journal of Medicine*, **311**, 552-559.

Siegrist, J. and Matschinger, H. (1985). Konzeptuelle und methodische Überlegungen zur Rolle sozialer Belastungen bei Spätkomplikationen nach Herzinfarkt. In Langosch, W. (Ed.), *Psychische Bewältigung der chronischen Herzerkrankung*. Springer, Berlin, pp. 231-239.

Cardiac Arrhythmia and Related Problems

INTRODUCTION TO SECTION IV

Cardiac arrhythmias often evoke serious cardiological and behavioural problems. Ventricular fibrillation has been shown to be the mechanism for most sudden deaths. This final state of electric instability can be elicited by a wide variety of different arrhythmic processes (e.g. extrasystoles, tachycardia).

Fortunately, not all episodes of cardiac arrhythmia result in cardiac arrest. Many of them end spontaneously within a relatively short period of time. This, however, does not imply that their termination prevents individuals from developing behavioural disorders. So far, it is not yet clear which individuals are highly susceptible either to life-threatening ventricular fibrillations or to emotional and behavioural disturbances such as panic attacks and generalized avoidance behaviour. In cardiologists' and general practitioners' offices, however, patients are very frequently seen who suffer both from cardiac arrhythmias and emotional disturbances. From a diagnostic point of view, it still remains a challenge for medical and behavioural professionals to determine the specific interaction between aberrant cardiac events and behavioural consequences. One of the reasons why this interdisciplinary approach in the field of behavioural medicine has not been driven forward in the past, is the availability of powerful antiarrhythmic drugs as well as the lack of promising empirical data from behavioural intervention studies (Cheatle and Weiss, 1982). Compared to hypertension and myocardial infarction, cardiac arrhythmias and their related emotional and behavioural problems seem to be a neglected area of behavioural medicine until now. Therefore, this section is devoted to some new aspects of cardiac arrhythmias and related problems which:

1. may shed light on the neural and behavioural components of arrhythmogenesis and lead to better understanding of the underlying mechanisms involved both in pharmacological and behavioural interventions;
2. illustrate the kind of behavioural intervention that might be helpful for ameliorating cardiac as well as emotional problems in patients who are at risk for both cardiovascular disorders and behavioural disturbances (e.g. cardiophobia, social isolation, depression).

With this in mind, the section is far from being comprehensive. Its main objective is to draw attention to a neglected area of behavioural medicine and to revive the discussion of new diagnostic and therapeutic approaches which are interdisciplinary in nature.

The first chapter by Skinner supports the notion that the brain is involved in the arrhythmogenesis in a very specific way. His animal model of how neocortex is modulating the conductivity in an ischemic heart is based upon experiments in pigs. An increase in cardiac vulnerability occurs through a learning-dependent process in frontocortical neurones. He postulates an increased responsivity of the frontal lobe to benign stimulus-events which is primarily due to a cerebral noradrenergic pathology. Because of this cerebral hyper-reactivity the modulating influences from the frontal cortex are remarkably reduced which may result in a dual autonomic tone during increased states of cardiac vulnerability. Dual tone in a resting heart is characterized by an increase of both sympathetic and parasympathetic tone while the sympathetic tone seems to predominate. The conclusions he has drawn from these findings concern primarily the pharmacological intervention by beta-blockers. Their cardioprotective function is not solely due to peripheral effects but primarily to central effects by which the processing of stressful events in the frontal lobe is reduced. With respect to behavioural interventions he concludes that those physiological and behavioural manipulations should be applied which favor parasympathetic predominance.

The question on whether and to what extent cardiac arrhythmias can be brought under voluntary control by behavioural strategies still remains open. One of the methods very frequently used is heart rate feedback. Despite the fact that its effects are very well documented in normals, its clinical usefulness has not yet been demonstrated. This is particularly due to the fact that there are only a few clinical outcome studies, most of which are single-case studies without any appropriate control conditions. According to the critical review by Cheatle and Weiss (1982) there are clinically relevant results in sinus tachycardia. Bringing heart rate into the normal range by a training for heart rate slowing is aimed directly at the rapid heart rate involved in sinus tachycardia.

Janssen and Berger (Chapter 18) followed this reasoning and developed a biofeedback training for 7 patients with sinus tachycardia. They could show that patients' heart rates decreased gradually and remained at this level during follow-up sessions. Beside these cardiac changes significant ameliorations of emotional and behavioural disturbances did occur which by themselves are of clinical relevance. A sample of 33 patients who have been characterized as cardiophobics were studied by Vaitl, Kuhmann, and Ebert–Hampel (Chapter 19). In these patients, cardiac arrhythmia and their modification was not the primary goal of intervention but the investigation of different heart rate feedback parameters involved in a training (ten sessions) for heart rate stabilization.

Clinically relevant changes could be obtained in all of the three response modalities measured: physiological responses (heart rate variability, cardiac-respiratory coherence), control strategies used, and symptom amelioration. The patterns of positive changes observed can primarily be explained by psychological factors involved (success, attention-placebo) rather than by cardiac control achieved by the aid of feedback given.

Patients with cardiophobic reactions or heart-related disorders were in the past clinically described with various diagnoses such as 'Da Costa syndrome', 'effort syndrome' or 'neuro-circulatory asthenia'. Very recently it became clear that this kind of emotional and physical disturbance resembles panic disorders as they have been classified by DSM III. Until now, there is still a controversy on the etiological relationship between cardiac dysfunctions and panic reactions. Chapter 17 by Ehlers, Margraf, Taylor, and Roth reviews the literature on this issue. It is mainly focused at the possible specificity of cardiovascular disorders (e.g. elevated cardiac arrhythmia, tonic heart rate level, mitral valve prolapse) involved in the pathogenesis of panic attacks. Surprisingly, their specific influences are moderate or low. The higher resting heart rate very frequently found in panic disorder patients as well as their somewhat poorer physical condition is far from being specific. The same is true for mitral valve prolapse which has been overemphasized in the past, compared to other cardiac conditions.

REFERENCE

Cheatle, M. D. and Weiss, T. (1982). Biofeedback in heart rate control and the treatment of cardiac arrhythmias. In *Clinical Biofeedback: Efficacy and Mechanisms*, Guilford Press, New York, pp. 164–194.

Behavioural Medicine in Cardiovascular Disorders
Edited by T. Elbert, W. Langosch, A. Steptoe and D. Vaitl
©1988 John Wiley & Sons Ltd

16

Brain Involvement in Cardiovascular Disorders

James E. Skinner

Neurophysiology Section, Neurology Department and Neuroscience Program, Baylor College of Medicine, Houston, TX 77030

CARDIAC ARRHYTHMOGENESIS: CEREBRAL FACTORS

Psychosocial stress is known to be a risk factor for sudden cardiac death (Cannon, 1942; Burrell, 1963; Wolf, 1967; Neurotech, 1987; Rees and Lutkins, 1967; Wolf, 1969; Parkes, 1976; Jenkins, 1976; Rissanen *et al.*, 1978; Reich *et al.*, 1981). In animals, our laboratory has shown that operationally defined stressor-events must be present for coronary artery occlusion to result in ventricular fibrillation (Skinner *et al.*, 1975a). Each stressor-event (e.g. novel stimulus, tone forewarning cutaneous shock, unexpected cutaneous shock, physical restraint) has been found to evoke an identical pattern of electrochemical responses in the frontal granular cortex. These event-related responses include: norepinephrine release followed by cyclic AMP accumulation (Skinner *et al.*, 1987), negative-polarity slow potentials (Skinner and Yingling, 1976, 1977), and extracellular potassium-reduction (Skinner and Molnar, 1983). The magnitude of each cerebral response is related to the animal's experience with the stressors (i.e. to learning and habituation). Three independent interventions have been found, each of which will prevent stress from evoking lethal cardiac arrhythmias:

1. learned adaptation to the stressor (Skinner *et al.*, 1975a);
2. blockade of frontocortical projections to the brainstem cardiovascular nuclei (Skinner and Reed, 1981);
3. the intracerebral (but not intravenous) injection of levo-propranolol (0.05 mg kg^{-1}) (Skinner, 1985a, 1985b).

We conclude that psychosocial stressors increase cardiac vulnerability through a *learning-dependent noradrenergic process in frontocortical neurons*. The neurophysiological model is presented in Figure 1 and the implications of this

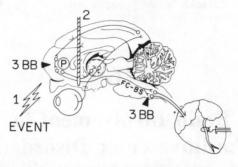

Figure 1. A theoretical model for the cerebral mechanism that mediates the deleterious effects of psychosocial stressors on cardiac vulnerability. An environmental stressor (EVENT) evokes a cerebral process in the frontal lobes (P) that determines whether or not activity occurs in the frontocortical-brainstem pathway (FC-BS). The activity in this pathway results in dual autonomic outflow (+ / −) and inhibits homeostatic reflexes. The projected autonomic activity, either alone or in combination with myocardial ischemia, triggers the initiation of ventricular fibrillation. Three independent interventions will prevent the lethal consequence of coronary artery occlusion in the psychologically stressed pig: (1) learned adaptation to the stressful event; (2) cryogenic blockade of the FC-BS pathway; and (3) intracerebral (but not intravenous) injection of a beta-receptor antagonist (i.e. a beta-blocker, BB). The composite cerebral response to the stressor-event (P) is composed of a series of electrochemical correlates which include: norepinephrine release (NE), cyclic AMP activation (cAMP), extracellular potassium activity decrease (K +), slow membrane potential shift (s-Vm), and the event-related slow potential (ERSP). How these cerebral activities are related to process-P is not yet understood. A noradrenergic mechanism, however, is known to enable long-term potentiation of synaptic efficacy (LTP) in a cortical model system. A beta-receptor antagonist and a muscarinic agonist, compounds which block the noradrenergic system by separate mechanisms, have in common the disabling of cortical LTP (anti-LTP) and the suppression of ventricular ectopy. Thus blocking the noradrenergic mechanism for the enhancement of synaptic efficacy in the FC-BS neurons may lead to the inactivation of process-P. Blockade of the FC-BS pathway also reduces blood pressure elevations in several models of hypertension, a finding which suggests a link between process-P and the maintenance of hypertension.

theoretical framework to the problem of sudden cardiac death will be discussed below; special emphasis is placed on (1) identification of the patient at risk and (2) pharmacologic treatment.

CENTRAL MODE OF ACTION OF
BETA-RECEPTOR ANTAGONISTS

When the beta-receptor antagonist, propranolol, is delivered intravenously (0.2–2.0 mg/kg), it has no effect on the prevention of lethal cardiac arrhythmogenesis in a psychologically stressed pig experiencing acute coronary artery occlusion (Skinner *et al.*, 1975a; Skinner, 1985a, 1985b). This lack of effect occurs, presumably, because the highest subtoxic dose administered

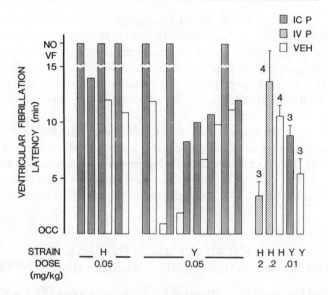

Figure 2. Intracerebral levo-propranolol prevents the initiation of ventricular fibrillation following acute coronary occlusion in the conscious unadapted pig. Hampshire (H) and Yorkshire (Y) pigs were operated and implanted with intrathoracic coronary artery occluders and intracranial injection cannulae. Following 4 to 6 days of recovery each animal was brought into the laboratory for the first time (i.e. was unadapted, to evoke psychological stress). Each animal was then injected with either intracranial (IC) or intravenous (IV) propranolol or with a vehicle (VEH) control. Intracerebral injections were either 0.05 or 0.01 mg/kg of levo-propranolol or were matched volumes of saline. Intravenous injections were either 2 or 0.2 mg/kg of the racemic mixture of propranolol or matched volumes of saline. Ten minutes after completing each injection, the animals' left anterior descending coronary artery was completely occluded (OCC). The latency to the onset of ventricular fibrillation was then observed. In some pigs in which intracerebral propranolol had been injected, VF did not occur within the expected 14-min interval; in several of these cases the animal had its coronary artery disoccluded prior to the maximum period of reversible ischemia so that the next day, after complete recovery of the heart, a subsequent vehicle control experiment could be carried. In most cases reperfusion VF occurred and extrathoracic electroconversion was performed. In all cases, however, cardiac recovery was complete, as assessed by the normalization of contractility, coronary flow, left ventricular pressure and the ECG. These within-subject experimental results are shown at the left, and for each animal the results are linked by a common baseline. The first H and the second Y pigs (from the left) each had their coronary occlusion maintained for 24 h without VF occurring. The individual bar graphs to the right show the means, numbers, and standard deviations of between-subject control groups, in which only a single experiment was conducted in each animal. These control groups, when compared to the group comprised of first experiment of each animal shown to the left, show that intracerebral injection of 1-propranolol results in 4 out of 6 animals failing to manifest VF within 18 min to 24 h min, whereas in the case of the controls, 0 out of 17 show this effect ($p < 0.01$, binomial test). (Preliminary unpublished data of Cunningham, Parker and Skinner.)

peripherally does not result in an effective cerebral concentration, a dose level which apparently can be achieved, as shown in Figure 2, through direct intracerebral administration. Since all beta-receptor antagonists cross the blood-brain barrier, including the less lipophilic ones (Goodman and Gillman, 1970), it may be that the central action of this family of drugs best explains at least this one type of clinical efficacy, i.e. the reduction of ischemia-induced mortality during psychological stress.

In the Beta-blocker Heart Attack Trials, a 26% decline in mortality was found to occur in survivors of acute myocardial infarction (Beta-blocker Research Group, 1982). Those victims who failed to respond to clinical therapy (i.e. the remaining 74%) may, like the pigs, have had an insufficient cerebral concentration of the drug to overcome the effect of high levels of psychologic stress.

CEREBRAL ORIGIN OF DUAL
AUTONOMIC TONE DURING ARRHYTHMOGENESIS

Manning and Cotten (1962) showed in the anesthetized dog that the stimulation of the distal cut ends of sympathetic and parasympathetic cardiac nerves individually did not elicit ventricular ectopy, but that the stimulation of both together did produce ventricular arrhythmias. In confirmation, our laboratory (Skinner et al., 1975b) showed in the unanesthetized pig that the state of slow-wave sleep, a state in which high dual autonomic-tones exist (Baust and Bohnert, 1969), is associated with increased arrhythmogenesis and more rapid onsets of lethal ectopy following coronary artery occlusion. In the heart of the unadapted or psychologically stressed pig, we showed (Skinner et al., 1983) that high sympathetic tone occurs (i.e. activation of phosphorylase enzyme activity) during hemodynamic rest. A resting heart under sympathetic drive implies that parasympathetic tone must also be high. Thus, high dual autonomic tone, measured by several independent means, seems to exist during increased states of vulnerability to arrhythmogenesis.

Psychologic stress is known to inhibit reflexive parasympathetic tone (i.e. baroreceptor reflexes) (Bard, 1960). Therefore it may be the case that the high dual autonomic tones associated with increased vulnerability to arrhythmogenesis may manifest a sympathetic predominance. In support of this hypothesis, Verrier and associates (Verrier and Lown, 1981) have shown in the psychologically stressed dog that vagal electric stimulation reduces vulnerability to arrhythmogenesis.

Further support for the hypothesis that failure of parasympathetic predominance leads to increased vulnerability is seen in the work of Schwartz and associates (Billman et al., 1982, 1984; Schwartz et al., 1984). They demonstrated that dogs with permanent occlusion of a small coronary artery will usually manifest lethal ventricular fibrillation (VF), not during exercise, but immediately following it, at a time when sympathetic tone is high due to the previous exercise and parasympathetic tone starts to climb to high levels due to the stopping. They then found a near perfect predictor of which dogs would manifest lethal arrhythmogenesis after the exercise was started. Those dogs which failed to show a baroreceptor reflex before they were run on a treadmill were found to be at higher risk of VF following exercise than dogs which initially manifested this reflex. In the reflex-inhibited group, daily experiences with running on a treadmill resulted in the reappearance of the reflex and a marked reduction in the exercise-induced vulnerability. Whether this reduced vulnerability was the result of increased vagal tone due to the exercise-conditioning or to the release of the baroreceptor reflex by stress-reduction (i.e. adaptation to the laboratory during the exercise sessions) is not yet established. In either case, however, a relative increase in parasympathetic tone would be expected. Thus physiological and behavioral manipulations favoring parasympathetic predominance appear to reduce risk of legal arrhythmogenesis.

Electric stimulation in either the frontal cortex (Delgado, 1960) or the hypothalamus (Hilton, 1980; Ulyanisky et al., 1977), where the frontocortical-brainstem pathway projects, will also produce inhibition of the baroreceptor reflex. Stimulation along this pathway will also evoke ventricular ectopy (Manning and Cotten, 1962; Weinberg and Fuster, 1960; Melville et al., 1963; Mauck et al., 1964; Hockman et al., 1966; Garvey and Melville, 1969; Hall et al., 1974, 1977; Ulyanisky et al., 1977), including VF (Garvey and Melville, 1969). Both of these phenomena are illustrated in Figure 3, in which it is seen that brief stimulation of a specific part of the frontal lobe of the pig results in ventricular ectopy within a few minutes; the initial effect, however, is bradycardia and suppression of the QRS complexes that normally follow a P-wave. Such stimulations can also produce a pathological insult (myofibrillar degeneration); this tissue damage is similar to that seen following intracoronary catecholamine injection (Hall et al., 1974, 1977; Ulyanisky et al., 1977). A similar pattern of cardiomyopathy also appears to be evoked by intense psychologic stress in both animals (Johansson et al., 1974; Corley et al., 1973) and humans (Cebelin and Hirsch, 1980). Thus electric stimulation of the parts of the brain that are known to be reactive to environmental stressors will produce the same physiological effects and pathological results that the environmental stressors themselves evoke (e.g. baroreceptor inhibition, myofibrillar degeneration, and ventricular ectopy).

In conclusion, it appears that environmental events which can be defined as psychosocial stressors evoke specific electrochemical activities in the frontal lobes that result in a descending projection to the brainstem cardiovascular centers. This projection evokes dual autonomic tones accompanied by homeostatic inhibition, with the result that, if intense enough, ventricular ectopy and cardiomyopathy may result. Behavioral and physiological influences which favor a shift toward parasympathetic predominance seem to reduce risk in the stressed subject. Producing this shift by the reduction of sympathetic tone alone, e.g. by the peripheral administration of propranolol, does not seem to achieve the desired effect if psychological stress is high.

DETECTION OF THE PATIENT AT RISK BY A NON-INVASIVE CEREBRAL MEASURE

Even if one had the most 'perfect' antiarrhythmic drug, that is, one which would prevent the lethal arrhythmia under all conditions, including high stress, this compound alone would not have much impact upon the problem of sudden cardiac death. This is because the majority of persons who suddenly die from ventricular fibrillation have had no prior symptoms to warrant medical attention. They expire unexpectedly and suddenly without a chance for resuscitation. Even though a strong familial (i.e. genetic) background for sudden cardiac death might lead a cardiologist to examine a patient more frequently and thoroughly, until some detectable physiological symptom is apparent good medical practice dictates that no medication be prescribed.

The theoretical model presented in Figure 1 shows that all environmental stressors evoke electrochemical activities in the frontal lobes which, collectively, are referred to as process-P. Evoking this specific cerebral perturbation at high intensity, either behaviorally or by electric stimulation (as in Figure 3), will cause severe arrhythmogenesis in the normal healthy heart; at a lower intensity this

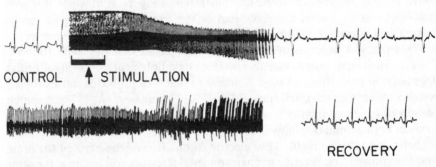

CONTROL   ↑ STIMULATION

RECOVERY

Figure 3. Electric stimulation of specific regions of the frontal lobes in the pig produces, in sequence, bradycardia, QRS-suppression, ST-alterations, and then ventricular ectopic beats. Bipolar electric stimulation (0.5 ms negative-polarity pulses delivered at 30 Hz for 10 s) on the surface of each gyrus anterior to the genu of the corpus callosum was carried out in the lightly anesthetized pig (methoxyflurane anesthesia) via electrodes inserted manually through a unilateral crainectomy the right frontal bone. Stimulation of the anterior cingulate gyrus and the C-shaped crescent of tissue on the mesial surface that extends anterior to the genu of the callosum and ventral toward the basal forebrain area were all effective in eliciting ventricular extopic beats, such as those illustrated. Stimuli of the surrounding gyri were without effect on ectopy. Note that the 10 s train of stimuli resulted in electrocardiographic alterations at a latency of some 10 s and ventricular ectopic beats at a latency of nearly 1 min.

process can trigger lethal arrhythmogenesis in the ischemic heart. One of the correlates of this set of electrochemical processes is the event-related slow potential (ERSP), which can be recorded non-invasively in humans. The detection of a cerebral pathology associated with process-P, perhaps via the ERSP, might present a symptom that for some physicians warrants clinical treatment prior to the sudden unexpected occurrence of VF and death. This is essentially the same logic that leads cardiologists to treat borderline hypertension and occurrence of single episodes of ventricular ectopy.

Before examining whether or not a cerebral pathology can in fact be detected in the ERSP, and then treated medically to prevent sudden death, it should first be asked whether or not this measure is a reasonable candidate for a physiological entity that a physician would feel compelled to treat, as are, for example, borderline high blood-pressures and single premature ventricular beats. Since stressors evoke process-P, something must be said about the behavior concept, 'stress'.

Firstly, it is known that what constitutes a stressful stimulus for one subject is not always the same as that for another. That is, is the ERSP sensitive to individual differences, especially when these can be attributed to differences in previous experience? The answer seems to be 'yes'. As discussed above, learning and habituation experiences determine the magnitude of the set of electrochemical responses (Skinner and Yingling, 1977; Skinner *et al.*, 1978; Skinner and Molnar, 1983) that stand between a stressor-event and cardiac vulnerability. Whether or not a given environment stressor-event increases cardiac vulnerability for a particular individual is presumably determined by these experiences (Skinner *et al.*, 1975a). 'Stress' is a cerebral reaction to a stimulus-event and not an inherent feature of it, like, say, its mass or color. Such a concept seems to explain why dogs (Gray *et al.*, 1984; Schaper, 1971) and pigs (Skinner *et al.*, 1975a) that have been laboratory pets or have been conditioned to the laboratory are at lower risk for fatal arrhythmogenesis than mongrels or those unfamiliar with the laboratory or its personnel. The mongrels have had different experiences and therefore have different cerebral reactions to the laboratory, with the consequence that their cardiac vulnerabilities are increased.

Secondly, does the ERSP represent a quantitative measure of 'stress' or is it qualitative? The former seems to be the case. In humans, it has been shown that tones which forewarn strong electric shocks evoke larger negative slow-potentials (i.e. ERSPs) than tones which forewarn mild shocks (Irwin *et al.*, 1966). After successive acquisitions of the two tone-shock pairings, the same psychological stressor (i.e. the same tone) in the same subject can be shown to evoke different response-amplitudes. Thus by measuring the amplitude of the ERSP in this individual, and at a particular moment in time, it can be established how 'stressful' he or she perceives the stimulus to be.

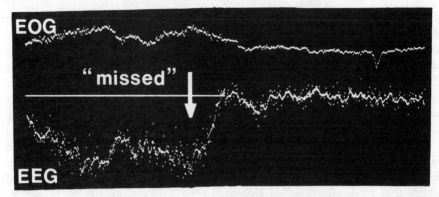

Figure 4. Event-related slow potential evoked while playing a video game. The EEG record was obtained from the CZ position on the vertex of the scalp of a normal subject using conventional DC-amplifiers and signal averaging (10-trial average). The superimposed EEG and EOG averages were synchronized relative to the time the subject missed returning the ball ('missed') while playing the progressively more difficult version of the game 'Breakout' (Atari, Inc.). The level of difficulty was set so that the subject generally missed after 5 s of play. The subject was instructed not to blink while playing the game and for at least 2 s after a 'missed' ball. The EOG record was from a pair of electrodes above and below the right eye and was used to reject automatically the inclusion of any data in the signal average if an eyeblink occurred during acquisition. A single eyeblink is observed in the record on the righthand part of the EOG trace. The time interval for the traces is 10 s. The amplitude of the peak negative (i.e. downward) EEG potential recorded just before the 'missed' ball is approximately 100 μV relative to the succeeding baseline. The amplitude of this peak is approximately 10-fold greater than the peak evoked in this same subject during the omitted-stimulus paradigm described in the next figure. Paradigms evoking larger event-related potentials may prove to be useful in investigating *within*-subject effects.

Persons with large cerebral ERSPs evoked by a benign stimulus-event would, from the above, be expected to have had a background of negative reinforcement associated with the evoking event. If no apparent negative reinforcer can be identified, then how could the potential be enlarged? From the chemical studies in animals, it seems that a noradrenergic basis exists for the generation of this potential (Figure 1). Thus if more norepinephrine is released in the cortex, then a larger potential would be expected to result. The question then becomes, is there any evidence that a cortical noradrenergic pathology could exist? The answer again is 'yes'. Levitt and Noebels (1981) have shown in the brain of the 'tottering-mouse' that hypertrophy of noradrenergic terminal growth exists, a genetic abberation which they believe could be the basis for the electrocortical pathology they have observed in these same subjects.

Finally, there is the matter that any type of stimulus situation in which the behavior of the subject is engaged will result in the evocation of an ERSP. Are all of these situations really 'stressful', at least as far as the heart is concerned? The answer seems to be that 'stress' is all around us. For example, playing a video game results in the evocation of an ERSP, as shown in Figure 4. Is this form of the ERSP associated with cardiovascular functions and perhaps dysfunctions? Again, the answer seems to be 'yes'. The particular video game used to evoke this ERSP (i.e. *Breakout* by Atari, Inc.) has been found by Eliot and associates (Eliot and Buell, 1985) to evoke cardiac hemodynamic reactions that are larger in amplitude in the subject at risk of cardiovascular disorder than in those subjects not at risk.

Now that the ERSP seems to be a reasonable candidate for a physiological symptom in need of treatment, can an association be found between it and a measure of cardiovascular pathology? In preliminary studies in 35 randomly selected cardiac patients with more than 30 ventricular arrhythmias per hour, we have demonstrated a linear regression between the amplitude of a scalp-recorded ERSP evoked by a benign stimulus-task ('Omitted-stimulus' task) and the degree of cardiac vulnerability measured by the rate of ventricular arrhythmias (24-hour Holter monitoring of the ECG). This particular paradigm was originally developed because its simplicity was thought to enable uniform administration, free of language, cultural, and previous-experience biases. Both the between-subject and within-subject regressions have been determined, the former using randomly selected patients under placebo treatment and the latter using, within the same individual, placebo plus two antiarrhythmic drugs of varying efficacy (double-blinded observations, randomized treatment order). The linear regressions in both studies were statistically significant ($p < 0.02$) and the slopes were nearly identical (Skinner *et al.*, 1982; Skinner 1985b).

Screening data is also available from normal populations. In a double-blind study, performed by Neurotech Laboratories, Inc. (1987), it was determined that family history of sudden cardiac death could be detected by measuring the amplitude of the ERSP evoked in the Omitted-stimulus paradigm ($p < 0.01$). That is, pre-clinical individuals who had a parent or grandparent die of sudden cardiac death before the age of 55 had, as a group, significantly larger ERSPs than those individuals who had no such family history. Since family history is known to be a good predictor of future cardiovascular disorder, some of those individuals with large ERSPs are expected, eventually, to have hypertension and/or dangerous cardiac arrhythmias. Those with family history are already on notice of the possibility for future cardiovascular disorders. Those normals with large ERSPs who have no family history, however, are not on notice, and it may be that early treatment of these individuals could have an important impact on the prevention of sudden cardiac death.

Figure 5 illustrates the treatment of a cardiac patient using the only cardiac drug, propranolol, which has been proven to have an anti-death effect in humans (Beta-blocker Research Group, 1982) and to prevent death in stressed animals by a cerebral action (Skinner, 1985a). This patient had an unusually large Omitted-stimulus ERSP, as compared to that of the normals in the Neurotech study; it was more than two standard deviations above the mean of the normals

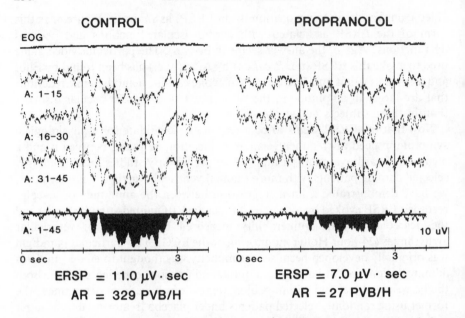

Figure 5. Effects of oral propranolol (60 mg kg^{-1}, t.i.d.) on the event-related slow potential (ERSP) in a cardiac patient with very high ventricular ectopy. The task used to evoke the ERSP was the detection of an omitted stimulus. That is, once every $10 + 2$ s a series of four tones was presented (50 ms each, separated by 500 ms, onsets indicated by vertical lines); the subject was told that in 10% of the trials the 3rd tone would be missing; in this case the subject was instructed to press a button, but at least 500 ms after the 4th tone; the subject was told not to move, blink or swallow during the 1 s before and after any of the 4-tone series because this would be detected (i.e. by the electro-occulogram, EOG) and data acquisition would be excluded. A:1–15, computer average of trials 1 through 15, etc. The baseline drawn through A:1–45 is the least-squares best fit of a line through the 1 s of data points before the 1st tone (left hand vertical line) and those 375 ms after the 4th tone. The voltage × time integral (area under the baseline, indicated by shading) between the 1st and 4th tones is the measure of the ERSP. This task was chosen because its simplicity makes it suitable for *between*-subject comparisons; furthermore, it evokes a large number of other endogenous event-related potentials (e.g. N1, P3, etc.), which can serve as controls because they do not change significantly between conditions. Note that the large initial negative potential that follows the 1st tone (N1) is not significantly altered by the propranolol, while the ERSP is reduced by almost 50%. Negative polarity is downward.

(Neurotech Laboratories Inc., 1987). Thus a pathological electrocortical potential, its pharmacologic treatment, and its treatment outcome have all been predicted from the neurophysiological model presented in Figure 1, which is based primarily on results from animal research.

If the enlarged ERSP (i.e. cerebral overreaction) that is detected in the highest ectopy patients existed pre-clinically, as appears to be the case in the normals with large ERSPs and family history of cardiovascular disease (Neurotech

Laboratories, Inc., 1987), then perhaps this brain potential could have been treated (i.e. with an antiadrenergic antiarrhythmic drug) to prevent clinical manifestations from developing. Furthermore, since severe environmental events can lead to some small amounts of 'stress cardiomyopathy' in normals, both human (Cebelin and Hirsch, 1980) and animal (Johansson, 1974), might it not be the case that less severe events combined with the cerebral pathology (i.e. over-reaction) could also produce cardiomyopathy? Only a well-controlled long-term prospective study of normals with large ERSPs can provide the answer to this interesting hypothesis.

Support for the hypothesis that the brain can evoke ventricular ectopy in the normal heart during intense psychological stress is observable in data from normal human subjects. NASA-astronauts, who do not show signs of ventricular ectopy on the ground, often do manifest ventricular arrhythmias during maneuvers that are associated with high psychological stress (Bungo and Johnson, 1983; Bungo, 1986). During extra-ventricular activity, ectopy has been found to be present in 40% of the 15 astronauts studied; such arrhythmias were not present while exercising inside the mother ship. During the critical period of re-entry, 33% of the 6 pilots and co-pilots studied had premature ventricular beats; such ectopy was not present during blast-off. These observations support the animal studies (Johansson, 1974) which demonstrated that acute psychological stressors can evoke cardiac ectopy in the normal healthy heart.

It is not yet known whether or not the astronauts manifesting space-evoked arrhythmias have larger ERSPs than those free of such ectopy (these studies are currently in progress at NASA and Neurotech Laboratories, Inc., in Houston). It would be of interest to know whether or not the mean ERSP amplitude of the astronauts with ectopy is significantly different from that of the highest ectopy patients observed in the clinical study. If the ERSP distinguishes which astronauts had ectopy, and if the mean ERSP amplitude of those with ectopy is similar to that of the cardiac patients with the highest ectopy, then support would occur for the possibility that a pre-clinical pathology existed in the astronauts with ectopy that, combined with the strong psychological stresses of orbital flight, resulted in the space-induced ectopy. It is significant that one astronaut who did manifest ventricular ectopy in space continued to manifest ventricular ectopy at least until the 21st post-flight day (Smith et al., in Bungo, 1986), and another who showed ventricular ectopy during extra-ventricular activity had a documented myocardial infarction a decade later (Bungo and Johnson, 1983).

We conclude that at least one EEG measure (ERSP) is predictive of at least one type of cardiac vulnerability (ectopy rate). The observation that a benign stimulus-event evokes a large cerebral response suggests that a cerebral pathology may exist. Since the ERSP is known to be accompanied by norepinephrine-release and cyclic AMP accumulation, this pathology may be related to a cerebral noradrenergic mechanism. This proposition is supported by clinical data, as illustrated in Figure 5, in which a subject with very high ectopy and very large ERSPs had both the cerebral and cardiac measures reduced by the noradrenergic receptor-inhibitor, propranolol. An implication of the brain–heart hypothesis is that persons with larger than normal ERSPs may be at pre-clinical risk for developing cardiovascular disorders; the occurrence of such abnormally large potentials is able to detect family history of sudden cardiac death, a risk factor which is known to be a pre-clinical predictor. Another implication of the theory is that the antiarrhythmic drug of choice in many applications may be the one that most effectively reduces the amplitude of the ERSP. Clearly, the previous *in vitro* approaches which have selected antiarrhythmic drugs because of their peripheral cardiac actions alone have precluded detection of a possible centrally mediated effect of the compound on the heart.

CORTICAL LEARNING MECHANISMS
AND CARDIAC VULNERABILITY

The raison d'être for brain regulation of the heart seems to be inherent in what Walter B. Cannon called the 'cerebral defense system'. He argued in his classical 1931 theory (Cannon, 1931) that an orchestrator of sensory input and autonomic output would be found to lie in the higher cerebral centers. This system, he postulated, evolved to enable an organism to prepare autonomic support in advance or in anticipation of somatic behaviors. Such autonomic priming is subject to habituation, he argued, for those input stimuli which do not result in behavior will not, after repetition, evoke the autonomic output responses.

Our laboratory has confirmed several features of Cannon's hypothesis. The frontal lobes, the most highly evolved region of the vertebrate brain, seem to be where the orchestration occurs. The ERSP, a cerebral reaction which has an anticipatory or 'expectancy' component (Levitt and Noebels, 1981), is primarily of frontal lobe origin (Skinner, 1971; Skinner and Yingling, 1977; Yingling and Skinner, 1977). The frontal lobes have output pathways that project to the brain stem to control autonomic support for anticipated behaviors and to the thalamus to control the ascent of sensory information from the periphery to the respective primary cortices (Skinner and Yingling, 1977; Yingling and Skinner, 1977). The neurophysiological analysis of this sensory gating mechanism shows that the frontal lobes selectively inhibit the thalamic relay of irrelevant sensory input, a finding which suggests that *selective perception is the result of selective inattention*. How this transaction is carried out (i.e. how the frontal lobes know what is irrelevant) is not yet known; it may be related to process-P.

Knowing that the frontocortical event-related slow potential is associated with a learning-dependent noradrenergic process (Skinner, 1984; Skinner *et al.*, 1987) led us to examine the effects of pharmacologic manipulations in a simple *in vitro* model of vertebrate cortical tissue. Long-term potentiation of synaptic efficacy (LTP) is currently thought to be a useful model for synaptic learning

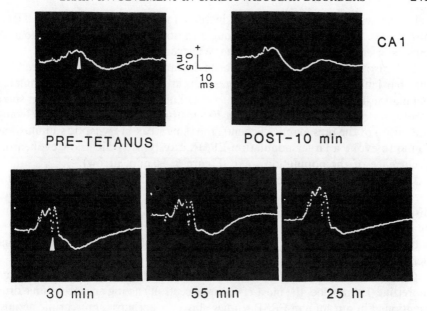

Figure 6. Long-term potentiation of synaptic efficacy (LTP) in the CA1 subfield of the hippocampus of the conscious behaving rat. Upper left: prior to the high frequency stimulus (pre-tetanus), excitatory postsynaptic potentials were elicited in the population of neurons surrounding the recording electrode in the CA1 cell-body layer (pop-EPSP); these responses were evoked by a low-frequency presynaptic stimulus delivered to the Schaeffer-collaterals; the intensity of the presynaptic stimulus was set to be just subthreshold for eliciting action potentials (pop-spikes) in the surrounding neuronal population (note the lack of a potential at the arrow). Upper right: 10 min following the brief high frequency stimulation of the presynaptic fibers (0.5 ms pulses, 100 Hz for 1 s) no change has yet occurred in the pop-EPSP, but the slow negative wave following it has become enlarged. Lower left: by 30 min following the tetanizing stimulus the pop-EPSP is markedly enhanced in amplitude and now a pop-spike is observed in response to the previously subthreshold stimulus (arrow). The enhancement of these responses is seen to be unchanged an hour later (lower middle) and to persist for at least one day (lower right). These data illustrate use-dependent enhancement of synaptic efficacy, a phenomenon which is inhibited by at least two different cardiac antiarrhythmic drugs, propranolol and Ethmozine; the later drug-effect is illustrated in Figure 7. (Unpublished data from Mitra and Skinner.)

and memory (Swanson *et al.*, 1982; Andersen and Wigstrom, 1980). Because the architecture of the hippocampal slice lends itself so easily to this type of synaptic study, it was the preparation of choice.

In the hippocampus it is possible to stimulate presynaptic axons at a low frequency and observe their postsynaptic responses with electrodes placed in the extracellular space. The population-EPSP (excitatory post-synaptic potential) and population-spike (action potential) evoked by the low-frequency stimuli are increased in amplitude following a brief high-frequency shift in the stimulus train being delivered. This use-dependent increase in synaptic efficacy (i.e. LTP) is observed to be maintained for very long durations, ranging from hours to days (Swanson et al., 1982; Andersen and Wigstrom, 1980).

LTP also occurs in the conscious behaving animal, as shown in Figure 6. In this particular example, a weak presynaptic stimulus evoked a summated population-EPSP; this response occurred without evoking the population-spike (arrow in Pretetanus control). Within 30 min after a brief high-frequency tetany (i.e. 'use') of the presynaptic elements, the same weak presynaptic stimulus was found to evoke a larger population-EPSP, a response which now evoked the occurrence of the population-spike (Figure 6, 30 min, arrow).

In the hippocampal slice Hopkins and Johnston (1984) showed that beta-receptor antagonists applied to the bath during the high-frequency stimulus disables the development of LTP, whereas the application of norepinephrine enables LTP, that is, to a high-frequency stimulus that was previously at a subthreshold intensity. Hippocampal LTP can also be disabled by catecholamine depletion (Bliss et al., 1983).

Our laboratory (Krontiris-Litowitz et al., 1985, 1987) has shown that morcizine/Ethmozine, the most efficacious centrally acting antiarrhythmic drug mentioned in our human ERSP studies above, is perhaps a muscarinic agonist with an LTP-effect opposite to that of norepinephrine and similar to that of propranolol. Some of this data is presented in Figure 7. The presence of Ethmozine during the high-frequency stimulus will prevent LTP, for at least 3 hours after the drug has been removed from the medium. This physiological effect is observed at very low concentrations of Ethmozine (1–10 nM) and occurs only if it is applied during the high-frequency stimulus. Ethmozine has a weak affinity for the muscarinic receptor in which ^{3}H-QNB displacement has $K_d = 10^{-6}$M; its physiological effect is weakly mimicked by the non-hydrolyzible muscarinic antagonist, carbachol; its strong anti-LTP effect, however, is reversed by co-perfusion with atropine. Thus, this weakly cholinergic compound, has a use-dependent effect, and, like propranolol, it disables or prevents LTP.

The biochemical mechanism for the interaction of cholinergic and beta-adrenergic receptor functions has several possibilities. First, the cholinergic effect could be mediated through the inhibitory regulatory protein (Birnbaumer et al., 1985; Watanabe et al., 1978) to turn off the accumulation of cyclic AMP, a second messenger which controls the phosphorylations of membrane-bound and/or cytoplasmic proteins that normally occur following beta-receptor stimulation. Secondly, among yet other possibilities, cholinergic effects on phosphotidylinositol metabolism could alter the calcium second-messenger to control the enzymatic cascade and protein phosphorylations underlying beta-receptor stimulation (Berridge and Irvine, 1984; Nishizuka, 1984). The point here is that although propranolol and Ethmozine both prevent LTP, each achieves its effect by a different receptor mechanism: competitive inhibition

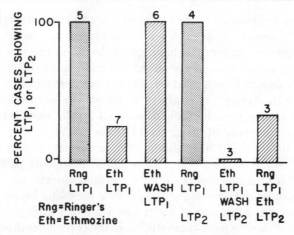

Figure 7. The cardiac antiarrhythmic drug, Ethmozine, produces use-dependent block of long-term potentiation of synaptic efficacy (LTP) in the hippocampal slice. Numbers at top indicate total number of slices in the group. Vertical scale: percent of total slices in group that met the criteria for LTP of the pop-spike (i.e. more than 20% increase in amplitude 15 min after the tetanizing stimulus; no change in the duration of the pop-spike; no change in the variance of the pop-spike relative to its mean). RNG: slices perfused with modified Ringer-solution (extracellular ions, 10% dextrose, saturated with 95% oxygen and 5% CO_2) during the high frequency stimulus (HFS). ETH: slices perfused with Ethmozine (1 nM) in the Ringer solution during the HFS. WASH: slices first perfused with Ethmozine (1 μM) for 15–20 min and then perfused with Ringer solution for 60 min before giving the HFS. LTP_1: the first episode of LTP attempted in a given slice. LTP_2: the second episode of LTP attempted in the same slice. Comparison of columns 3 and 6 (from the left) show that the effects of Ethmozine are use-dependent (i.e. require the HFS) and persist for at least 1 h after drug-washout. (Adapted from Krontiris-Litowitz et al., 1987.)

of an excitatory receptor for propranolol and use-dependent excitation of a receptor with an inhibitory consequence for Ethmozine. In the case of propranolol, it must be present to prevent LTP, whereas for Ethmozine it does not.

The concept of 'competitive-inhibition of LTP' is not isomorphic with that of 'use-dependent block of LTP' (i.e. 'anti-LTP'), but there does seem to be an important common ground—it is what synapses are and are not potentiated that sets the figure/ground form of the information in the system. When sculpting a statue from a block of stone, it is the pieces removed, not the remaining stone, that results in the form. This concept of selective suppression of the background was introduced in the discussion of the thalamic gating system (Skinner and Yingling, 1977; Yingling and Skinner, 1977); it also seems to pertain to the present case for hippocampal modification of synaptic efficacy (Krontiris-Litowitz et al., 1985, 1987). The principle will again be encountered when considering learned patterns of electric activity in the olfactory bulb, as described below.

The olfactory bulb has all of the basic cell types and neurochemicals known to be present in neocortex, but it has a much simpler and better understood neurophysiological structure (Shepherd, 1970). In this simple system model of the cortex, using a novel odor, we observed that habituation of an event-related pattern of EEG-activity is prolonged when exogenous norepinephrine is perfused locally through the bulb (Gray et al., 1984, 1986). The learned acquisition of a similar event-related pattern during odor-shock conditioning is prevented by the intrabulbar infusion of propranolol (Gray et al., 1984, 1986). Our interpretation of this data is that norepinephrine enables learning by *blocking habituation*. It is the failure to suppress or move the activity pattern into the background that seems to account for the learning process, that is, selective forgetting (habituation), not selective memory seems to be the underlying biological process for this spatial pattern measure of learning.

It is important to note from these studies in the cortical model-systems that a muscarinic agonist and a beta-receptor antagonist, each of which has a documented effect on the heart that is *antiarrhythmic*, also has an effect in neural tissues that appears to block learning. How the higher cerebral effects of these cardiac drugs (i.e. use-dependent anti-LTP for Ethmozine and block of LTP for propranolol) might lead to the expression of their antiarrhythmic properties is not yet known. Based on existent data, however, it is logically possible to speculate that a noradrenergic over-reaction in the frontal lobes, which blocks habituation of autonomic reactivity, might be the mechanism by which the noradrenergic learning-dependent increase in cardiac vulnerability to arrhythmogenesis occurs, as described at the outset of this chapter.

COMMON CEREBRAL ORIGINS OF ARRHYTHMOGENESIS AND HYPERTENSION

Hypertension is often regarded as a risk factor for sudden cardiac death, but the double dissociation leaves many cardiologists unconvinced (i.e. not all persons dying suddenly have hypertension and not all persons with hypertension die suddenly). The elusive relationship between these two variables may occur because both have a common origin in the brain, perhaps in the same frontocortical-brainstem system, as the accumulated data presented below seem to suggest.

Reis and associates (Doba and Reis, 1973) showed that transection between the diencephalon and mesencephalon would reverse the blood-pressure elevations that had been produced by lesions in the nucleus of the tractus solitarius. This observation indicated that the blood-pressure elevation was maintained by a descending projection from the level of the diencephalon. This interpretation was confirmed by Brody and associates (Brody and Johnson 1980), who found that lesions confined to the anteroventral portion of the hypothalamus near the third ventricle (AV3V) reverse blood-pressure elevations in several models

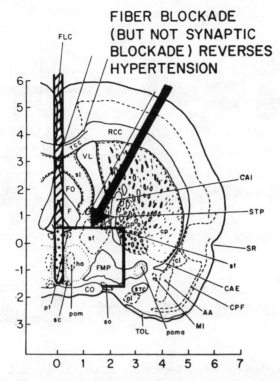

Figure 8. Diagram illustrating the limits of the spatial temperature gradient in the anterior hypothalamus (box) created by cooling the cryoprobe tip located at the midline. The region indicated by the box is between 10 and 20 °C when the tip temperature is at 5 °C; this same region is between 0 and 10 °C when the tip is at 0 °C. The 10–20 °C gradient is known to block synaptic activity, but not axonal transmission, whereas the 0–10 °C gradient blocks both types of neural activity. Blockade of synaptic activity alone in this anteroventral region of the third ventricle (i.e. AV3V) does not alter blood pressure elevations, as shown in Figure 8, whereas blockade of the fibers-of-passage through the AV3V normalizes blood pressure elevations.

of hypertension (mineralocorticoid, renovascular, salt sensitive); only the genetic model (spontaneously hypertensive rats, SHR) was not effected by this intervention. Lesions in the amygdala, however, were found to prevent the development of hypertension in the SHR (Galeno *et al.*, 1982).

Recently our laboratory has explored the possibility that the AV3V lesions might have disrupted fibers passing through the area rather than the local neural functioning. Cryoblockade has been shown to block synaptic function without altering axonal propagation when the tissue temperature range is between 20 and 10 °C and to block both neural activities when the gradient is between 10 to 0 °C (Benita and Conde, 1972; Brooks, 1983). Using cryoblockade of the AV3V tissue in rats, as illustrated in Figure 8, we determined that blockade of

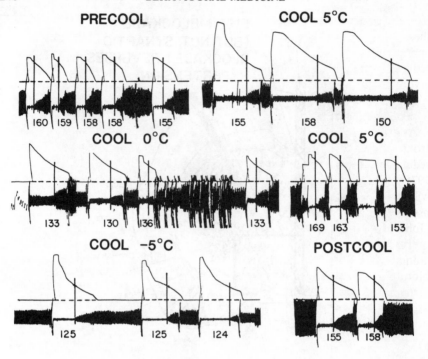

Figure 9. Effects of cryoprobe surface temperature on peak systolic blood pressure in the aldosterone-model of hypertension. Blood pressure was measured using the tail-cuff method in the warmed conscious rat. Hypertension developed slowly over a 4-week period of continuous administration of aldosterone by a subcutaneous Alzet Mini-pump; a total of 2 mg was delivered over the 4-week interval. The cryoprobe surface temperature is indicated above each pair of traces. The top trace shows the cuff pressure, the lower trace shows the systolic beats recorded from the distal tail, and the number below each trace-pair indicates the peak arterial pressure (mmHg) determined at the verticle line. (Unpublished data of Szilagyi and Skinner.)

local synaptic activity did not reverse blood-pressure elevations in two independent models of hypertension (mineralocorticoid and renovascular) but that blockade of both synaptic and axonal transmission did; furthermore cryoblockade in the frontal lobes was found to produce a similar effect (Szilagyi et al., 1987). As shown in Figure 9, we have also accumulated evidence that blockade along the trajectory of the frontocortical-brainstem pathway normalizes aldosterone-induced hypertension; this latter model of experimental hypertension is commonly thought to be purely peripheral in origin.

The origin of the fibers passing through the AV3V seems to be from the frontal cortex (mesoventral cortex anterior to the genu of the corpus callosum) as well as the amygdala, for cryoblockade of synaptic activity in either structure, between 10 and 20 °C, will reduce the blood-pressure elevations (Szilagyi and

Skinner, 1985; Szilagyi *et al.*, 1985, 1987). Synaptic cryoblockade in each of these two telencephalic locations reduces the blood-pressure elevations by approximately 50%, whereas cooling in AV3V at the fiber-blocking temperature reduces systolic blood pressure to normotensive levels. The fact that neither cryoblockade was found to have an affect on blood pressure in normotensive control rats is important; that is, the neurophysiological interventions reduce hypertension, not blood pressure.

As mentioned previously, our laboratory has shown that blockade of the frontocortical-brainstem pathway, which passes through the AV3V region, will reduce cardiac vulnerability to arrhythmogenesis in stressed pigs (Skinner *et al.*, 1975a). We also have preliminary evidence to show that amygdaloid blockade will also prevent the lethal consequence of coronary artery occlusion in psychologically stressed pigs (Skinner, 1985b). Johansson and associates (Johansson *et al.*, 1981) have shown that such amygdaloid lesions in pigs will prevent the myofibrillar degeneration found in the hearts of severely stressed animals. Thus blockade of the same two telencephalic structures that reduce blood-pressure elevations in hypertensive animals also blocks lethal arrhythmogenesis.

OTHER BRAIN SYSTEMS THAT REGULATE CARDIOVASCULAR DISORDERS

Why both the frontal cortex and amygdala are involved in the same types of cardiovascular disorders has an explanation in comparative anatomy, physiology, and behavior. MacLean's classical theory (MacLean, 1970) of human brain encephalization is based upon the studies of the brains and behaviors of various species. He has focused his theory by dwelling upon three species stereotypes and then arguing that the human brain is composed of a layered encephalization of these three brains, each controlling its own type of somatic behavior and autonomic support of that behavior. These layered structures are arranged in a hierarchical order so that each newer (i.e. more evolved) brain component can gain expression by inhibiting the functional outputs of the older ones below it. The diencephalic structures embody the behavioral and autonomic repertory characteristic of the reptiles. The limbic structures underlie the additional behavioral and autonomic activities typical of the rodents. The hypertrophy of the neocortex, especially that of the frontal lobes, is the cerebral component thought to mediate the characteristic human behaviors and the autonomic support that they require, both in actuality and as an anticipated behavior. The three layered components of the triune brain, in ascending hierarchical order are: reptilian, paleo-mammalian, and neo-mammalian.

The behavioral repertory of the paleo-mammalian (limbic) brain has been characterized primarily as a controller of stereotypical behavior associated with emotional affect (e.g. feeding, fleeing, fighting, and mating behavior). In contrast to these simple behaviors, those mediated by the neo-mammalian brain depend upon the degree of neocortical encephalization. For example, some environmental stimulus-situations will evoke behaviors in humans that can be characterized as 'bereavement, job insecurity, marital strife, being in an unfamiliar environment'; only the latter, however, could be expected to be evokable in the pig. Each of the stimulus-situations in this example is a proven psychosocial stressor that has been shown to place the human at higher risk of sudden cardiac death (Parkes, 1967). Only the latter stressor has been demonstrated, or could be expected to be demonstrated, for the pig (Skinner *et al.*, 1975a).

Although rats suffer various forms of hypertension, including that induced by at least one psychosocial stimulus-situation (Alexander, 1974), these animals do not seem to suffer lethal arrhythmogenesis, as do pigs and humans. Rodents have very little frontal cortex, a result which could be an explanation for why they don't manifest sudden cardiac death; that is, they do not have the perceptual and emotional apparatus to enable increased cardiac vulnerability to be evoked by the psychosocial stressors that uniquely activate the neo-mammalian brain. The more traditional argument that rodents have small hearts (a biological situation mitigating against re-entrant arrhythmogenesis), cannot explain the stress-evoked myofibrillar degeneration and arrhythmogenic deaths suffered by squirrel monkeys (Corley *et al.*, 1973), whose hearts are smaller than those of large rats.

The point expressed by these comparative animal studies is that psychosocial stress is a cerebral reaction that depends not only upon the psychological history of the organism (i.e. upon learning and memory), but also upon the *structure* of the brain systems involved. In the human and higher mammals (e.g. pigs), parallel sources of autonomic support activities descend from both the frontal cortex and amygdala and project to the brainstem cardiovascular centers: each system singly, or in combination with the other, could therefore contribute to the development and maintenance of cardiovascular diseases of cerebral etiology.

CONCLUSIONS

The primary trigger and/or cause of unexpected sudden death may be related to a cerebral noradrenergic over-reaction (i.e. pathology) that transmits a pattern of dual autonomic output to the heart to increase its vulnerability to arrhythmogenesis. The location of this cerebral dysfunction appears to be the frontal lobes (for psychosocial situations that evoke activity in the neo-mammalian cerebrum) and the amygdala (for simpler stimulus environments that evoke reactions in the paleo-mammalian brain). These two cerebral systems together normally orchestrate autonomic support and sensory inflow during and in anticipation of the unique behaviors that each one mediates. The cerebral defensive reactions are elicited by obvious psychosocial stressors, but perhaps in addition they are evoked by seemingly benign environmental situations to which the normally functioning brain readily habituates or adapts.

In cardiac patients with very high ectopy, an apparent cerebral dysfunction is detected as an enlarged cerebral response to a benign stimulus-event. Competitive inhibitors of beta-receptors as well as weak cholinergic muscarinic agonists have central actions, each of which suppresses the neuromodulation of synaptic throughput in cortical tissues (i.e. disables LTP). This central action, presumably in the frontal lobes and/or amygdala, reduces in concert the event-related cerebral potentials, dual autonomic tones, myofibrillar pathologies and cardiac ectopies that are evoked by stressors. The dysfunction is tentatively characterized as a *hyper-reactive noradrenergic* process that prevents learned habituation to stimulus-events that initially activate the cerebral defense system. This prevention of habituation results in the *inappropriate mobilization of autonomic responses*, an action which in turn and over time increases cardiac vulnerability to arrhythmogenesis. These same paleo- and neo-mammalian cerebral systems also appear to maintain the blood-pressure elevations in most models of experimental hypertension.

REFERENCES

Alexander, N. (1974). Psychosocial hypertension in members of a Wistar rat colony. *Proceedings of the Society of Experimental Biology in Medicine*, **146**, 163–169.

Andersen, P. and Wigstrom, H. (1980). In Tsukod, Y. and Aghawoff, B. W. (Eds), *Neurobiological Basis of Learning and Memory*. Wiley, New York, pp. 17–47.

Bard, P. (1960). Anatomical organization of the central nervous system in relation to control of the heart and blood vessels. *Physiology Reviews*, **40** (suppl. 4), 3–26.

Baust, W. and Bohnert, B. (1969). The regulation of heart rate during sleep. *Experimental Brain Research*, **7**, 169–180.

Benita, M. and Conde, H. (1972). Effects of local cooling upon conduction and synaptic transmission. *Brain Research*, **35**, 133–151.

Berridge, M. J. and Irvine, R. F. (1984). Review of: Inositol trisphosphate, a novel second messenger in cellular signal transduction. *Nature*, **312**, 315–321.

Beta-blocker Heart Attack Trials Research Group (1982). A randomized trial of propranolol in patients with acute myocardial infarctions. *Journal of the American Medical Association*, **247**, 1707–1714.

Billman, G. E., Schwartz, P. J. and Stone, H. L. (1982). Baroreceptor reflex control of heart rate: a predictor of sudden cardiac death. *Circulation*, **66**, 874–880.

Billman, G. E., Schwartz, P. J. and Stone, H. L. (1984). Effects of daily exercise on susceptibility to sudden cardiac death. *Circulation*, **69**, 1182–1189.

Birnbaumer, L., Codina, J., Mattera, R. *et al.* (1985). Regulation of hormone receptors and adenylyl cyclases by guanine nucleotide binding proteins. In Greep, R. D. (Ed.), *Recent Progress in Hormone Research. Proceedings of the 1984 Laurentian Hormone Conference*, vol. 41. Academic Press, 41–99.

Bliss, T. V. P., Goddard, G. V. and Rives, M. (1983). Reduction of long-term potentiation in the dentate gyrus of the rat following selective depletion of monoamines. *Journal of Physiology, London*, **334**, 475–491.

Brody, M. J. and Johnson, A. K. (1980). Role of forebrain structures in models of experimental hypertension. In Abboud, F. M., Fozzard, H. A., Gilmore, J. P. and Reis, D. J. (Eds), *Frontiers in Neuroendocrinology*, vol. 6. American Physiological Society, Bethesda, pp. 105-117.

Brooks, V. B. (1983). Study of brain function by local reversible cooling. *Reviews of Physiology, Biochemistry and Pharmacology*, **95**, 1-109.

Bungo, M. W. (1986). Personal communication from the Director of the Space Biomedical Research Institute of the Johnson Space Center, Houston. The composite updated data reported were from the entire Shuttle program to date. Additional supporting data from the Sky Lab program are to be found in Smith, R. F., Stanton, K., Stoop, D., Brown, D., Janusz, W. and King, P. Vectorcardiographic changes during extended space flight (M093): observations at rest and during exercise. In Johnston, R. S. and Dietlein, R. S. (Eds), *Biomedical Results from Skylab*, NASA SP-377, 1977, pp. 399-350.

Bungo, M. W. and Johnson, P. C., Jr. (1983). Cardiovascular examinations and observations. In Pool, S. L., Johnson, P. C. Jr. and Mason, J. A. (Eds), *Shuttle OFT Medical Report: summary of medical results from STS-1, STS-2, STS-3 and STS-4*, NASA Technical Memorandum 58252, 1983, pp. 17-22.

Burrell, R. J. W. (1963). The possible bearing of curse death and other factors in Bantu culture on the etiology of myocardial infarction. In James, T. N. and Keys, J. W. (Eds), *The Etiology of Myocardial Infarction*. Henry Ford Hospital International Symposium, Little Brown and Co., Boston, 1963, pp. 95-100.

Cannon, W. B. (1931). Again the James-Lange and the thalamic theories of emotion. *Psychology Reviews*, **38**, 281-295.

Cannon, W. B. (1942). 'Voodoo' death. *American Anthropology*, **44**, 169-181.

Cebelin, M. S. and Hirsch, C. S. (1980). Human stress cardiomyopathy: myocardial lesions in victims of homicidal assaults without internal injuries. *Human Pathology*, **11**, 123-132.

Corley, K C., Shiel, F. O. M., Mauck, H. P. and Greenhoot, J. (1973). Electrocardiographic and cardiac morphologic changes associated with environmental stress in squirrel monkeys. *Psychosomatic Medicine*, **35**, 361-364.

Delgado, J. M. R. (1960). Circulatory effects of cortical stimulation. *Physiology Reviews*, **40** (suppl. 4), 146-171.

Doba, N. and Reis, D. J. (1973). Acute fulminating neurogenic hypertension produced by brainstem lesions in rat. *Circulation Research*, **32**, 584-593.

Eliot, R. S. and Buell, J. C. (1985). Role of emotions and stress in the genesis of sudden death. *Journal of the American College of Cardiology*, **5**, 95H-98H.

Galeno, T. M., Van Hoesen, G. W., Maixner, W., Johnson, A. K. and Brody, M. J. (1982). Contribution of the amygdala to the development of spontaneous hypertension. *Brain Research*, **246**, 1-6.

Garvey, J. L. and Melville, K. I. (1969). Cardiovascular effects of lateral hypothalamic stimulation in normal and coronary-ligated dogs. *Journal of Cardiovascular Surgery*, **10**, 377-385.

Goodman, L. S. and Gillman, A. (1970). *The Pharmacological Basis of Therapeutics*. Macmillan, New York, p. 569.

Gray, C. M., Freeman, W. J. and Skinner, J. E. (1984). Associative changes in the spatial amplitude patterns of rabbit olfactory EEG are norepinephrine-dependent. *Society for Neuroscience Abstracts*, **10**, 121.

Gray, C. M., Freeman, W. J. and Skinner, J. E. (1986). Chemical dependencies of learning in the rabbit olfactory bulb: acquisition of the transient spatial pattern change depends on norepinephrine. *Behavioral Neuroscience*, **100**, 585-596.

Gregg, D. E. (1971). Sudden cardiac death. In Wolf, S. (Ed.), *The Artery and the Process of Arteriosclerosis*, Plenum Press, New York, p. 273.

Hall, R. E., Sybers, H. D., Greenhoot, J. H. and Bloor, C. M. (1974). Myocardial alterations after hypothalamic stimulation in the intact conscious dog. *American Heart Journal*, **88**, 770–776.

Hall, R. E., Livingstone, R. R. and Bloor, M. D. (1977). Orbital cortical influences on cardiovascular dynamics and myocardial structure in conscious monkeys. *Journal of Neurosurgery*, **46**, 638–647.

Hilton, S. M. (1980). Inhibition of the baroreceptor reflex by the brainstem defense centre. In Sleight, P. (Ed.), *Arterial Baroreceptors and Hypertension*. Oxford University Press, Oxford, pp. 318–323.

Hockman, C. H., Mauck, H. P. and Hoff, E. C. (1966). ECG changes resulting from cerebral stimulation. II. A spectrum of ventricular arrhythmias of sympathetic origin. *American Heart Journal*, **71**, 695–701.

Hopkins, W. F. and Johnston, D. (1984). Frequency-dependent noradrenergic modulation of long-term potentiation in the hippocampus. *Science*, **226**, 350–352.

Irwin, D. A., Knott, J. R., McAdam, D. W. and Rebert, C. S. (1966). Motivational determinants of the 'contingent negative variation'. *Electroencephalography and Clinical Neurophysiology*, **21**, 538–543.

Jenkins, C. D. (1976). Recent evidence supporting psychosocial risk factors for coronary disease. *New England Journal of Medicine*, **294**, 987 and 1033.

Johansson, G., Johnson, L., Lannek, N., Blomgren, L., Lindberg, P. and Pouph, O. (1974). Severe stress-cardiopathy in pigs. *American Heart Journal*, **87**, 451–457.

Johansson, G., Olsson, K., Haggendal, J., Johnson, L. and Thoren-Tolling, K. (1981). Effect of amygdalectomy on stress-induced myocardial necroses and blood levels of catecholamines in pigs. *Acta Physiology Scandinavica*, **113**, 553–555.

Krontiris-Litowitz, J., Skinner, J. E. and Birnbaumer, L. (1985). A muscarinic agonist (Ethmozine) prevents long-term potentiation in the hippocampal slice. *Society for Neuroscience Abstracts*, **11**, 781.

Krontiris-Litowitz, J., Skinner, J. E., Mattera, R. and Birnbaumer, L. (1987). Use-dependent block of synaptic plasticity is enabled by the cardiac drug, Ethmozine (submitted).

Levitt, P. and Noebels, J. L. (1981). Mutant mouse tottering: selective increase of locus ceruleus axons in a defined single-locus mutation. *Proceedings of the National Academy of Science*, USA, **78**, 4630–4634.

Loveless, N. E. and Sanford, A. J. (1974). Slow potential components of preparatory set. *Biology and Psychology*, **1**, 303–314.

MacLean, P. D. (1970). The triune brain, emotion and scientific bias. In Schmitt, F. O. (Ed.), *The Neurosciences, Second Study Program*. Rockefeller University Press, New York, pp. 336–348.

Manning, J. W. and Cotten, M. de V. (1962). Mechanism of cardiac arrhythmias induced by diencephalic stimulation. *American Journal of Physiology*, **203**, 1120–1124.

Mauck, H. O., Hockman, C. H. and Hoff, E. C. (1964). ECG changes after cerebral stimulation of the mesencephalic reticular formation. *American Heart Journal*, **68**, 98–101.

Melville, K. I., Blum, B., Shister, H. E. and Sliver, M. D. (1963). Cardiac ischemic changes in arrhythmias induced by hypothalamic stimulation. *American Journal of Cardiology*, **12**, 781–791.

Nishizuka, Y. (1984). Turnover of inositol phospholipids and signal transduction. *Science*, **225**, 1365–1370.

Neurotech Laboratories, Inc. (1987). Supporting data for the 'Stress-analyzer'. Neurotech Laboratories, Inc., The Woodlands, Texas, 77381.

Parkes, C. M. (1967). Bereavement. *British Medical Journal*, **3**, 232–233.

Rahe, R. H., Bennett, L., Romo, M., Seltanen, P. and Arthur, R. S. (1973). Subject's recent life changes and coronary heart disease in Finland. *American Journal of Psychiatry*, **130**, 1222–1226.

Rees, W. D. and Lutkins, S. G. (1967). Mortality of bereavement. *British Medical Journal*, **4**, 13–16.

Reich, P., DeSilva, R. A., Lown, B. and Murawski, J. (1981). Acute psychological disturbances preceding life-threatening ventricular arrhythmias. *Journal of the American Medical Association*, **246**, 233–235.

Rissanen, V., Romo, M. and Seltanen, P. (1978). Premonitory symptoms and stress factor preceding sudden death from ischemic heart disease. *Acta Medica Scandinavica*, **204**, 389.

Shaper, W. (1971). *The Collateral Circulation of the Heart*. North-Holland Biomedical Press, Amsterdam.

Schwartz, P. J., Billman, G. E. and Stone, H. L. (1984). Autonomic mechanisms in ventricular fibrillation induced by myocardial ischemia during exercise in dogs with healed myocardial infarction. *Circulation*, **69**, 790–800.

Shepherd, G. M. (1970). The olfactory bulb as a simple cortical system: Experimental analysis and functional implications. In Schmitt, F. O. (Ed.), *The Neurosciences: Second Study Program*. Rockefeller University Press, New York, pp. 539–552.

Skinner, J. E. (1971). Abolition of a conditioned, surface-negative, cortical potential during cryogenic blockade of the nonspecific thalamo-cortical system. *Electroencephalography and Clinical Neurophysiology*, **31**, 197–209.

Skinner, J. E. (1984). Central gating mechanisms that regulate event-related potentials and behavior. In Elbert, T., Rochstroh, B., Lutzenberger, W. and Birnbaumer, N. (Eds), *Self-Regulation of the Brain and Behavior*. Springer-Verlag, New York, pp. 42–58.

Skinner, J. E. (1985a). The regulation of cardiac vulnerability by the cerebral defense system. *Journal of the American College of Cardiology*, **5**, 88B–94B.

Skinner, J. E. (1985b). Psychosocial stress and sudden cardiac death: brain mechanisms. In Beamish, R. E., Singal, P. K. and Dhalla, N. S. (Eds), *Stress and Heart Disease*. Martinus Nijhoff, Boston, pp. 44–59.

Skinner, J. E., Beder, S. D. and Entman, M. L. (1983). Psychological stress activates phosphorylase in the heart of the conscious pig without increasing heart rate and blood pressure. *Proceedings of the National Academy of Sciences*, USA, **80**, 4513–4517.

Skinner, J. E., Caplan, J. P., Welch, K. M. A. and Helpern, J. A. (1987). Event-related noradrenergic responses and slow potential shifts in the cortex of the conscious rat (submitted).

Skinner, J. E., Lie, J. T. and Entman, M. L. (1975a). Modification of ventricular fibrillation latency following coronary artery occlusion in the conscious pig: the effects of psychological stress and beta-adrenergic blockade. *Circulation*, **51**, 656–667.

Skinner, J. E., Mohr, D. N. and Kellaway, P. (1975b). Sleep-stage regulation of ventricular arrhythmias in the unanesthetized pig. *Circulation Research*, **37**, 342–349.

Skinner, J. E. and Molnar, M. (1983). Event-related extracellular potassium-ion activity changes in the frontal cortex of the conscious cat. *Neurophysiology*, **49**, 204–215.

Skinner, J. E., Montaron, M-F. and Pratt, C. M. (1982). Efficacy of antiarrhythmic drugs in cardiac patients is proportional to their ability to reduce the amplitude of the cerebral event-related slow potential. *Society for Neuroscience Abstracts*, **8**, 428.

Skinner, J. E. and Reed, J. C. (1981). Blockade of a frontocortical-brainstem pathway prevents ventricular fibrillation of the ischemic heart in pigs. *American Journal of Physiology*, **240**, H156–H163.

Skinner, J. E., Welch, K. M. A., Reed, J. C. and Nell, J. H. (1978). Cyclic 3′,5′-adenosine monophosphate level in conscious rat. *Journal of Neurochemistry*, **30**, 691–698.

Skinner, J. E. and Yingling, C. D. (1976). Regulation of slow potential shifts in nucleus reticularis thalami by the mesencephalic reticular formation and the frontal cortex. *Electroencephalography and Clinical Neurophysiology*, **40**, 288–296.

Skinner, J. E. and Yingling, C. D. (1977). Central gating mechanisms that regulate event-related potentials and behavior: a neural model for attention. In Desmedt, J. E. (Ed.), *Progress in Clinical Neurophysiology*, vol. I. Karger-Basel, Brussels, pp. 30–69.

Swanson, L. W., Teyler, T. J. and Thompson, R. F. (Eds) (1982). Hippocampus long-term potentiation: mechanisms and implications for memory. *Neuroscience Research Progress Bulletin*, **20**, 613–769.

Szilagyi, J. E. and Skinner, J. E. (1985). Blockade of the amygdaloid nuclei partially reverses doca-salt hypertension. *Society Neuroscience Abstract*, **11**, 996.

Szilagyi, J. E., Skinner, J. E., Taylor, A. A. and Mitchell, J. R. (1985). Evidence that the frontal cortex maintains elevated blood pressure in hypertension. *Federal Proceedings*, **44**, 629.

Szilagyi, J. E., Taylor, A. A. and Skinner, J. E. (1987). Cryoblockade of ventromedial frontal cortex reverses hypertension in the rat. *Hypertension* (in press).

Ulyanisky, L. S., Stepanyan, E. P. and Krymsky, I. P. (1977). Cardiac arrhythmias of hypothalamic origin in sudden death. In *Proceedings USA–USSR Joint Symposium on Sudden Death*, DHEW No. (NIH) 78-1472. US Government Printing Office, Washington, D.C., pp. 417–429.

Verrier, R. L. and Lown, B. (1981). Autonomic nervous system and malignant cardiac arrhythmias. In Weiner, H., Hofer, M. A. and Stunkard, A. J. (Eds), *Brain, Behavior, and Bodily Disease*. New York, Raven, pp. 273–291.

Watanabe, A. M., McConnaughey, M. M., Strawbridge, R. A., Fleming, J. W., Jones, L. R. and Besch, H. R. Jr. (1978). Muscarinic cholinergic receptor modulation of beta-adrenergic receptor affinity for catecholamines. *Journal of Biological Chemistry*, **253**, 4833–4836.

Weinberg, S. J. and Fuster, J. M. (1960). Electrocardiographic changes produced by localized hypothalamic stimulations. *Annals of Internal Medicine*, **53**, 332–341.

Wolf, S. (1967). Neural mechanisms in sudden cardiac death. The Jeremiah Metzger Lecture. *Transactions of the American Clinical Climatology Association*, **79**, 158–176.

Wolf, S. (1969). Psychosocial forces in myocardial infarction and sudden death. *Circulation* (suppl. IV), **30–40**, 74–81.

Yingling, C. D. and Skinner, J. E. (1977). Gating of thalamic input to cerebral cortex by nucleus reticularis thalami. In Desmedt, J. E. (Ed.), *Progress in Clinical Neurophysiology*, vol. I. Karger-Basel, Brussels, 70–96.

Behavioural Medicine in Cardiovascular Disorders
Edited by T. Elbert, W. Langosch, A. Steptoe and D. Vaitl
©1988 John Wiley & Sons Ltd

17

Cardiovascular Aspects of Panic Disorder

Anke Ehlers*, Jürgen Margraf*,
C. Barr Taylor[†] and Walton T. Roth[†]

*Department of Psychology, Philipps-University, Marburg, Gutenbergstr.
18, D-3550 Marburg, FRG, [†]Department of Psychiatry and
Behavioral Sciences, Stanford University School of Medicine, USA*

INTRODUCTION

The purpose of this chapter is to review the relationship of panic disorder and the cardiovascular system from a psychophysiological perspective. Panic disorder leads the list of psychiatric disorders for which people seek professional help (Boyd, 1986). Recent large-scale epidemiological studies establish a high prevalence of the disorder (Robins et al., 1984; Wittchen, 1986). Lifetime prevalence rates reported for panic disorder without agoraphobia range from 1.4 or 1.5% in the United States to 2.4% in Germany. Even higher rates are found for panic disorder with agoraphobic avoidance behavior.

The relationship of panic attacks and cardiovascular physiology and pathology has attracted considerable interest for a number of reasons. First, panic disorder patients experience a multitude of somatic symptoms during their anxiety attacks. At the beginning of the disorder, they usually do not present to psychiatrists or psychologists, but to emergency rooms, primary care physicians, or cardiologists. Second, cardiovascular complaints number among the patients' most frequent and distressing symptoms (Barlow et al., 1985; Margraf et al., 1987b). The physiological changes that correspond to these symptoms are yet unclear. Third, many panic patients suffer from intense fear of having a heart attack during a panic episode. They usually undergo a series of elaborate diagnostic tests and are then reassured that their condition is not medically dangerous. Fourth, on the other hand, there have been reports of excessive cardiovascular mortality in patients with panic disorder. And finally, it has been hypothesized that panic disorder is causally related to a particular cardiovascular condition, mitral valve prolapse.

We will begin our review of the relationship of panic disorder and the cardiovascular system with some historical remarks on this topic and a discussion of differential diagnoses. We will then review studies of the cardiovascular physiology of panic patients in the laboratory and in their natural environment. In particular, we will address the following questions:

—What are the cardiovascular changes during panic attacks?
—Are there cardiovascular differences between panic patients and control subjects?
—What is the role of physical conditioning in panic disorder?
—What is the relationship of panic disorder and mitral valve prolapse?
—Is there an elevated cardiovascular mortality in panic patients?

We will not deal with the role of anxiety in cardiovascular disease like myocardial infarction (see Section III of this book for discussions of this topic).

PANIC AND THE CARDIOVASCULAR SYSTEM: A HISTORICAL PERSPECTIVE

The *Diagnostic and Statistical Manual of Mental Disorders* (third edition, revised, DSM-III-R) of the American Psychiatric Association (APA, 1987) defines panic attacks as discrete episodes of intense fear or discomfort with symptoms such as dyspnea, palpitations, chest pain, faintness, sweating, hot flushes or chills, feelings of unreality, or fear of dying or going crazy. Panic attacks have a sudden onset and occur at times unpredictably. Many patients with panic disorder develop phobic avoidance behavior.

Interest in the panic syndrome as a separate diagnostic entity is very recent. Although Freud had described the phenomenon of panic attacks already in 1895, they were given explicit diagnostic relevance only 85 years later with the publication of DSM-III (APA, 1980). The renewed interest is associated with medical models of panic attacks (for a review, see Margraf et al., 1986a). DSM-III-R emphasizes the role of panic attacks within the anxiety disorders even more than DSM-III. For example, the DSM-III diagnosis 'agoraphobia with panic attacks' has been changed to 'panic disorder with agoraphobia' because panic attacks are considered the primary phenomenon.

Cardiovascular manifestations of anxiety have been known in the medical and psychological sciences for a long time. The clinical descriptions of patients with various diagnoses such as 'Da Costa's syndrome', 'soldier's heart', 'effort syndrome', 'neuro-circulatory asthenia', or 'cardiac neurosis' bear many similarities to the diagnostic criteria for panic disorder (Skerritt, 1983). As Skerritt points out in his review, interest in these syndromes was always stimulated in times of war when it became apparent that some young men were incapacitated by functional cardiac complaints. In times of peace, similar syndromes were also described for civilians (mostly women), but the focus was on symptoms from other organ systems. Perhaps due to the wide variations in symptom patterns between the different patient groups, experts in the 19th century did not reach agreement as to the etiology of the conditions designated by these labels.

Not much has changed since then. There still is much controversy on the etiology of what is now called panic disorder (cf. Margraf *et al.*, 1986a). It is interesting that many of the current research ideas on panic disorder that we will review in this chapter, such as the relationship with hyperventilation syndrome, blood acid–base balance, or exercise intolerance, were already mentioned in the scientific literature of the 19th and early 20th century. Similarly, in a thoughtful editorial entitled 'Where are the diseases of yesteryear?' Wooley (1976) pointed out the close relationship between the historical diagnoses mentioned above and the mitral valve prolapse syndrome (see p. 269 ff.).

DIAGNOSTIC CONSIDERATIONS

Research in psychiatry used to be hampered by a low reliability of psychiatric diagnoses. Inter-rater agreement on neurotic disorders tended to be very low (cf. Jablensky, 1985). In recent years, significant progress has been made in improving diagnostic reliability. DSM-III has contributed to this development by specifying symptoms and criteria for each diagnostic category. Another important contribution was the development of structured diagnostic interviews. With these interviews, inter-rater and test-retest reliabilities for panic disorder now reach moderate to high levels (Di Nardo *et al.*, 1983; Wittchen and Semler, 1986).

The diagnostic criteria for panic disorder in DSM-III required that panic attacks were not 'due to a physical disorder or another mental disorder, such as major depression, somatization disorder, or schizophrenia' (APA, 1980, p. 232). However, DSM-III-R no longer requires the exclusion of other mental disorders. Only organic causes of panic attacks have to be ruled out. This differential diagnosis, however, is quite complex. The majority of the patients undergo several specialty consultations with lengthy work-ups and many diagnostic tests before receiving the diagnosis of panic disorder (Katon, 1984).

Many diverse medical conditions can present with symptoms of anxiety (McCue and McCue, 1984; Jacob and Rapport, 1984; Lesser and Rubin, 1986). They range from abnormalities in endocrine hormone function (like hyperthyroidism, Cushing's syndrome, or pheochromocytoma) to neurologic disorders (like temporal lobe epilepsy, Meniere's disease, or labyrinthitis). It has to be ruled out that panic symptoms result from substance abuse (e.g., amphetamines, cocaine, appetite suppressants, or caffeine) or from substance withdrawal (e.g., benzodiazepines or alcohol). In addition, hypoglycemia, allergies, and several cardiovascular and respiratory conditions may present with panic-like symptoms. Among the cardiological diagnoses, the overlap of panic disorder and mitral valve prolapse has received the most attention. We will discuss the relationship of these syndromes later.

There is converging evidence for a significant overlap of panic disorder and hyperventilation (Lum, 1981; Garssen *et al.*, 1983; Rapee, 1986; Salkovskis and Clark, 1986). Symptoms like dizziness, paresthesias, chest pain, and even S-T segment changes in the ECG can be caused by habitual and acute hyperventilation (Katon, 1984). Respiratory training has been shown to be beneficial in the treatment of panic attacks (for a summary see Salkovskis and Clark, 1986). Furthermore, evidence from our laboratory shows that there is a substantial overlap between panic and somatization disorder (King *et al.*, 1986; cf. Katon, 1984).

The *International Classification of Diseases, Injuries and Causes of Death* (ICD-9, World Health Organization, 1977) distinguishes between anxiety states (300.0) and functional respiratory and cardiovascular complaints (Respiratory or cardiovascular malfunction arising from mental factors, 306.1 or 306.2). In Europe, a diagnosis of cardiac neurosis is often given to patients who would be classified as panic disorder according to DSM-III (cf. Jablensky, 1985). Buller *et al.* (1987), using structured interview techniques, found that the diagnosis 'cardiac neurosis' can be considered a subtype of the DSM-III diagnosis 'panic disorder'. Other authors argue, however, that not all cardiac neurotics meet diagnostic criteria for panic disorder (e.g., Beunderman *et al.*, 1987).

The subgroup of panic patients that would be diagnosed as cardiac neurotics according to ICD-9 is especially likely to undergo extensive and expensive diagnostic work-ups to rule out cardiological disorders. Between 43 and 57% of patients referred for coronary angiography with angiographically normal coronary arteries have panic attacks (Beitman *et al.*, 1987; Hall *et al.*, 1987). It would be desirable to develop more efficient methods for differential diagnoses.

Beunderman *et al.* (1987) compared patients with non-cardiac chest pain attending an emergency coronary care unit with patients hospitalized because of myocardial infarction. On the basis of self-reported symptom patterns alone, Beunderman *et al.* were able to classify 76% of the patients correctly using discriminant analyses. When sex, age, and help-seeking behavior were added, the number of correct classifications rose to 94%. In a recent study (Margraf *et al.*, in preparation), we have replicated Beunderman's finding that patients with functional cardiac complaints (the majority of whom had panic attacks) experience pain primarily at the left upper part of the body, whereas patients with organic cardiac syndromes report bilateral pain. Similar findings were reported by Mukerji *et al.* (1987) (cf. Hayward *et al.*, in press).

In summary, recent methodological advances enable us to diagnose panic disorder with greater reliability. The development of more economic methods for differentiating between panic disorder and organic syndromes remains an important task for future research. A step in this direction are recent studies that systematically compared the symptom patterns of panic disorder patients and patients with heart disease.

LABORATORY STUDIES OF PANIC DISORDER

Physiology of panic attacks: case reports

The DSM-III-R definition and clinical reports emphasize the abruptness of panic attack symptoms. Since panic attacks are rare events, naturally occurring attacks are seldom observed in the laboratory. The few published reports of such observations all find evidence for abrupt changes in physiological parameters. Lader and Mathews (1970) observed panic attacks in three anxiety patients during psychophysiological recording sessions. Heart rate and skin conductance levels increased in all three patients. Heart rate increases of 40 to 50 beats per minute (bpm) occurred within 30 to 90 seconds. The maximum heart rates reached during the attacks were about 120, 130, and 138 bpm, respectively. The electromyogram and number of skin conductance fluctuations showed less consistent changes. Cohen *et al.* (1985) reported two cases of relaxation-associated panic attacks observed in their laboratory. In both patients, heart rate and frontalis EMG increased abruptly within 1 or 2 minutes. Heart rate accelerated by roughly 50 bpm and reached maxima of about 100 and 115 bpm, respectively. In addition, there were small increases in hand temperature. In our laboratory, we observed a panic attack associated with false heart rate feedback (Margraf *et al.*, 1987a). The patient's heart rate rose more than 50 bpm in less than a minute (maximum heart rate 123 bpm). Her systolic and diastolic blood pressure and skin conductance level also increased during the attack.

Physiology of panic attacks: group studies

It is unclear whether the abrupt physiological changes described in the cited case reports are representative of naturally occurring panic attacks. A study by Cameron *et al.* (1987) suggests they are not. These authors had patients with frequent panic attacks staying in bed for extended periods of time. Several biochemical and physiological measures were taken at frequent intervals and whenever patients reported panic. This study failed to find any pattern of physiological changes during panic attacks that was consistent across all patients.

Another, much more widely used approach to studying the physiology of panic attacks in the laboratory is to induce them experimentally with pharmacologic agents like sodium lactate, carbon dioxide, caffeine, isoproterenol or yohimbine (for reviews, see Guttmacher *et al.*, 1983; Ehlers *et al.*, 1986a; Shear, 1986). Researchers use such panic induction methods to gain insights into the pathophysiology of panic attacks. Furthermore, reliable panic challenges are considered useful tools in the evaluation of treatments.

The status of lactate infusion studies is representative of this line of research since lactate is the most widely used substance to elicit panic attacks in the laboratory (for a review, see Margraf *et al.*, 1986b). Current research elaborates on older studies from the 1960s and early 1970s that related sodium lactate to anxiety in general. The first study by Pitts and McClure (1967) was inspired by reports that patients with anxiety neurosis showed excessive lactate production and anxiety symptoms during exercise. Pitts and McClure developed the idea that the lactate ion itself could produce anxiety attacks in susceptible persons. In a double-blind study, they found lactate infusion to produce anxiety attacks in 13 of 14 anxiety neurotics but only in 2 of 10 normal controls. Interest in lactate infusions vanished temporarily when Pitts' and McClure's original explanation for lactate's panic-inducing effects was rejected. The recent revival of interest in the method came with the focus on panic attacks in anxiety research. Several studies have reported that lactate produces panic attacks in panic disorder patients, but not in normal controls.

However, as we have outlined elsewhere (Margraf et al., 1986b), these reports are inconclusive because of severe methodological shortcomings. The sensitivity and specificity of lactate as a panic challenge is low. Furthermore, the mechanism by which lactate induces anxiety remains unclear (Margraf et al., 1986b; Liebowitz et al., 1986). Psychological factors such as expectancy affect the outcome of laboratory panic induction methods. The lack of attention to such methodologic detail limits their usefulness in understanding panic.

The results of our review of lactate infusion studies (Margraf et al., 1986b) and two studies from our laboratory showed that baseline levels of anxiety and cardiovascular arousal have to be taken into account in the interpretation of panic induction studies. Using lactate infusion (Ehlers et al., 1986b) and carbon dioxide inhalation (Ehlers et al., 1988a), we found that the major difference between panic disorder patients and normal controls was in their tonic levels of anxiety and heart rate throughout the laboratory sessions. The pattern of response to the 'panic challenges', however, was similar in both groups. Both groups showed increases in anxiety and cardiovascular arousal. Furthermore, the results indicated that it is inappropriate to use a simple dichotomy panic/non-panic to describe the effects of panic provocation methods.

As of today, it is unclear how similar the effects of lactate infusions and other so-called panic induction methods are to naturally occurring panic attacks. Based on the patients' reports and some of the induced physiological changes, we can expect at least some degree of similarity. Consistently across all studies, the anxiogenic effects of lactate infusions were found to be accompanied by increases in heart rate (of about 20 beats/min), blood pressure, skin conductance level, and forearm blood flow. The electromyogram and respiration rate failed to show consistent changes. The electroencephalogram showed increased beta and delta, and decreased alpha. In contrast to self-report and psychophysiological variables, biochemical measures did not consistently indicate heightened arousal or stress-related hormonal changes. Interestingly, there were no consistent changes of peripheral catecholamines in lactate-induced anxiety.

Similar results were obtained with another anxiety-induction technique, a 20-minute inhalation of 5% carbon dioxide (CO_2). We have by now tested some 80 patients and 40 controls with this paradigm. Like lactate infusions, this procedure leads to increases in anxiety, heart rate (about 10 beats/min), blood pressure and skin conductance level.

While the pattern of changes in some of the variables resembles the results of the case reports reviewed earlier (p. 259), there is one important difference: the physiological changes induced by lactate or carbon dioxide in our laboratory were usually gradual and smooth, and lacked the abruptness described for naturally occurring attacks. As we will outline in section 5, however, we have to know more about the physiological changes during naturally occurring panic before we can reach a final conclusion on the similarity of pharmacologic panic provocation and natural panic. Thus, conclusions on cardiovascular changes during panic attacks drawn from these studies have to be considered preliminary.

Physiology of panic attacks in feared situations

Another approach in studying the physiology of panic attacks is to expose patients to anxiety-provoking situations or stimuli, either *in vivo* or by phobic imagery. This approach is restricted to patients who are able to identify such stimuli. There is a large amount of literature on physiological changes during exposure to phobic stimuli that we are unable to review here (see Curtis *et al.*, 1982; Weiner, 1985). However, the results of most of the older studies do not apply directly to our topic since patients were not selected for a history of panic attacks. It is uncertain to what degree the panic that phobics experience during exposure resembles the panic attacks of patients with panic disorder.

Recently, researchers have started to systematically recruit agoraphobics with panic attacks to study their physiology during exposure. Ko *et al.* (1983) studied 6 patients with panic disorder. As a part of a treatment study, they measured plasma levels of MHPG (3-methoxy-4-hydroxyphenylethylene glycol), as an indicator of brain noradrenergic neuronal activity, 30 minutes after the patients had exposed themselves to phobic situations. After exposure-induced panic attacks, plasma MHPG was significantly elevated compared to days without exposure. The MHPG levels correlated significantly with a questionnaire measure of 'subjective and somatic anxiety'. Although the absolute increase of MHPG after exposure was smaller when subjects had been treated with imipramine and clonidine, the absence of a statistical interaction in the analysis of variance employed does not allow to interpret this change. Since less than 30% of plasma MHPG comes from the CNS, it is also unclear if the elevations in MHPG were not caused by peripheral catecholamines. Unfortunately, the study did not include a comparison group to control for effects of physical activity during exposure.

A recent study by Woods *et al.* (1987) used this control strategy and failed to find larger increases in plasma MHPG in the patient group. Eighteen medication-free panic patients were exposed to their phobic situations. Their responses were compared with those of 13 matched controls. Patients that reported panic attacks showed larger increases in mean heart rate (by 23 bpm) than controls (12 bpm). Increases in blood pressure, plasma MHPG, cortisol, and growth hormone were similar in both groups. Plasma prolactin increased slightly more in the control group. Patients had higher levels of systolic blood pressure prior to the exposure.

In a study from our laboratory (Roth *et al.*, 1986), the heart rates of 37 agoraphobics with panic attacks and 19 matched non-anxious controls were compared before and during a standard test walk in a shopping mall. Thirty-five patients were unable to complete the test walk because of overwhelming anxiety. The patients' heart rates were significantly higher both before and during the test walk. The increase in mean heart rate from baseline to the test walk was equal in both groups (16 vs 14 bpm for patients and controls, respectively). Differences in walking speed did not account for the lack of difference in heart rate increases. When walking heart rates were adjusted for sitting heart rates by analysis of covariance, some evidence for higher reactivity in the patient group emerged. Öst (1987) reported similar findings. Agoraphobics (with and without panic attacks) showed similar increases in heart rate as social and simple phobics when patients were exposed to their phobic situations. They had, however, higher heart rates than the clinical control groups before and during the exposure test.

It is unclear why the results of Roth *et al.* and Öst differ from those of Woods *et al.* One possible explanation is the law of initial values (Wilder, 1931). Higher baseline heart rates may have downscaled the agoraphobics' reactivity in the studies of Roth *et al.* and Öst. Woods *et al.* did not find such baseline differences in heart rate. The average baseline heart rate in their patient group was 17 to 18 bpm lower than in the studies of Roth *et al.* and Öst. However, Woods' control group also showed less reactivity than Roth's controls. Furthermore, there is little evidence in the psychophysiological literature that the law of initial values as formulated by Wilder applies to heart rate reactivity (Myrtek, 1984). It is possible that Roth's and Öst's patients, in contrast to Woods', already differed from controls in their anticipatory heart rate responses.

Thus, as of today, the evidence for distinct physiological patterns during situational panic attacks is limited. Further research should explore possibilities to induce panic by exposure to situations that do not involve significant physical activity of the subjects (for instance, driving). The results may be more conclusive if the effects of anxiety and physical activity are not confounded.

Cardiovascular reactivity and hypertension during panic-free periods

Katon (1984) reported an elevated rate of hypertension (15%) among 46 panic disorder patients referred for psychiatric consultation by primary care physicians.

This is in keeping with Noyes *et al.* (1978) who found an increased rate of hypertension in anxiety neurotics. However, these results might not be representative for all panic disorder patients since most laboratory studies, including our own, did not find evidence for hypertension in panic patients.

In the same vein, panic disorder patients were usually not found to be more reactive to standard cardiovascular stress tests than are controls. Grunhaus *et al.* (1983) compared the responses of 6 panic disorder patients and 7 normal controls to the cold pressor test. No differences were found in blood pressure and prolactin levels and responses. In our laboratory, we have tested large numbers of subjects with the cold pressor test or mental arithmetic and have also found that panic disorder patients are not more responsive than matched controls on measures of self-reported anxiety and excitement, heart rate, blood pressure, skin conductance level, and skin conductance fluctuations (Ehlers *et al.*, 1988a). Other authors have even found smaller heart rate reactivity to mental arithmetic in anxious patients (Kelly *et al.*, 1970).

In another study from our laboratory, little evidence was found for differences in reactivity and habituation to neutral and startling auditory stimuli between agoraphobics with panic attacks and normal controls on heart rate and skin conductance measures (Roth *et al.*, 1986). The major difference between the groups was the patients' higher skin conductance and heart rate levels. The results were different from Lader's reports of slower habituation of the skin conductance response in agoraphobics and anxiety neurotics (Lader and Wing, 1964; Lader, 1967). This discrepancy may be due to the fact that Lader used tones of a higher intensity likely to elicit 'defense' rather than 'orienting' responses. Thus, reactivity differences, if they exist, are at least considerably less general than assumed in much of the earlier work.

In our laboratory, we have observed reactivity differences between panic patients and controls under two different conditions, both of which involve cognitive processes. First, patients responded stronger to the anticipation of an anxiety induction procedure (carbon dioxide inhalation) than control subjects (Ehlers *et al.*, 1988a). Before the CO_2-inhalation, subjects were given room air through a gas mask for 15 minutes. They knew that CO_2 would be given at some time during a longer inhalation period, but were not informed about when exactly CO_2 would be given. Patients showed larger blood pressure and heart rate responses than controls during the anticipation period. In contrast, on a previous test day when subjects did not expect CO_2, wearing the mask did not lead to any changes in cardiovascular measures.

In another experiment, 25 patients and 25 controls were given false feedback of an abrupt heart rate increase. On all measures (self-reported anxiety and excitement, skin conductance level, heart rate, systolic and diastolic blood pressure), patients responded stronger to the false feedback than controls (Ehlers *et al.*, 1988c). The patients' response pattern was consistent with the idea of a positive feedback loop between physiological anxiety symptoms and the patient's anxious cognitive reaction to them postulated by psychophysiological models of panic attacks (e.g., Margraf et al., 1986a; Ehlers et al., 1988b). The results of these two experiments are in line with an old hypothesis that considers 'fear of fear' an essential feature of anxiety neurosis and agoraphobia. It postulates that patients with these anxiety disorders suffer from a fear of being anxious, in contrast to patients with simple or social phobia who are afraid of certain stimuli or situations. In keeping with the 'fear of fear' hypothesis, panic patients seem to be more anxious about, and more responsive to, stimuli or situations associated with their own anxiety responses.

In summary, when panic attack patients and control subjects are compared on various laboratory tests including so-called panic induction methods, the patients' tonically higher levels of heart rate and anxiety usually emerge as the most prominent difference (Ehlers et al., 1986b, 1988a; Roth et al., 1986). Panic patients are not generally more responsive to stressful or neutral stimulation. However, they seem to be more responsive to internal or external stimuli that signal the possibility that they might be becoming anxious.

Physical conditioning

For a long time, clinicians have noted that certain patients with mixed anxiety and depression syndromes tend to complain that they tire quickly with physical exertion. The diagnostic labels 'neurocirculatory asthenia' and 'effort syndrome' illustrate the importance given to the notion of 'exercise intolerance'. In the 1940s and 1950s, a series of studies tested this hypothesis in patients with diagnoses such as anxiety neurosis, neurasthenia, and effort syndrome (for example Cohen and White, 1950). Patients performed poorer in exercise testing than controls or showed higher blood lactate levels. In fact, these observations led Pitts and McClure (1967) to hypothesize a relationship between serum lactate levels and anxiety (see p. 260). Thus, the relationship of exercise and anxiety was the starting point of the lactate infusion model of anxiety and, more recently, of panic attacks (cf. Margraf et al., 1986b).

Recent data support a poorer physical condition of panic attack patients. Crowe et al. (1981) compared 20 patients with panic disorder and 20 age- and sex-matched hospital employees on a treadmill protocol. Subjects were exercised to at least 80% of their maximum age-predicted heart rate. The patient group showed a significantly lower maximum oxygen consumption (estimated from the amount of work required to reach the target heart rate). The difference between patients and controls was attributable to a subgroup of 8 patients who also had mitral valve prolapse (see p. 269 ff.).

An earlier study from our laboratory did not find differences in the treadmill responses of 12 female panic patients and 12 female controls (Taylor et al., 1986). None of the subjects had mitral valve prolapse. However, in this study, subjects were only tested up to four metabolic equivalents, which represents a moderate level of effort. More recently, we used a standard maximal treadmill test to compare physical fitness in 40 patients with panic disorder, 20 unselected age-matched controls free of any history of psychiatric disorders, and another 20 controls selected for their sedentary lifestyles (Taylor *et al.*, 1987). All subjects were female. The results showed that panic patients are not generally 'exercise intolerant'. They reached the same peak workload as non-exercising control subjects (11.2 METs), whereas the unselected control group demonstrated better physical fitness (13.5 METs). Patients showed higher heart rates at submaximal test levels and upon standing than both control groups. An analysis of covariance showed that the heart rate elevation was independent of differences in physical fitness.

In summary, there is some evidence that, on the average, panic disorder patients are in poorer physical condition than unselected controls. These results have to be taken into account when interpreting heart rate differences obtained from samples not matched for physical conditioning.

AMBULATORY MONITORING OF PANIC DISORDER

Heart rates during naturally occurring panic attacks

Since laboratory results on the physiology of panic attacks are inconclusive, researchers have recently started to systematically monitor panic attacks as they occur in the patients' natural environment. Ambulatory monitoring has the advantage of greater ecological validity.

Taylor *et al.* (1983) studied the question whether panic attacks occur at heart rates disproportionate of physical activity levels. In ten panic attack patients, 1-minute averages of heart rate and physical activity were recorded continuously with a portable microcomputer (Vitalog). Patients rated their anxiety, level of panic, and level of physical activity every 15 minutes. Computer programs were used to determine high heart rate levels disproportionate to Vitalog-determined physical activity levels. Three of eight panic attacks occurring during the recording period met the criteria. Maximum heart rates ranged between 115 and 148 bpm. During one other attack, the patient had a high heart rate, but was also physically active. Four (50%) of the panic attacks occurred at heart rates between 80 and 100 bpm that were not higher than expected from activity levels.

In a more recent study, we approached the same question by rater evaluation of heart rate and activity patterns (Taylor *et al.*, 1986). During six days of recording, 33 panic attacks and eight other anxiety episodes were reported by 12 panic patients. During 19 of the 33 panic attacks (57.6%), a heart rate increase of at least 20 bpm occurred that was greater than expected from concurrent levels of activity. The mean maximum heart rate during these attacks was 117 bpm. The attacks were rated by the patients as more intense than the 14 panic attacks without heart rate changes. However, symptom patterns including cardiovascular complaints were not different.

Freedman *et al.* (1985) monitored heart rates, finger temperature, and ambient temperature in 12 panic patients for two consecutive days. Five of these patients had a total of eight panic attacks. All panic attacks were accompanied by heart rate increases larger than during high-anxiety control periods (range 18 to 38 bpm). Peak heart rates ranged between 80 and 120 bpm. Unfortunately, physical activity was not controlled in this study. In addition to the heart rate increases, there was some evidence of increases in finger temperature prior to the panic attacks.

We have recently analyzed another sample of 44 panic attacks that occurred while 27 patients were wearing the heart rate and activity monitor (Margraf *et al.*, 1987b). The approach in this study differed slightly from those described above (Taylor *et al.*, 1983, 1986) in that we studied the average pattern of heart rate changes in panic attacks. For both mean and peak heart rates, only the subgroup of panic attacks occurring in feared situations were accompanied by heart rate elevations compared to matched periods. The mean peak heart rate during these 27 situational panic attacks was 109 bpm. Interestingly, heart rates were already elevated during the 15-minute period preceding the actual situational attacks. The average heart rate elevation was relatively small (mean: 5 bpm), but could be interpreted as an effect of anxiety rather than of physical workload. The 17 panic attacks classified by the patients as spontaneous were, on the average, not characterized by heart rate elevation. The mean peak heart rate during these attacks was 95 bpm.

Thus, data from our ambulatory monitoring studies show consistently that heart rate increases occur in a *subgroup* of panic attacks. Shear and colleagues (cited from Shear, 1986), recently reported similar results. In addition, Shear *et al.* and White and Baker (1986) found evidence for blood pressure elevation during panic attacks.

However, a substantial proportion of panic attacks recorded ambulatorily is not accompanied by heart rate changes, or the heart rate changes observed are most probably consequences of elevated physical activity. This lack of consistent heart rate increases is in contrast to the patients' self-reports: palpitations were reported for nearly 70% of a sample of 175 panic attacks recorded by Margraf *et al.* (1987b). Furthermore, the magnitude of heart rate changes is smaller than expected from case reports of panic attacks recorded in the laboratory (see p. 259). The mean peak levels recorded during panic attacks in the natural environment are far below heart rate levels during exercise.

There are several possible explanations for these discrepancies. Most likely, case reports represent a publication bias towards more dramatic effects. In addition, there are some methodological problems inherent in ambulatory monitoring studies, such as the exact timing of panic attacks. Furthermore, maximum heart rates reported in ambulatory monitoring studies are based on minute-averages whereas peak heart rates reported in laboratory studies usually lasted for less than a minute. Finally, it is possible that patients' reports of palpitations reflect their perception of changes in stroke volume rather than heart rate changes (for a discussion on the relationship of interoception and panic attacks, see Ehlers et al., 1988b).

Cardiac arrhythmias and panic attacks

Little is known about the relationship of cardiac arrhythmias and panic attacks. In the study of Taylor et al. (1986), six of the panic attacks occurred during simultaneous electrocardiogram monitoring. During these attacks the heart rhythm, when elevated, was a sinus tachycardia rather than any other type of atrial or ventricular arrhythmia. There was no difference in the overall frequency of arrhythmias between panic patients and controls. Similarly, no arrhythmias were observed during treadmill tests of the same subjects. There was, however, some evidence that panic patients had periods of activity-independent heart rate increases (in the absence of panic attacks) more frequently than controls, but this trend did not reach statistical significance.

The latter observation resembles findings of Tzivoni et al. (1980) who recorded the electrocardiogram of 67 patients with 'neurocirculatory asthenia' during their everyday activities. Nearly all patients showed episodes of sinus tachycardia in the absence of self-reported unusual physical effort, even during sleep. There was also evidence for a higher frequency of sinus arrhythmias and other cardiac arrhythmias compared to controls, although apparently this was not tested statistically. It is, however, unclear whether these results can be generalized to patients with panic disorder. The pattern of somatic complaints of the patients studied by Tzivoni et al., resembles those of panic disorder patients, but only a minority (39%) reported anxiety.

Shear et al. (1986) recently observed a low 24-hour mean frequency of arrhythmias in 23 panic patients. However, the frequency of atrial and ventricular premature beats was elevated compared to values previously reported for normal controls. During periods of panic and anxiety, these arrhythmias were more frequent than during asymptomatic periods. The arrhythmias were not clinically significant. The results remain preliminary since this study did not include a control group.

Results from a controlled study by Harbauer-Raum (1987) are in contrast to Shear's conclusions. Harbauer-Raum recorded 24-hour electrocardiograms of 23 patients with cardiac neurosis, 21 patients with mitral valve prolapse, and 16 healthy controls. Patients with cardiac neurosis did not show more cardiac arrhythmias than controls. In contrast, patients with mitral valve prolapse had more frequent ventricular premature beats. Since there is at least some overlap of panic disorder and cardiac neurosis, these results, as well as those of Taylor et al. (1986), contradict a higher frequency of arrhythmias in panic disorder.

Similarly, the laboratory study of Roth *et al.* (1986), found that differences between agoraphobics with panic attacks and normal controls on measures of heart rate variability could entirely be explained by differences in heart rate levels.

Thus, while the results are too preliminary to draw final conclusions, there is so far no firm evidence for an elevated frequency of cardiac arrhythmias in panic disorder patients. However, a more reliable answer to this question will have to await surveys of more representative and larger patient samples.

Tonic heart rate levels

One of the most consistent results of the laboratory studies reviewed in the previous sections was that panic disorder patients show tonically higher levels of heart rate and anxiety than controls. The average heart rate difference found in our studies ranges from 5 to 12 bpm. The question remains whether these differences are also present in the natural environment. Alternatively, the finding could just reflect differential responses to the laboratory setting.

Ambulatory monitoring allows study of this question. Freedman *et al.* (1985) did not find evidence for elevated heart rates in panic patients based on hourly 1-minute averages during 2 days of recording. Periods of sleep were not included. Unpublished data of Shear (Shear, 1986) also failed to show differences in overall heart rate and blood pressure between patients and controls.

One problem in comparing daytime heart rates is they are generally much more influenced by physical activity than by anxiety. In a study of Taylor *et al.* (1987), we therefore distinguished between sleeping and waking heart rates. Heart rate and physical activity were measured ambulatorily with a Vitalog monitor for 2 consecutive days and 1 night. Subjects were 37 female patients with panic disorder and 20 female controls free of any history of psychiatric disorders. Average physical activity and waking and sleeping heart rates were calculated from minute-averages stored by the microcomputer. Consistent with the results of laboratory studies, patients had significantly higher daytime and sleeping heart rates (average difference 5 and 7 bpm). In addition, patients, especially the agoraphobic subgroup, were physically less active. The control group demonstrated better physical fitness in a treadmill test (see p. 264 ff.). However, heart rate elevations at submaximal effort seemed to be independent of fitness level.

In this context it is interesting to note that Nesse *et al.* (1985) reported higher night-time catecholamine excretion in panic disorder patients. In addition, Uhde and colleagues (cited from Uhde *et al.*, 1985) found increased movement time during sleep in 9 panic patients compared to 9 control subjects. The mean total time awake, sleep latency, or sleep efficiency, however, were not different. REM latency and density was decreased. The sleep architecture, however, was different from that observed in depressed patients. Adams *et al.* (1985) recently reported abnormal sleep polygraphic recordings in 61 patients with panic disorder that resembled those of 28 narcoleptic patients. In an ongoing sleep study of panic disorder patients, Zarcone *et al.* (1986) found an abnormal polysomnographic recording in a 41-year-old male panic patient with frequent night-time panic attacks. At all sleep stages, his sleep was frequently interrupted (about 11 times per hour) by high amplitude K complexes and alpha. This abnormal EEG pattern was not of epileptic nature. Sleep apnea, periodic leg movements, and hyperventilation were also ruled out. The results were interpreted as evidence of heightened arousal.

The results of these studies indicate that the laboratory finding of heightened arousal in panic patients is at least to some degree representative of their state in the natural environment. The results also point to a possible relationship between anxiety and disturbed sleep (Williams and Karacan, 1984).

MITRAL VALVE PROLAPSE AND PANIC DISORDER

The relationship of panic disorder and mitral valve prolapse (MVP) has received much attention over the past years. DSM-III-R explicitly states that a diagnosis of MVP is not an exclusion criterion for panic disorder. The clinical symptomatology of MVP may show considerable overlap with that of panic disorder: palpitations, chest pain, dyspnea, fatigue, lightheadedness, dizziness, and actual or near syncope may occur in both syndromes (Liberthson *et al.*, 1986). This has lead to speculation that panic disorder may in some cases be 'caused' by mitral valve prolapse, or conversely that panic disorder may lead to mitral vale prolapse (Pariser *et al.*, 1979; Kantor *et al.*, 1980; Klein and Gorman, 1980). Studies of the possible overlap of MVP and panic disorder, however, have yielded surprisingly inconsistent results.

The mitral valve prolapse syndrome

Although the auscultatory signs of MVP have been known for over 100 years (Wooley, 1976), it was not until the 1960s that mid-systolic clicks and late systolic murmurs were related to the mitral valve. Reid's (1961) and Barlow's (Barlow *et al.*, 1963, 1968) confirmation of the intracardiac origin of these sounds marked the recognition of the prolapsed mitral valve as a cardiac syndrome. Since the publication of the influential review by Devereux *et al.* (1976), this syndrome is commonly designated by the term MVP. In the past decade MVP has become the most frequently diagnosed cardiac valvular abnormality.

The mitral valve separates the left atrium from the left ventricle. It consists of an anterior and a posterior leaflet that are attached to the papillary muscles of the left ventricular wall by the chordae tendineae. Normally, the mitral valve closes completely when blood is ejected into the aorta during ventricular systole, thus preventing back-flow into the left atrium. In the case of MVP, however, the mitral valve bows back into the left atrium during systole as shown

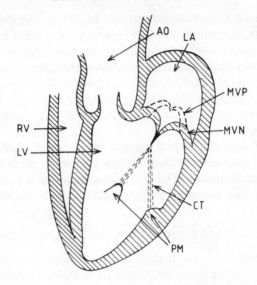

Figure 1. Schematic representation of the left heart showing a normal (solid lines) and a prolapsed mitral valve (broken lines). AO aorta, LA left atrium, MVP mitral valve prolapse, MVN Mitral valve (normal), CT chordae tendineae, PM papillary muscles, LV left ventricle, RV right ventricle.

in Figure 1. Typically, this involves the posterior leaflet or both leaflets, but only rarely the anterior leaflet alone (Devereux *et al.*, 1976). Rarely, the bulging of the leaflets is sufficient to disrupt their normal apposition and regurgitation of the blood back into the left atrium occurs.

Diagnostic issues

The syndrome was originally diagnosed by auscultation. The abrupt tensing during systole of the leaflets and the chordae tendineae generally produces a characteristic clicking sound. This occurs most often during mid-systole. In addition, if blood leaks back into the left atrium, a typical late systolic murmur can often be heard. Today the diagnosis of MVP is usually based on echocardiography which allows non-invasive visualization and thus measurement of the mobility of the mitral valve. While echocardiography is generally more sensitive than auscultation, there is also great variability in the criteria used to detect MVP by this method. Although there are published criteria (e.g., Weiss *et al.*, 1975; Markiewicz *et al.*, 1976; Wann *et al.*, 1983), their application is still fairly subjective. This may in part explain the widely discrepant findings obtained from different studies.

Even within the same study, the prevalence of MVP may drop from 13% to 0.5% with the adoption of more stringent criteria (Warth *et al.*, 1985).

An estimate of the retest and inter-rater reliability of raters from the same laboratory using the same criteria was attempted by Wann et al. (1985). This study demonstrated a lack of diagnostic precision that the authors found disconcerting: the percent agreement between the three independent raters ranged from 52% to 80% for one- and two-dimensional echocardiography, the mean being a low 64%. Intraindividual agreement (a measure of retest reliability) ranged from 80% to 90% (mean: 88%). Reliability seemed to be highest when the most stringent and conservative criteria were used. It can be expected that agreement between raters from different institutions may be even less satisfactory. This is in fact indicated by the recent study of Gorman et al. (1986) who investigated a series of 15 patients with panic disorder. Here, two experienced echocardiogram readers agreed in no single case on the positive diagnosis of MVP. The lack of diagnostic precision demonstrated in these studies has to be taken into consideration when evaluating the following sections on the prevalence and relevance of MVP and its possible relationship to panic disorder.

Epidemiology of MVP

The estimated prevalence of MVP varies widely with the populations studied and the diagnostic methods employed. Until recently, estimates ranged from 4% to 21% of the population (cf. Devereux et al., 1976; Markiewicz et al., 1976). However, these studies of clinical series, ad hoc samples, or samples of referred patients are unlikely to yield reliable and representative results. The recent data from the Framingham Heart Study (Savage et al., 1983a) allow a more satisfactory estimation of the prevalence of MVP in the general community. The overall rate of MVP was 5% in this sample of 4967 subjects. There was a striking interaction with age and sex: while the prevalence in men ranged from 2% to 4% at all ages, the rates in women decreased strongly with increasing age. The rate for women between 20 and 29 years was 17%, for women over 70 years less than 2%. The strongest drop in frequency of MVP appeared from middle age (40s and 50s) to older age (60s and 70s). Since other studies suggest that MVP does not decrease the average life span (see below for details), this age dependence in the female population does not seem to be an artifact of cross-sectional sampling.

Until recently, most studies of associated pathology in MVP were done on patients referred with cardiac complaints or other diseases. While the majority of patients in these studies did not show significant cardiac pathology, MVP was associated in some subjects with anatomical abnormalities such as thickening of the leaflets or elongated, thin, and attenuated chordae tendineae (Devereux et al., 1976). Most important of the rare complications of MVP are infective endocarditis, spontaneous rupture of the chordae tendineae, and progressive mitral regurgitation (cf. Devereux et al., 1976; Wynne, 1986). In addition, there have so far been 17 documented cases of sudden death in MVP patients (Pocock et al., 1984). A small minority of MVP patients also show other cardiac conditions such as the Marfan and Ehlers-Danlos syndromes (Devereux et al., 1976). MVP patients from clinical series also have often shown a higher prevalence of cardiovascular and general neuropsychiatric symptoms as well as dysrhythmias (Young et al., 1979; Schweizer et al., 1979; Liberthson et al., 1986). Other reported findings from such samples include higher plasma levels and urinary excretion of catecholamines (DeCarvalho et al., 1979; Boudoulas et al., 1980; Pasternac et al., 1982; Gaffney et al., 1983; Puddu (1983); Boudoulas et al., 1984).

However, the results from studies of clinical subjects may not be representative of the MVP syndrome in general. There is reason to expect that people actually searching professional help may have more pathology than asymptomatic subjects. This problem can only be solved by large scale community surveys. The Framingham Heart Study is such a study and its clinical results support the notion that MVP in general is a harmless condition. In this study, subjects with and without MVP were not significantly different with respect to the prevalence of the Marfan or Ehlers-Danlos syndromes, significant cardiac disease (including inherited connective tissue syndromes and coronary artery disease), left ventricular function, cardiovascular symptoms (including chest pain, dyspnea, and syncope), abnormal standard 12-lead EKG findings (including ST-T and QT_c changes), response to treadmill exercise testing, or dysrhythmias during 24-hour ambulatory EKG monitoring or treadmill exercise (Savage et al., 1983b, 1983c). With respect to the previous associations with specific cardiovascular conditions these results indicate that MVP may be an integral feature of such conditions rather than their cause.

These findings from the Framingham Heart Study are quite consistent with the reported long-term outcome of MVP: retrospective as well as first prospective studies show premature mortality to be uncommon in people with MVP (Allen et al., 1974; Appelblatt et al., 1975; Koch and Hancock, 1976; Mills et al., 1977; Belardi et al., 1981; Nishimura et al., 1985).

Clinical relevance of MVP

The clinical relevance of MVP is not yet fully established. This may be due to the lack of diagnostic reliability or to the discrepancies between studies of clinical series and community surveys discussed above. Another possible explanation for the lack of complications in the majority of cases is that the syndrome may represent a heterogeneous entity.

In a recent editorial in the New England Journal of Medicine, Wynne (1986) suggests that the advent of the more sensitive echocardiographic methods have led to the inclusion of normal variants into the MVP syndrome. He points out that the diagnosis is based on the mobility of the mitral valve which is a continuous, not a dichotomous variable. Therefore, the findings of the Framingham study can be interpreted as meaning that the diagnosis of MVP is applied to two groups of individuals. The first contains subjects that are not more symptomatic and have no more arrhythmias than their peers without MVP. They are at low risk for complications. In general, their diagnosis is based on echocardiography, while the typical auscultatory signs are missing. The second group contains subjects who in addition to the echocardiographic findings also show evidence of mitral regurgitation (often with the auscultatory signs). These subjects have more symptoms and appear to be at greater risk for complications. Additional evidence for this is presented by Nishimura *et al.* (1985) who found that in almost every case complications occurred in subjects with anatomical abnormalities.

It is thus possible that the majority of the cases diagnosed by echocardiography alone are basically variants of normal functioning or have a functional, perhaps state-dependent, abnormality. Only a minority of cases may represent anatomical abnormalities of perhaps greater pathological significance. Given this background, what is the relationship of MVP and panic disorder? The question has been approached from two perspectives. Most researchers studied the prevalence of MVP in patients that were diagnosed as having panic attacks. A smaller number of studies investigated the opposite question, namely the prevalence of panic attacks in samples of MVP patients. The two strategies have yielded different results as we will present in the following sections.

Prevalence of MVP in panic attack patients

After Pariser *et al.* (1978) first described a case of combined MVP and panic disorder, several studies reported high prevalences of MVP in panic attack patients. These studies have led to the claim that MVP may be one frequent cause of panic attacks (Pariser *et al.*, 1979; Kantor *et al.*, 1980). Among the more recent studies are several, however, that report no elevated frequency of MVP. A summary of the 17 studies of MVP in patients with panic disorder or agoraphobia is given in Table 1. Not all studies used homogeneous patient samples. Pariser *et al.* (1979) included 10 patients with major depression (MDE), Kathol *et al.* (1980) included three with generalized anxiety disorder (GAD) or simple phobias, and out of the 31 chest pain patients with normal coronary arteries studied by Bass *et al.* (1983), only 12 met criteria for anxiety or phobic neurosis. All of the studies have at least been published as abstracts with the exception of study 17. These data come from an as yet unpublished study done in our laboratory (Taylor *et al.*, in preparation).

Only five studies included 'normal' control subjects (*n* from 3 to 25), most of whom were 'professionals' (e.g., hospital employees). This limits the interpretability of the findings, considering the great variability in the diagnosis and the published prevalence of MVP in the general population. In addition,

Table 1. Prevalence of MVP in panic attack patients.

Study	Panic patient sample	Control sample	'Blind' ratings?	Criteria for MVP	Number of subjects with MVP
1. Pariser et al., 1979	5 PD, 10 MDE, 2 undiagnosed; 9F/8M, 21–53 yrs	none	?	ausc./echo.	PD: 1 (20%), MDE: 3 (30%), undiagnosed: 2 (100%)
2. Venkatesh et al., 1980	21 anxiety neurosis (Feighner); 15F/6M, 37 yrs	20 hospital employees; 9F/8M, 37 yrs	yes	ausc./echo. (Markiewicz)	patients: 5 only met ausc. (24%), 3 only echo. (14%) 5 ausc.+ echo. criteria (24%); controls: 5 (25%), 1 (5%), 1 (5%), respectively
3. Kantor et al., 1980	25 PD/AG, history of palpitations; all F, 42 yrs	23 hospital employees; all F, same age	yes	ausc./echo.	patients: 2 only met ausc. (8%), 3 (12%) ausc. and echo. criteria; controls: 2 (9%) met only echo. criteria
4. Kathol et al., 1980	18 PD, 5 AG, 3 GAD or simple phobia; 12F/14M, 36 yrs	none	?	ausc./echo. (Markiewicz)	PD: 1 (4% of PD/AG)
5. Gorman et al., 1981a	20 PD/AG; 15F/5M, 40 yrs	none	1 of 2 raters blind	ausc./echo. (Markiewicz)	non-blind rater: 10 (50%) blind rater: 7 (35%)
6. Grunhaus et al., 1982	23 PD/AG; 15F/8M, 35 yrs	none	?	ausc./echo. (Weiss)	2 only ausc. (9%), 7 (30%) ausc. and echo. criteria
7. Bass et al., 1983	31 chest pain with normal coronary arteries, includes 12 anxiety neurosis 17F/14M, 44.5 yrs	none	yes	ausc./echo. (Wann)	none
8. Hickey et al., 1983	50 AG; 42F/8M, 36 yrs	none	?	ausc./echo. (Markiewicz)	none
9. Mavissakalian et al., 1983	54 AG; 46F/7M, 37.6 yrs	none	?	ausc./echo. (Markiewicz)	3 definite (6%), 4 probable (7%)

Study	Patient sample	Control sample	Blind	Method	Results
10. Chan et al., 1984	10 PD, 4 AG, 4 GAD, 1 social phobia	none	?	ausc./echo. (Wann)	none
11. Shear et al., 1984	25 PD/AG; 14F/11M, 35.8 yrs	25 spouses of MVP patients, 14F/11M, 37 yrs	yes	echo.	patients: 2 definite (8%), 2 probable (8%); controls: 2 probable (8%)
12. Harbauer-Raum 1987 Strian, 1987	27 PD	none	?	ausc./echo.	2 definite (7%)
13. Nesse et al., 1985	20 PD/AG; 16F/4M, 32 yrs	3 volunteers	yes	ausc./echo. (Markiewicz)	patients: 7 (35%) controls: 0
14. Ballenger et al., 1986	78 PD/AG	none	?	ausc./echo.	9 ausc. and echo. (12%) 19 echo only (24%)
15. Dager et al., 1986	24 PD, 11 AG, 9 GAD with panic attacks; 30F/14M, 35.4 yrs	20 GAD; 10F/10M, 36.6 yrs	yes	echo.	panic patients: 15 definite (34%), 4 probable (9%), 7 possible (16%); GAD: 3 definite (15%), 3 probable (15%)
16. Liberthson et al., 1986	131 PD/AG; 84F/47M, 38 yrs	none	?	ausc./echo.	44 definite (34%) (includes 22 = 17% ausc. and echo.), 7 probable (5%)
17. Taylor et al. (in prep.)	12 PD/AG; all F, 39.8 yrs	12 volunteers, all F, 35.5 yrs	yes	ausc./echo.	none

Note: 'Blind' ratings refer to whether the cardiologist was aware of the subjects' psychiatric status. The study of Hickey et al. (1983) is the same as that listed in Table 2, where only the results for the MVP and cardiac control samples are reported. The descriptions of the samples list the number and type of patients or controls, the ratio of female and male subjects, and mean ages (if available).

Abbreviations ausc.: auscultation, echo.: echocardiogram, yrs: years, F: female, M: male, PD: panic disorder, PA: panic attacks, AG: agoraphobia with panic attacks, GAD: generalized anxiety disorder, MDE: major depressive episode, MVP: mitral valve prolapse.

in a number of the studies cardiological diagnoses were performed by raters with knowledge of the psychiatric status of the patients (ratings not 'blind'). That 'blind' ratings are important is emphasized by the study of Gorman *et al.* (1981a) in which one blind rater found 35% MVP while the non-blind rater found 50% MVP among their panic attack patients.

Most of the studies used two sets of criteria for the diagnosis of MVP, usually termed definite and probable criteria. Averaged across those 589 patients in the 17 studies that had panic disorder or agoraphobia, 18% (106) met criteria for definite MVP and 27% (157) criteria for probable or definite MVP. (These numbers do not include the small samples of depressive, GAD, or undiagnosed patients that several studies contained). In one study (Dager *et al.*, 1986), a clinical control group of patients with generalized anxiety disorder was tested. Their rates of definite or probable/definite MVP were 15% and 30%, respectively. In the 81 normal controls the average rate of definite MVP was 1% (1). Probable and/or definite MVP was diagnosed in 12% (10). This rate of definite MVP is lower than that reported for the general population, which may be related to the lack of representativeness of 'professional' control subjects. In this context it is interesting to note that the two studies using community volunteers rather than professionals as control subjects found no difference in the prevalence of MVP (studies 11 and 17). The pooled differences between panic disorder, GAD, and normals are significant for both the definite ($\chi^2 = 15.15$, df = 2, $p < 0.0005$) and probable criteria for MVP ($\chi^2 = 10.71$, df = 2, $p < 0.0047$).

Eleven studies allow an estimate of the percentage of subjects that met both auscultatory and echocardiographic criteria for MVP. This was the case for only 10% (45) of the 464 panic attack patients in these reports (studies 2-4, 7-10, 12, 14, 16, 17). For control subjects this prevalence is 2% (1 of 57, studies 2, 3, 17). Again this difference is statistically significant (Fisher's exact probability test, $p < 0.0000$).

The methodological problems discussed above (studies of clinical series of highly symptomatic referred patients, lack of adequate control groups, non-blind ratings, unreliable diagnosis of MVP) and the great variations in published results allow at present no final judgment of the overlap of MVP and panic disorder. The reported prevalences are not distributed continuously. One group of studies reports low frequencies of 0% to 8%, the other high frequencies of 24% to 35% for 'definite' MVP. This suggests the operation of other factors that are as of yet undetected. Until these factors have been identified, the computation of averages across the two groups of studies as performed above must remain tentative. These caveats have to be kept in mind when we interpret the average findings as indicating a possible elevated prevalence of MVP in panic attack patients studied in clinical settings.

Could such a result be due to the sex and age characteristics of the panic attack samples studied? The average age of the patients across all studies was 37.6 years and 68% were women. As discussed above, the prevalence of MVP is indeed highest in women under age 50. Calculated from the Framingham Heart Study we can expect to see a prevalence of 13.1% (with stringent echocardiographic criteria) for this group of subjects. Two reasons, however, argue against this tempting explanation for an elevated prevalence of MVP in panic attack patients. First, the control groups were matched for age and sex. Second, the proportion of female subjects and their average ages are not different in studies with a low frequency of MVP (38 years and 67% women) from those in studies with a high frequency (37.3 years and 69% women).

Is the possible higher prevalence of MVP specific to panic disorder or does it exist in other psychiatric populations as well? Dager *et al.* (1986), in the only direct study of this question, found a higher prevalence in panic than in generalized anxiety disorder. However, their rate of MVP in GAD is comparable to the mean rate for all panic disorder samples calculated above. In addition, a recent study by Giannini *et al.* (1984) reported a high prevalence (44%) in bipolar affective disorder as well. These authors used the simultaneous presence of positive echocardiographic and auscultatory findings as the criterion for MVP.

A definite answer to the question of overlap of MVP and panic disorder will only be possible after unselected panic disorder patients from community surveys will have been screened for MVP and compared with controls from the same population. Until then we can only say that at least 80% of the panic attack patients studied so far do not show 'definite' MVP and about 90% do not meet both echocardiographic and auscultatory criteria.

Prevalence of panic attacks in MVP patients

The results from the six studies of this topic are summarized in Table 2. Overall there seems to be no elevated prevalence of panic attacks in MVP patients compared to subjects with other cardiac complaints. The figures in MVP patients range from 0% to 24% with an average of 14% with panic attacks (63 of 440 patients, based on studies 2 through 6). For cardiac control subjects the average prevalence of panic attacks is 15% (5 of 33, study 2), and for normal controls, many of which were hospital employees, 8% (11 of 141, based on studies 2, 4, 6). The differences between the three groups are not significant ($\chi^2 = 4.21$, df = 2, $p > 0.05$). The mean prevalence of panic disorder was 7% among MVP patients (29 of 390, based on studies 2, 4–6), 6% among cardiac control subjects (2 of 33, study 2), and 2% among normal controls (3 of 141, studies 2, 4, 6). Again, these differences are not significant ($\chi^2 = 5.15$, df = 2, $p > 0.05$). Finally, there were no significant differences between MVP and cardiac control patients in the prevalence of 'phobic disorder' or agoraphobia (studies 2, 5, 6).

Patients with MVP generally scored higher than normal controls but similar to cardiac control subjects on questionnaire measures of hypochondriasis (Whitely Index), avoidance behavior (Maudsley-Oxford Fear Questionnaire),

Table 2. Prevalence of panic attacks in MVP patients.

Study	MVP patient sample	Control sample	'Blind' ratings?	Criteria for MVP/panic	Number of subjects with panic and other results
1. Uretsky, 1980	45 medical outpatients (includes 29 without any other disease); 49.9 yrs	927 medical outpatients (includes 184 without any disease = the 'worried well') 46.7 yrs	no	aus.; symptom reports	neuropsychiatric symptoms: MVP = 'worried well' (10%); chronic anxiety: MVP = 'worried well' (8.8%); both groups more symptoms than med. outpatients in general (4.2%).
2. Kane et al., 1981	65 referrals for echocardiography; 45F/20M, 43 yrs	A: 33 cardiac controls ('CC', no MVP); 22F/11M, 40.9 yrs B: 22 hospital employees; 17F/5M, 40.3 yrs	yes	echo.; DSM-III, questionnaires	MVP: 5 PD (8%), 16 PA (25%), 6 AG (9%), A ('CC'): 2 PD (6%), 5 PA (15%), 4 AG (12%); B (hosp. empl.): 1 PD (5%), 1 PA (5%), 1 AG (5%) MVP = B ('CC') on questionnaires, both higher than hospital employees
3. Crowe et al., 1982	50 outpatients	none	?	ausc./echo.; DSM-III	MVP: 12 PA (24%)
4. Hartman et al., 1982	A: 141 referrals for echo.; 103F/38M, 16–76 yrs B: 33 family members of subjects from A; 22F/11M	70 family members without MVP; 27F/43M	?	ausc./echo. (Markiewicz); DSM-III	MVP-A: 22 PD (16%), 29 PA (21%); MVP-B: 1 PD (3%), 3 PA (9%); non-MVP family members: 2 PD (3%), 8 PA (10%)
5. Hickey et al., 1983	103 referrals for echo.; 55F/48M, 53 yrs	67 cardiac controls ('CC', no MVP); 34F/33M, 48 yrs	?	ausc./echo. (Markiewicz, 10 patients echo. only); DSM-III, questionnaires	MVP: 3 PA (3%), 1 AG (1%); CC: no PA, no AG; MVP = CC on neuroticism and neurotic symptoms
6. Mazza et al., 1986	48 referrals for echo.; 36F/12M, 42.9 yrs	49 hospital employees and volunteers (no MVP); 36F/13M, 42.4 yrs	yes	ausc./echo.; DSM-III questionnaires	MVP and controls: no PD/AG. MVP more anxious than controls (Zung Scale), but lower than norms for anxiety disorder patients

Note 'Blind' ratings refer to whether the psychiatric diagnostician was aware of the subjects' cardiological status. The study of Hickey et al. (1983) is the same as that listed in Table 1, where only the results for the agoraphobic sample are reported. The descriptions of the samples list the number and type of patients and controls, the ratio of female and male subjects, and the mean ages (if available). The numbers given for the diagnoses panic disorder, agoraphobia, and panic attacks are overlapping.

Abbreviations ausc.: auscultation, echo.: echocardiogram, yrs: years, F: female, M: male, PD: panic disorder, PA: panic attacks, AG: agoraphobia with panic attacks, MVP: mitral valve prolapse, CC: cardiac control subjects cardiac and neuropsychiatric symptoms, chronic anxiety, general neurotic symptoms (General Health Questionnaire), neuroticism (Eysenck Personality Inventory), the Zung Anxiety Scale, and the SCL-90 scales with exception of paranoid ideation (studies 1, 2, 4, 6). The scores on anxiety scales, while being higher than those of the normal controls, were considerably lower than the norms reported for patients with anxiety disorders (studies 2, 6).

All of these studies were done on clinical samples of MVP patients. However, studying referral populations in hospital settings may lead to the selection of highly symptomatic individuals. This has been termed 'ascertainment bias' by Motulsky (1978). In this context, two of the control groups employed by Uretsky (1980) and Hartman *et al.* (1982) are especially interesting. These authors looked for strategies allowing to circumvent or control the problem of biased selection. Uretsky (1980) separated his medical control group into those that had evidence of medical disease and those that had sought professional help, but did not show any identifiable disease (the 'worried well'). The second group scored just as high as the patients with MVP on his measures of neuropsychiatric symptoms, cardiac symptoms, and chronic anxiety. Using a different approach, Hartman *et al.* (1982) studied the family members of their MVP patients. These subjects had not sought professional help at that time and thus presumably represented a group with less selection bias. The family members with MVP were not different from those without MVP. Both groups had few panic attacks than the original sample of MVP patients who had been referred to the clinic.

These results are consistent with the lack of significant cardiovascular symptoms (including many typical panic attack symptoms) found in the Framingham Heart Study discussed above. These studies clearly illustrate the relevance of ascertainment bias for our topic. If this bias is eliminated or controlled, the prevalence of panic attacks or neuropsychiatric symptoms is not higher than among all patients in cardiologic practice. It is possible, however, that all of these groups have a higher prevalence of panic attacks than normal control subjects that are not searching for professional help.

Possible explanations for the findings

At present, a fair conclusion is that a higher prevalence of MVP in panic disorder patients is not well established but cannot be ruled out either. In addition, MVP patients do not experience more panic attacks than other cardiac patients or people who have been termed the 'worried well'. People with cardiovascular complaints may, however, show somewhat more panic attacks than non-clinical controls, but this is not specific to MVP.

If there is an overlap between panic disorder and MVP, it is small, affecting less than 8% of MVP and less than 20% of clinical (and thus presumably highly selected) samples of panic disorder patients. Such an overlap would consist primarily of subjects with milder variants of MVP that may represent functional and perhaps reversible rather than anatomical and permanent abnormalities. This is suggested by three lines of evidence. First, there is a low proportion of panic attack patients with both echocardiographic and auscultatory evidence for MVP. Second, it is possible to induce mild MVP experimentally in the context of high heart rate and low ventricular volume or to produce new arrhythmias by psychological stressors or direct programed ventricular stimulation (Coombs et al., 1977; Rosenthal et al., 1985; Ballenger et al., 1986). Third, Gorman (1986) recently presented data showing that evidence of MVP often disappears after remission of panic attacks has been achieved for at least 6 months. Unfortunately, we have no information about the retest reliability of the diagnostic methods used to determine MVP in this study.

Whether the relationship between panic disorder and MVP is of a causal or a purely correlational nature is unclear. There are no symptomatic differences between panic disorder patients with or without MVP (Mavissakalian et al., 1983; cf. Kane et al., 1981) and their responses to lactate are similar (Gorman et al., 1981b). In addition, the familial morbidity risk for panic disorder is not affected by the presence of MVP (Crowe et al., 1980). It remains possible that people with cardiac complaints, especially those that seek treatment, may more often develop panic attacks. One possible mechanism for this could be the perception and subsequent anxious appraisal of arrhythmias related to MVP. However, Strian (1987) was not able to show any differences in the accuracy of perception or the appraisal of arrhythmias between MVP patients and normals. On the other hand, panic disorder patients were better at perceiving their arrhythmias and responded to them with greater anxiety than either of the other groups.

Another possibility is that panic attacks or the stress associated with them leads to a functional variant of MVP. This would be consistent with the disappearance of MVP after successful treatment of panic attacks. Ballenger et al. (1986) recently suggested as the possible mechanism for such a relationship high levels of circulating catecholamines in the presence of a rapid heart rate. While a number of studies discussed above have reported increased levels of plasma and urinary catecholamines, this does not seem to be the case in panic disorder patients. Nesse et al. (1985) found elevated urinary catecholamine excretion only in panic patients without MVP. The patients with MVP showed significantly lower levels of norepinephrine and epinephrine and were not different from normal controls.

Neither of these explanations have thus been supported in a convincing way. This leaves us with two other possibilities. Both phenomena could be produced by a third factor such as an as yet unknown autonomic abnormality. If this explanation is accepted, one would still have to explain the probably elevated prevalence of MVP in other psychiatric disorders such as bipolar affective disorder. This observation is more easily explained by the second possibility, namely that we are dealing with a problem of co-morbidity. People with two disorders are more likely to seek treatment or to be detected in community surveys than people with one disorder alone. This explanation is a kind of null hypothesis. At the present state of our knowledge we suggest that this hypothesis cannot be refuted. A change in this assessment of the evidence probably must await the results of prospective longitudinal studies and community surveys of panic disorder patients.

CARDIOVASCULAR MORTALITY AND PANIC DISORDER

In two independent retrospective follow-up studies of 113 and 155 patients, Coryell et al. (1982, 1986) found an increased mortality for male panic disorder patients. The mortality rate was twice as high as predicted from vital statistics. The excess mortality was due to cardiovascular death and suicide. However, these results were based on very small numbers of expected and actual deaths in both studies. Martin et al. (1985) and Black et al. (1985) did not find evidence for increased mortality due to natural causes (including cardiovascular disease) in follow-ups of anxiety neurotics ($n = 62$) and neurotics with various diagnoses ($n = 348$, anxiety, somatization, and obsessive-compulsive disorders), respectively. Thus, results from retrospective studies are inconsistent. As of today, no prospective studies have been conducted.

Indirect evidence for an elevated cardiovascular risk in panic disorder is also largely lacking. One factor that may contribute to a higher risk is the patients' poorer physical fitness described above (p. 264 ff.). Among the cardiovascular parameters studied in panic disorder, tonically elevated blood pressures would have the greatest predictive validity for cardiovascular disease. However, in the studies reviewed above, there was little evidence for hypertension in the average panic patients. The most consistent cardiovascular result was a slight tonic elevation in heart rate. However, there are no data showing that this finding has significance for the prediction of cardiovascular disease. Finally, in a recent review, Hayward et al. (in press) report some evidence for increased cardiovascular risk factors in panic disorder such as hyperlipidemia, alcohol abuse, and cigarette smoking. Thus, as of today, any link between panic disorder and cardiovascular mortality has to be considered tentative at most.

CONCLUSIONS AND CLINICAL IMPLICATIONS

The studies described in this chapter have helped to clarify what cardiovascular changes accompany panic attacks. It appears that clinical descriptions and published case reports are misleading. Overall, laboratory and ambulatory monitoring studies of panic attacks have failed to find a consistent pattern of physiological changes that would distinguish panic attacks from anticipatory anxiety. The abrupt and dramatic physiological changes, especially in heart rate, described in case reports seem to represent the prototype of an extreme panic attack rather than the average panic attack. The first reason is that studies using ambulatory monitoring devices show heart rate increases only in a subgroup of panic attacks. Second, the average heart rate increase observed in laboratory and field studies is only moderate. Heart rate levels reached during panic attacks are, on the average, much lower than those during mild exercise.

This result is somewhat surprising given the fact that the great majority of panic patients report experiencing palpitations during their panic attacks. One is reminded of the discussion of discordance and desynchrony of different measures of fear (Hodgson and Rachman, 1974; Himadi et al., 1985). There are several possible explanations for the discrepancy. First, reported palpitations may correspond to changes in cardiac functions other than heart rate, for example to changes in stroke volume. Second, the results might partly be due to a recollection bias. Margraf et al. (1987b) showed that panic patients tend to endorse more symptoms in retrospective accounts of their panic attacks (in questionnaires or diagnostic interviews) than in concurrent diary reports.

However, we think that this question has to be approached on a more general level. At the very beginning of a panic attack, patients usually notice some kind of unpleasant body sensation (cf. Margraf et al., 1986a). It is possible that the symptom reports of panic patients reflect at least to some degree their appraisal of physiological changes rather than actual physiological responses. Therefore, the role of the accuracy of interoception and the appraisal of interoceptive cues needs to be studied in panic disorder (cf. Tyrer, 1976; Pennebaker, 1982; Ehlers et al., 1988b). Preliminary data show that such research provides valuable information. Harbauer-Raum (1987) found that patients with cardiac phobia perceived their heart beat more accurately than controls. On the other hand, premature ventricular beats were detected equally well by patients with cardiac phobia and normal controls, who both did better than patients with mitral valve prolapse. In contrast to normal controls, cardiac phobics responded to the perception of arrhythmias with anxiety increases. These results point to an enhanced sensitivity to cardiac sensations in patients with cardiac phobia that has both perceptual and appraisal components. However, it is uncertain to what degree these results can be generalized to all patients with panic disorder. Preliminary evidence from our laboratory shows more accurate heart rate perception in a subgroup of panic patients (Ehlers et al., 1988b). In addition, patients responded with larger increases in anxiety and physiological arousal when they believed that their heart rate had accelerated (Ehlers et al., 1988c).

A rather stable result that emerged from laboratory and field studies is that panic patients show tonically higher resting heart rates when compared to matched controls. In contrast, an enhanced cardiovascular reactivity to various stressors was not consistently found. It is yet unclear whether this slight heart rate elevation is of any clinical significance and whether it may be related to an increased risk for cardiovascular disease. Animal studies suggest that lower heart rates might retard coronary artherosclerosis (Beere *et al.*, 1985). Furthermore, tricyclic antidepressants that are used to treat panic disorder have severe cardiovascular side-effects (for a review see Vohra, 1977). In laboratory and ambulatory assessments of patients treated with imipramine, we found elevations in heart rate levels of 10 to 15 bpm compared to pre-treatment levels, even during sleep. It is possible that this side-effect is especially undesirable in patients with already elevated heart rates.

The relationship of the higher resting heart rate in panic disorder patients to their poorer physical condition remains to be clarified by future studies. One could speculate that systematic exercise programs might be beneficial for panic disorder patients. In some cases, we have observed that patients remitted completely from their panic attacks after starting a rigorous exercise regimen. Sturm *et al.* (1987) found that an inpatient program combining exercise and exposure to phobic situations was beneficial in the treatment of cardiac neurotics. The mechanism of these therapeutic effects, however, is unclear. Exercise may alter physiological response patterns or it may help patients to re-evaluate physiological changes like heart rate increases as natural and not dangerous.

The studies reviewed in this chapter have focused primarily on heart rate, blood pressure, and mitral valve prolapse. In addition, some studies recorded ECGs. For a more complete picture, other cardiovascular parameters such as stroke volume, contractility of the heart, renal blood flow, coronary artery status, retinal arterial status, coronary ischemia, and oxygen consumption would have to be studied.

The possible overlap of panic disorder and mitral valve prolapse has been overemphasized in the literature. If it exists, it is small and probably not specific to mitral valve prolapse compared to other cardiac conditions. In addition, the overlap is of limited clinical significance. Even if mitral valve prolapse is diagnosed in a panic disorder patient, this information does not have implications for clinical management. Unless significant cardiovascular complications are present, MVP does not require specific treatment in addition to antianxiety therapy. Shear *et al.* (1984, p. 303) suggest that 'routine screening of patients with panic disorder for MVP may not be warranted, and psychiatric treatment of panic disorder should not be different for a patient with MVP'. Thus, additional measures beyond the standard ECG for panic disorder patients with cardiovascular complaints do not seem to be necessary. Several studies have shown that MVP does not affect outcome of treatments for panic attacks (Gorman *et al.*, 1981a; Grunhaus *et al.*, 1982; Mavissakalian *et al.*, 1983). There are now effective behavioral as well as pharmacologic treatments available (Marks, 1983; Barlow *et al.*, 1984; Bonn *et al.*, 1984; Jacob and Rapport, 1984; Clark *et al.*, 1985; Fiegenbaum, 1986; Gitlin *et al.*, 1985; Hand *et al.*, 1986; Judd *et al.*, 1986; Margraf and Ehlers, 1986; Öst, 1988) that lead to clinically significant improvement or even complete remission in the great majority of cases.

Acknowledgements

Preparation of this chapter was supported by German Research Foundation grant Eh 97/1-1, the Medical Research Service of the Veterans Administration of the USA, and the Upjohn Company.

REFERENCES

Adams, J. R., Wahby, V. S. and Giller, E. L. (1985). EEG of panic disorder and narcolepsy. Paper presented at the 138th Annual Meeting of the American Psychiatric Association, Dallas, Texas.

Allen, H., Harris, A. and Leatham, A. (1974). Significance and prognosis of an isolated late systolic murmur: A 9- to 22-year follow-up. *British Heart Journal*, **36**, 525.

American Psychiatric Association (Ed) (1980). *Diagnostic and Statistical Manual of Mental Disorders*, 3rd edn, APA, Washington, D.C.

American Psychiatric Association (Ed) (1987) *Diagnostic and Statistical Manual of Mental Disorders*, 3rd edn revised. APA, Washington, D.C.

Appelblatt, N. H., Willis, P. W., Lenhart, J. A., Shulman, J. I. and Walton, J. A. Jr. (1975). Ten to 40 year follow-up of 69 patients with systolic click with or without late systolic murmur. *American Journal of Cardiology*, **35**, 119.

Ballenger, J. C., Gibson, R., Peterson, G. A. and Laraia, M. T., (1986). 'Functional' MVP in agoraphobia/panic disorder. Paper presented at the 139th Annual Meeting of the American Psychiatric Association, Washington, D.C.

Barlow, J. B., Pocock, W. A., Marchand, P. and Denny, M. (1963). The significance of late systolic murmurs. *American Heart Journal*, **66**, 443.

Barlow, J. B., Bosman, C. K., Pocock, W. A. and Marchand, P. (1968). Late systolic murmurs and non-ejection (mid-late) systolic clicks: An analysis of 90 patients. *British Heart Journal*, **30**, 203.

Barlow, D. H., Cohen, A. S., Waddell, M. T., Vermilyea, B. B., Klosko, J. S., Blanchard, E. B. and Di Nardo, P. A. (1984). Panic and generalized anxiety disorders: Nature and treatment. *Behavior Therapy*, **15**, 431–449.

Barlow, D. H., Vermilyea, J., Blanchard, E. B., Vermilyea, B. B., Di Nardo, P. A. and Cerny, J. A. (1985). The phenomenon of panic. *Journal of Abnormal Psychology*, **94**, 320–328.

Bass, C., Cawley, R., Wade, C., Ryna, K. C., Gardner, W. N., Hutchinson, D. C. S. and Jackson, G. (1983). Unexplained breathlessness and psychiatric morbidity in patients with normal and abnormal coronary arteries. *Lancet*, March 19, 605–609.

Beere, P. A., Glagov, S. and Zarins, C. K. (1985). Retarding effects of lowered heart rate on coronary atherosclerosis. *Science*, **226**, 180–182.

Beitman, B. D., Lamberti, J. W., Mukerji, V., De Rosear, L., Basha, I. M. and Schmid, L. (1987). Panic disorder in patients with angiographically normal coronary arteries. *Psychosomatics*, **28**, 480–484.

Belardi, J., Lardani, H. and Sheldon, W. (1981). Idiopathic prolapse of the mitral valve: Follow-up study of 136 patients studied by angiography. *American Journal of Cardiology*, **47**, 426.

Beunderman, R., van Dis, H. and Duyvis, D. (1987). Eine Vergleichsstudie somatischer und psychologischer Symptome bei Patienten mit nicht kardial bedingtem Brustschmerz, In: Nutzinger, D. O., Pfersmann, D., Welan, T. and Zapotoczky, H. G., (Eds), *Die Herzphobie*. Enke, Stuttgart, pp. 56–65.

Black, D. W., Warrack, G. and Winokur, G. (1985). The Iowa record-linkage study. III. Excess mortality among patients with 'functional' disorders. *Archives of General Psychiatry*, **42**, 82–88.

Bonn, J. A., Readhead, C. P. A. and Timmons, B. A. (1984). Enhanced adaptive behavioral response in agoraphobic patients pretreated with breathing retraining. *Lancet*, September, 665–669.

Boudoulas, H., Reynolds, J. C., Mazzaferri, E. and Wooley, C. F. (1980). Metabolic studies in mitral valve prolapse syndrome. A neuroendocrine-cardiovascular process. *Circulation*, 61, 1200–1205.

Boudoulas, H., King, B. D. and Wooley, C. F. (1984). Mitral valve prolapse: A marker for anxiety or an overlapping phenomenon? *Psychopathology*, 17, suppl. 1, 98–106.

Boyd, J. H. (1986). Use of mental health services for treatment of panic attacks. *American Journal of Psychiatry*, 143, 1569–1574.

Buller, R., Maier, W., Sonntag, A. and Knisel, M. (1987). Das Herzangstsyndrom—ein Subtyp des Panik-Syndroms. In: Nutzinger, D. O., Pfersmann, D., Welan, T. and Zapotoczky, H. G. (Eds), *Die Herzphobie*. Enke, Stuttgart, pp. 42–49.

Cameron, O. G., Lee, M. A., Curtis, G. C. and McCann, D. S. (1987). Endocrine and physiological changes during "spontaneous" panic attacks. *Psychoneuroendocrinology*, 12, 321–331.

Chan, M. P., Hibbert, G. A. and Watkins, J. (1984). Mitral valve prolapse and anxiety disorders. *British Journal of Psychiatry*, 145, 216–217.

Clark, D. M., Salkovskis, P. M. and Chalkley, A. J. (1985). Respiratory control as a treatment for panic attacks. *Journal of Experimental Psychiatry and Behavior Therapy*, 16, 23–30.

Cohen, M. E. and White, P. D. (1950). Life situations, emotions, and neurocirculatory asthenia (anxiety neurosis, neurasthenia, effort syndrome). *Annals of Research in Nervous and Mental Diseases*, 29, 832–869.

Cohen, A. S., Barlow, D. H. and Blanchard, E. B. (1985). Psychophysiology of relaxation-associated panic attacks. *Journal of Abnormal Psychology*, 94, 96–101.

Coombs, R., Shah, P. M., Shulman, R., Klorman, R. and Sylvester, N. (1977). Effects of psychological stress on click and rhythm in mitral valve prolapse. *American Heart Association Monograph*, no. 57, part II, vol. 56(4), III–111.

Coryell, W., Noyes, R. and Clancy, J. (1982). Excess mortality in panic disorder. *Archives of General Psychiatry*, 39, 701–703.

Coryell, W., Noyes, R. and House, J. D. (1986). Mortality among outpatients with panic disorder. *American Journal of Psychiatry*, 143, 508–510.

Crowe, R. R., Pauls, D. L., Slymen, D. J. and Noyes, R. (1980). A family study of anxiety neurosis. *Archives of General Psychiatry*, 37, 77–79.

Crowe, R. R., Pauls, D. L., Kerber, R. and Noyes, R. (1981). Panic disorder and mitral valve prolapse. In Klein, D. F. and Rabkin, J. (Eds), *Anxiety: New Research and Changing Concepts*. Raven Press, New York, pp. 103–114.

Crowe, R. R., Gaffney, G. and Kerber, R. (1982). Panic attacks in families of patients with mitral valve prolapse. *Journal of Affective Disorders*, 4, 121–125.

Curtis, G., Nesse, R., Cameron, O., Thyer, B. and Liepman, M. (1982). Psychobiology of exposure *in vivo*. In Dupont, R. L. (Ed.), *Phobia: A Comprehensive Summary of Modern Treatments*. Brunner & Mazel, New York.

Dager, S. R., Comess, K. A. and Dunner, D. L. (1986). Differentiation of anxious patients by two-dimensional echocardiographic evaluation of the mitral valve. *American Journal of Psychiatry*, 143, 533–535.

DeCarvalho, J. G. R., Messerli, F. H. and Frohlich, E. D. (1979). Mitral valve prolapse and borderline hypertension. *Hypertension*, 1, 518.

Devereux, R. B., Perloff, J. K., Reichek, N. and Josephson, M. E. (1976). Mitral valve prolapse. *Circulation*, 54, 3–14.

Di Nardo, P. A., O'Brien, G. T., Barlow, D. H., Waddell, M. T. and Blanchard, E. B. (1983). Reliability of DSM-III anxiety disorder categories using a new structured interview. *Archives of General Psychiatry*, **40**, 1070–1074.

Ehlers, A., Margraf, J. and Roth, W. T. (1986a). Experimental induction of panic attacks. In Hand, I. and Wittchen, H. U. (Eds), *Panics and Phobias*. Springer, Berlin, pp. 53–66.

Ehlers, A., Margraf, J., Roth, W. T., Taylor, C. B., Maddock, R. J., Sheikh, J., Kopell, M. L., McClenahan, K. L., Gossard, D., Blowers, G. H., Agras, W. S. and Kopell, B. S. (1986b). Lactate infusions and panic attacks: Do patients and controls respond differently? *Psychiatry Research*, **17**, 295–308.

Ehlers, A., Margraf, J. and Roth, W. T. (1988a). Interaction of expectancy and physiological stressors in a laboratory model of panic. In Hellhammer, D., Florin, I. and Weiner, H. (Eds), *Neurobiology of Human Diseases*. Huber, Toronto, pp. 379–384.

Ehlers, A., Margraf, J. and Roth, W. T. (1988b). Selective information processing, interoception, and panic attacks. In Hand, I. and Wittchen, H. U. (Eds), *Treatments of Panic and Phobias*. Springer, Berlin.

Ehlers, A., Margraf, J., Roth, W. T., Taylor, C. B. and Birbaumer, N. (1988c). Anxiety induced by false heart rate feedback in patients with panic disorder. *Behaviour Research and Therapy*, in press.

Fiegenbaum, W. (1986). Longterm efficacy of exposure *in-vivo* for cardiac phobia. In Hand, I. and Wittchen, H. U. (Eds), *Panic and Phobias*. Springer, Berlin, pp. 81–89.

Freedman, R. B., Ianni, P., Ettedgui, E. and Puthezhath, N. (1985). Ambulatory monitoring of panic disorder. *Archives of General Psychiatry*, **42**, 244–248.

Freud, S. (1895). Über die Berechtigung von der Neurasthenie einen bestimmten Symptomenkomplex als 'Angstneurose' abzutrennen, *Neurologisches Zentralblatt*, 2. In Freud, S., (1952) *Gesammelte Werke*. Band I, Imago, London.

Gaffney, F. A., Bastian, B. C., Lane, L. B., Taylor, W. F., Horton, J., Schutte, J. E., Graham, R. M., Pettinger, W., Blumquist, C. G. and Moore, W. E. (1983). Abnormal cardiovascular regulation in the mitral valve prolapse syndrome. *American Journal of Cardiology*, **52**, 316.

Garssen, B., van Veenendahl, W. and Bloemink, R. (1983). Agoraphobia and the hyperventilation syndrome. *Psychotherapy and Psychosomatics*, **33**, 573–577.

Giannini, A. J., Price, W. A. and Loiselle, R. H. (1984). Prevalence of mitral valve prolapse in bipolar affective disorder. *American Journal of Psychiatry*, **141**, 991–992.

Gitlin, B., Martin, J., Shear, M. K., Frances, A., Ball, G. and Josephson, S. (1985). Behavior therapy for panic disorder. *Journal of Nervous and Mental Disease*, **173**, 742–743.

Gorman, J. M. (1986). Panic disorder: Focus on cardiovascular status. Paper presented at the 139th Annual Meeting of the American Psychiatric Association, Washington, D.C.

Gorman, J. M., Fyer, A. F., Glicklich, J., King, D. L. and Klein, D. F. (1981a). Mitral valve prolapse and panic disorders: Effect of imipramine. In Klein, D. F. and Rabkin, J. (Eds), *Anxiety: New Research and Changing Concepts*. Raven Press, New York, pp. 317–326.

Gorman, J. M., Fyer, A. F., Glicklich, J., King, D. L. and Klein, D. F. (1981b). Effect of imipramine on prolapsed mitral valve of patients with panic disorder. *American Journal of Psychiatry*, **138**, 977–978.

Gorman, J. M., Shear, K., Devereux, R. B., King, D. L. and Klein, D. F. (1986). Prevalence of mitral valve prolapse in panic disorder: Effect of echocardiographic criteria. *Psychosomatic Medicine*, **48**, 167–171.

Grunhaus, L., Gloger, S., Rein, A. and Lewis, B. S. (1982). Mitral valve prolapse and panic attacks. *Israel Journal of Medical Sciences*, **18**, 221-223.

Grunhaus, L., Gloger, S., Birmacher, B., Palmer, C. and Ben-David, M. (1983). Prolactin response to the cold pressor test in patients with panic attacks. *Psychiatry Research*, **8**, 171-177.

Guttmacher, L. B., Murphy, D. L. and Insel, T. R. (1983). Pharmacologic models of anxiety. *Comprehensive Psychiatry*, **24**, 312-326.

Hall, M. L., Katon, W. J., Russo, J., Cormier, L., Hollifield, M. and Vitaliano, P. P. (1987). Chest pain and normal coronary arteriography predicts high prevalence of panic disorder. *Clinical Research*, **35**, 105.

Hand, I., Angenendt, J., Fischer, M. and Wilke, C. (1986). Exposure *in-vivo* with panic management for agoraphobia: Treatment rationale and longterm outcome. In Hand, I. and Wittchen, H. U. (Eds), *Panic and Phobias*. Springer, Berlin, pp. 104-128.

Harbauer-Raum, U. (1987). Wahrnehmung von Herzschlag und Herzarrhythmien — Eine Labor-Feldstudie an Patienten mit Herzphobie. In: Nutzinger, D. O., Pfersmann, D., Welan, T. and Zapotoczky, H. G. (Eds), *Die Herzphobie*. Enke, Stuttgart, pp. 84-91.

Hartman, N., Kramer, R., Brown, W. T. and Devereux, R. B. (1982). Panic disorder in patients with mitral valve prolapse. *American Journal of Psychiatry*, **139**, 669-670.

Hayward, C., Taylor, C. B. and Clark, D. (in press). Panic disorder, anxiety, and cardiovascular risk. In Ballenger, J. (Ed.), *Clinical Aspects of Panic Disorder*. Alan Liss Inc., New York.

Hickey, A. J., Andrews, G. and Wilcken, D. E. L. (1983). Independence of mitral valve prolapse and neurosis. *British Heart Journal*, **50**, 333-336.

Himadi, W. G., Boice, R. and Barlow, D. H. (1985). Assessment of agoraphobia: Triple response measurement. *Behaviour Research and Therapy*, **23**, 311-332.

Hodgson, R., and Rachman, S. (1974). Desynchrony in measures of fear. *Behaviour Research and Therapy*, **12**, 319-326.

Jablensky, A. (1985). Approaches to the definition and classification of anxiety and related disorders in European psychiatry. In Tuma, A. H. and Maser, J. (Eds), *Anxiety and the Anxiety Disorders*. Lawrence Erlbaum, Hillsdale, pp. 735-758.

Jacob, R. and Rapport, M. D. (1984). Panic disorder: Medical and psychological parameters. In Turner, S. M. (Ed.), *Behavioral Theories and Treatment of Anxiety*. Plenum Press, New York.

Judd, F. K., Norman, T. R. and Burroughs, G. D., (1986). Pharmacological treatment of panic disorder. *International Clinical Psychopharmacology*, **1**, 3-16.

Kane, J. M., Woerner, M., Zeldis, S., Kramer, R. and Saravay, S. (1981). Panic and phobic disorders in patients with mitral valve prolapse. In Klein, D. F. and Rabkin, J. (Eds), *Anxiety: New Research and Changing Concepts*. Raven Press, New York, pp. 327-340.

Kantor, J. S., Zitrin, C. M. and Zeldis, S. M. (1980). Mitral valve prolapse syndrome in agoraphobic patients. *American Journal of Psychiatry*, **137**, 467-469.

Kathol, R. G., Noyes, R., Slymen, D. J., Crowe, R. R., Clancy, J. and Kerber, R. (1980). Propanolol in chronic anxiety disorders. *Archives of General Psychiatry*, **37**, 1361-1365.

Katon, W. (1984). Panic disorder and somatization. *The American Journal of Medicine*, **77**, 101-106.

Kelly, D., Brown, C. C. and Shaffer, J. W. (1970). A comparison of physiological and psychological measurements of anxious patients and normal controls. *Psychophysiology*, **6**, 429-441.

King, R., Margraf, J., Ehlers, A. and Maddock, R. J. (1986). Panic disorder — overlap with somatization disorder. In Hand, I. and Wittchen, H. U. (Eds), *Panic and Phobias*. Springer, Berlin, pp. 72–80.

Klein, D. F. and Gorman, J. M. (1984). Panic disorders and mitral valve prolapse. *Journal of Clinical Psychiatry Monograph*, March, 14–17.

Ko, G. N., Elsworth, J. D., Roth, R. H., Rifkin, B. G., Leigh, H. and Redmond, D. E. (1983). Panic-induced elevation of plasma MHPG levels in phobic-anxious patients. *Archives of General Psychiatry*, **40**, 425–430.

Koch, F. H. and Hancock, E. W. (1976). Ten year follow-up of forty patients with the midsystolic click/late murmur syndromes. *American Journal of Cardiology*, **37**, 149.

Lader, M. H. (1967). Palmar skin conductance measures in anxiety and phobic states. *Journal of Psychosomatic Research*, **11**, 271–281.

Lader, M. H. and Mathews, A. (1970). Physiological changes during spontaneous panic attacks. *Journal of Psychosomatic Research*, **14**, 377–382.

Lader, M. H. and Wing, L. (1964). Habituation of the psycho-galvanic reflex in patients with anxiety states and in normal subjects. *Journal of Neurology, Neurosurgery and Psychiatry*, **27**, 210–218.

Lesser, I. M. and Rubin, R. T. (1986). Diagnostic considerations in panic disorder. *Journal of Clinical Psychiatry*, **47**, suppl. 4–10.

Liberthson, R., Sheehan, D. V., King, M. E. and Weyman, A. E. (1986). The prevalence of mitral valve prolapse. *American Journal of Psychiatry*, **143**, 511–515.

Liebowitz, M. R., Gorman, J. M., Fyer, A., Dillon, D., Levitt, M. and Klein, D. F. (1986). Possible mechanisms for lactate's induction of panic. *American Journal of Psychiatry*, **143**, 495–502.

Lum, L. C. (1981). Hyperventilation and anxiety state. *Journal of the Royal Society of Medicine*, **74**, 1–4.

Margraf, J. and Ehlers, A. (1986). Erkennung und Behandlung von akuten Angstanfällen. In Brengelmann, J. C. and Bühringer, G. (Eds), *Therapieforschung für die Praxis*, vol. 6. Röttger Verlag, Munich.

Margraf, J., Ehlers, A. and Roth, W. T. (1986a). Biological models of panic disorder and agoraphobia: A review. *Behaviour Research and Therapy*, **24**, 553–567.

Margraf, J., Ehlers, A. and Roth, W. T. (1986b). Lactate infusions and panic attacks: A review and critique. *Psychosomatic Medicine*, **48**, 23–51.

Margraf, J., Ehlers, A. and Roth, W. T. (1987a). Panic attack associated with perceived heart rate acceleration: A case report. *Behavior Therapy*, **18**, 84–89.

Margraf, J., Taylor, C. B., Ehlers, A., Roth, W. T. and Agras, W. S. (1987b). Panic attacks in the natural environment. *Journal of Nervous and Mental Disease*, **175**, 558–565.

Markiewicz, W., Stoner, J., London, E., Hunt, S. A. and Popp, R. L. (1976). Mitral valve prolapse in one hundred presumably healthy young females. *Circulation*, **53**, 464–473.

Marks, I. (1983). Are there anticompulsive or antiphobic drugs? Review of the evidence. *British Journal of Psychiatry*, **143**, 338–347.

Martin, R. L., Cloninger, R., Guze, S. B. and Clayton, P. J. (1985). Mortality in a follow-up of 500 psychiatric outpatients. *Archives of General Psychiatry*, **42**, 47–66.

Mavissakalian, M., Salerni, R., Thompson, M. E. and Michelson, L. (1983). Mitral valve prolapse and agoraphobia. *American Journal of Psychiatry*, **140**, 1612–1614.

Mazza, D. L., Martin, D., Spacavento, L., Jacobsen, J. and Gibbs, H. (1986). *American Journal of Psychiatry*, **143**, 349–351.

McCue, E. and McCue, P. (1984). Organic and hyperventilatory causes of anxiety-type symptoms. *Behavioural Psychotherapy*, **2**, 308-317.

Mills, P., Rose, J., Hollingsworth, J., Amara, I. and Craig, E. (1977). Long-term prognosis of mitral valve prolapse. *New England Journal of Medicine*, **297**, 13.

Motulsky, A. G. (1978). Biased ascertainment and the natural history of diseases. *New England Journal of Medicine*, **298**, 1196-1197.

Mukerji, V., Beitman, B. D., Alpert, M. A., Hewett, J. E. and Basha, I. M. (1987). Panic attack symptoms in patients with chest pain and angiographically normal coronary arteries. *Journal of Anxiety Disorders*, **1**, 41-46.

Myrtek, M. (1984). *Constitutional Psychophysiology*, Academic Press, Orlando.

Nesse, R. M., Cameron, O. G., Buda, A. J., McCann, D. S., Curtis, G. C. and Huber-Smith, M. J. (1985). Urinary catecholamines and mitral valve prolapse in panic-anxiety patients. *Psychiatry Research*, **14**, 67-74.

Nishimura, R. A., McGoon, M. D., Shub, C., Miller, F. A. Jr., Illstrup, D. M. and Tajik, A. J. (1985). Echocardiographically documented mitral-valve prolapse: Long-term follow-up of 237 patients. *New England Journal of Medicine*, **313**, 1305-1309.

Noyes, R., Clancy, J. and Hoenk, P. R. (1978). Anxiety neurosis and physical illness. *Comprehensive Psychiatry*, **19**, 407-413.

Öst, L. G. (1987). Age of onset in different phobias. *Journal of Abnormal Psychology*, **96**, 223-229.

Öst, L. G. (1988). Applied relaxation vs. progressive relaxation in the treatment of panic disorder. *Behaviour Research and Therapy* **26**, 13-22.

Pariser, S. F., Pinta, E. R. and Jones, B. A. (1978). Mitral valve prolapse syndrome and anxiety neurosis/panic disorder. *American Journal of Psychiatry*, **135**, 246-247.

Pariser, S. F., Jones, B. A., Pinta, E. R., Young, E. A. and Fontana, M. E. (1979). Panic attacks: Diagnostic evaluations of 17 patients. *American Journal of Psychiatry*, **136**, 105-106.

Pasternac, A., Tubau, J. F., Puddu, P. E., Krol, R. B. and DeChamplain, J. (1982). Increased plasma catecholamine levels in patients with symptomatic mitral valve prolapse. *American Journal of Medicine*, **73**, 783.

Pennebaker, J. W. (1982). *The Psychology of Physical Symptoms*, Springer, New York.

Pitts, F. N. and McClure, J. N. (1967). Lactate metabolism in anxiety neurosis. *New England Journal of Medicine*, **227**, 1329-1336.

Pocock, W. A., Bosman, C. K., Chesler, E., Barlow, J. B. and Edwards, J. E. (1984). Sudden death in primary mitral valve prolapse. *American Heart Journal*, **107**, 378-382.

Puddu, P. E. (1983). QT interval prolongation and increased plasma catecholamine levels in patients with mitral valve prolapse. *American Heart Journal*, **105**, 441.

Rapee, R. (1986). Differential response to hyperventilation in panic disorder and generalized anxiety disorder. *Journal of Abnormal Psychology*, **95**, 24-28.

Reid, J. V. O. (1961). Midsystolic clicks. *South African Medical Journal*, **135**, 353-355.

Robins, L. N., Helzer, J. E., Weissman, M. M., Orvaschel, H., Gruenberg, E., Burke, J. D. and Regier, D. A. (1984). Lifetime prevalence of specific psychiatric disorders in three sites. *Archives of General Psychiatry*, **41**, 949-958.

Rosenthal, M. E., Hamer, A., Gang, E. S., Oseran, D. S., Mandel, W. J. and Peter, T. (1985). The yield of programmed ventricular stimulation of mitral valve prolapse patients with ventricular arrhythmias. *American Heart Journal*, **110**, 970-976.

Roth, W. T., Telch, M. J., Taylor, C. B., Sachitano, J. A., Gallen, C., Kopell, M. L., McClenahan, K., Agras, S. and Pfefferbaum, A. (1986). Autonomic characteristics of agoraphobia with panic attacks. *Biological Psychiatry*, **21**, 1133-1154.

Salkovskis, P. M. and Clark, D. M. (1986). Cognitive and physiological processes in the maintenance and treatment of panic attacks. In Hand, I. and Wittchen, H. U. (Eds), *Panic and Phobias*. Springer, Berlin, pp. 89–103.

Savage, D. S., Garrison, R. J., Devereux, R. B., Castelli, W. P., Anderson, S. J., Levy, D., McNamara, P. M., Stokes, J., Kannel, W. B. and Feinleib, M. (1983a). Mitral valve prolapse in the general population. 1. Epidemiologic features: The Framingham study. *American Heart Journal*, **106**, 571–576.

Savage, D. S., Devereux, R. B., Garrison, R. J., Castelli, W. P., Anderson, S. J., Levy, D., Thomas, H. E., Kannel, W. B. and Feinleib, M. (1983b). Mitral valve prolapse in the general population. 2. Clinical features. The Framingham study. *American Heart Journal*, **106**, 577–581.

Savage, D. S., Levy, D., Garrison, R. J., Castelli, W. P., Kligfield, P., Devereux, R. B., Anderson, S. J., Kannel, W. B. and Feinleib, M. (1983c). Mitral valve prolapse in the general population. 3. Dysrhythmias: The Framingham study, *American Heart Journal*, **106**, 582–586.

Schweizer, P., Hanrath, P., Merx, W., Henning, B., Saal, M., Schaefer, P., Bleifeld, W. and Effert, S. (1979). Ventrikuläre Rhythmusstörungen beim Mitralklappenprolaps-syndrom. *Deutsche Medizinische Wochenschrift*, **104**, 85–89.

Shear, M. K., (1986). Pathophysiology of panic: A review of pharamacologic provocative tests and naturalistic monitoring data. *Journal of Clinical Psychiatry*, **47**, suppl. 18–26.

Shear, M. K., Devereux, R. B., Kramer-Fox, R., Mann, J. J. and Frances, A. (1984). Low prevalence of mitral valve prolapse in patients with panic disorder. *American Journal of Psychiatry*, **141**, 302–303.

Shear, M. K., Kligfield, P., Harshfield, G., Devereux, R. B., Pickering, T. and Frances, A. J. (1986). Cardiac arrhythmias in panic patients. Paper presented at the 139th Annual Meeting of the American Psychiatric Association, Washington, D.C.

Skerritt, P. W. (1983). Anxiety and the heart—a historical review. *Psychological Medicine*, **13**, 17–25.

Strian, F. (1987). Psychiatrische Aspekte des Mitralklappenprolaps-Syndroms. In Nutzinger, D. O., Pfersmann, D., Welan, T. and Zapotoczky, H. G. (Eds), *Die Herzphobie*. Enke, Stuttgart, pp. 66–74.

Sturm, J., Ehrhardt, M. and Müller, C. (1987). Ein multimodales verhaltensmedizinisches Gruppenkonzept für die Behandlung von Herzphobikern. In Nutzinger, D. O., Pfersmann, D., Welan, T. and Zapotoczky, H. G. (Eds), *Die Herzphobie*. Enke, Stuttgart, pp. 136–144.

Taylor, C. B., Telch, M. J. and Havvik, D. (1983). Ambulatory heart rate changes during panic attacks. *Journal of Psychiatric Research*, **17**, 261–266.

Taylor, C. B., Skeikh, J., Agras, W. S., Roth, W. T., Margraf, J., Ehlers, A., Maddock, R. J. and Gossard, D. (1986). Ambulatory heart rate changes in patients with panic attacks. *American Journal of Psychiatry*, **143**, 478–482.

Taylor, C. B., King, R., Ehlers, A., Margraf, J., Clark, D., Roth, W. T. and Agras, W. S. (1987). Treadmill exercise test and ambulatory measures in patients with panic attacks. *American Journal of Cardiology* **60**, 48J–52J.

Tyrer, P. J. (1976). *The Role of Bodily Feelings in Anxiety*. Oxford University Press, London.

Tzivoni, D., Stern, Z., Keren, A. and Stern, S. (1980). Electrocardiographic characteristics of neurocirculatory athenia during everyday activities. *British Heart Journal*, **44**, 426–432.

Uhde, T. W., Roy-Byrne, P. P., Vittone, B. J., Boulenger, J. P. and Post, R. M. (1985). Phenomenology and neurobiology of panic disorder. In Tuma, A. H. and Maser, J. (Eds), *Anxiety and the Anxiety Disorders*. Erlbaum, Hillsdale.

Uretsky, B. F. (1980). Does mitral valve prolapse cause nonspecific symptoms? *Circulation*, **62**, suppl. 3, 206.

Venkatesh, A., Pauls, D. L., Crowe, R., Noyes, R., Van Valkenburg, C., Martins, J. B. and Kerber, R. (1980). Mitral valve prolapse in anxiety neurosis (panic disorder). *American Heart Journal*, **100**, 302–305.

Vohra, J. K. (1977). Tricyclic antidepressants and cardiac function. In Burrows, G. D. (Ed.), *Handbook of Studies on Depression*. Excerpta Medica, Amsterdam, pp. 405–410.

Wann, L. S., Groves, J. R. and Hess, T. R. (1983). Prevalence of mitral valve prolapse by 2D echocardiography in healthy young women. *British Heart Journal*, **49**, 334–340.

Wann, L. S., Gross, C. M., Wakefield, R. J. and Kalbfleisch, J. H. (1985). Diagnostic precision of echocardiography in mitral valve prolapse. *American Heart Journal*, **109**, 803–808.

Warth, D. C., King, M. E., Cohen, J. M., Tesoriero, V. L., Marcus, E. and Weyman, A. E. (1985). Prevalence of mitral valve prolapse in normal children. *Journal of the American College of Cardiology*, **5**, 1173–1177.

Weiner, H. (1985). The psychobiology and pathophysiology of anxiety and fear. In Tuma, A. H. and Maser, J. (Eds), *Anxiety and the Anxiety Disorders*, Erlbaum, Hillsdale, New Jersey.

Weiss, A. N., Mimbs, J. W., Ludbrook, P. A. and Sobel, B. E. (1975). Echocardiographic detection of the mitral valve prolapse. *Circulation*, **52**, 1091–1096.

White, W. B. and Baker, L. H. (1986). Episodic hypertension secondary to panic disorder. *Archives of Internal Medicine*, **146**, 1129–1130.

Wilder, J., (1931). Das 'Ausgangswert-Gesetz' — ein unbeachtetes biologisches Gesetz; seine Bedeutung für Forschung und Praxis. *Klinische Wochenschrift*, **10**, 1889–1893.

Williams, R. L. and Karacan, I. (1984). Anxiety and sleep. In Pasnau, R. O. (Ed.), *Diagnosis and Treatment of Anxiety Disorders*. American Psychiatric Press, Washington.

Wittchen, H. U. (1986). Epidemiology of panic attacks and panic disorders. In Hand, I. and Wittchen, H. U. (Eds), *Panic and Phobias*. Springer, Berlin, pp. 18–28.

Wittchen, H. U. and Semler, G. (1986). Diagnostic reliability of anxiety disorders. In Hand, I. and Wittchen, H. U. (Eds), *Panic and Phobias*. Springer, Berlin, pp. 7–17.

Woods, S. C., Charney, D. S., McPherson, C. A., Gradman, A. H. and Heninger, G. R. (1987). Situational panic attacks: Behavioral, physiological, and biochemical characterization. *Archives of General Psychiatry*, **44**, 365–375.

Wooley, C. F. (1976). Where are the diseases of yesteryear? DaCosta's syndrome, soldier's heart, the effort syndrome, neurocirculatory asthenia — And the mitral valve prolapse syndrome. *Circulation*, **53**, 749–751.

World Health Organization (Ed.) (1977). *Manual of the International Statistical Classification of Diseases, Injuries, and Causes of Death*, 9th revision, WHO, Geneva.

Wynne, J. (1986). Mitral-valve prolapse. *New England Journal of Medicine*, **314**, 577–578.

Young, J. B., Kumpuris, A. G., Bagby, C., Cos, M. D., Quinones, M. A., Winters, W. L. and Miller, R. R. (1979). Psychologic profile of mitral valve prolapse patients. *Clinical Research*, **27**, 218.

Zarcone, V. P., Maddock, R. and Slegel, D. (1986). Atypical polysomnographic features in the sleep of a panic disorder patient. Paper presented at the Annual Meeting of the Professional Sleep Societies, Columbus, Ohio.

Behavioural Medicine in Cardiovascular Disorders
Edited by T. Elbert, W. Langosch, A. Steptoe and D. Vaitl
©1988 John Wiley & Sons Ltd

18

Treatment of Sinus Tachycardia with Heart Rate Feedback: A Group Outcome Study

Kees H. L. Janssen* and Martijn P. F. Berger[†]

*Tilburg University, The Netherlands

[†]University of Twente, The Netherlands

SUMMARY

After cardiological examination 7 patients with elevated heart rate and related symptoms were diagnosed as having psychosomatic sinus tachycardia. During a 2½-week baseline period initial heart rate levels were assessed in two separate recording sessions. Treatment consisted of twelve heart rate feedback sessions twice weekly. Sessions comprised four feedback periods of 6 minutes, in which the subject trained to lower heart rate with analogue auditory and visual signals. Three months after treatment patients returned for a follow-up session. Patients charted their complaint every 4 hours throughout baseline and treatment period, and again 2 weeks prior to follow-up session. Analysis of results indicates a clear improvement over treatment in the chartings of 5 patients. Likewise significant decreases in heart rate values were observed. These effects on heart rate and on complaint endured at follow-up. The clinical utility of heart rate feedback for sinus tachycardia is further substantiated by significant changes in neuroticism and neurosomatization, and reports by patients on positive effects of treatment on their life situation. These findings will be discussed in terms of the possible specificity of the treatment applied, and hence the role of respiratory factors and neurophysiological mechanisms in explaining these results.

*Address for correspondence: Martijn P. F. Berger, Department of Education, University of Twente, P.O. Box 217, 7500 AE Enschede, The Netherlands.

INTRODUCTION

There is a large body of evidence that human subjects can learn to influence their heart rate when given exteroceptive feedback of their cardiac activity (Blanchard and Young, 1973; Williamson and Blanchard, 1979). There have been numerous reports on subjects producing significantly large changes in heart rate as a result of learned cardiac acceleration training (e.g. Clemens and Shattock, 1979). Positive results of biofeedback-assisted heart rate deceleration have not been as numerous or of the same magnitude (e.g. Stoney et al., 1986), but this contrast with acceleration studies may well be explained by biological constraints of the cardiovascular system. The subjects in these studies typically have been young (college age) and free of disease. Since the normal resting heart rate is usually about 70 bpm, the potential range of change to be expected for heart rate acceleration and deceleration would be on the order of 100 bpm and 15 bpm, respectively (Cheatle and Weiss, 1982). Therefore no definite inferences on the therapeutic potential of heart rate feedback can be drawn from these studies with non-clinical populations.

The limitations of the above studies with normals become clear if one considers the several reports that demonstrate the potential of learned deceleration of heart rate for sinus tachycardia (Engel and Bleecker, 1974; Scott et al., 1973; Vaitl, 1975; Janssen, 1983). Sinus tachycardia refers to an abnormally increased heart rate in which the rhythm is still generated from the S-A node. Hence the electrocardiogram has normal QRS complexes except that the rate of heart beat is considerably higher than normal. Three independent general causes of tachycardia are increased body temperature, toxic conditions of the heart, and stimulation of the heart by the autonomic nerves (Guyton, 1981). In healthy individuals sinus tachycardia occurs as an adaptation mechanism to adjust cardiac output to the demands of the body, e.g. in physical exercise or emotion (Robles de Medina et al., 1980), or in cognitive-informational tasks (Mulder and Mulder, 1981). In cases of persistent sinus tachycardia, if differential diagnosis excludes organic pathology, psychosocial or psychodynamic factors can be found to be involved. Symptoms that often accompany the tachycardia include strong precordial pulsation, respiratory distress, chest symptoms, and jerking pulse (Garnier, 1981). Thus tachycardia may constitute a frightening, burdensome and taxing experience to the person, and one way for it to persist is when its interpretation (or cognitive attribution) induces in the subject a state of anxiety. The physiological changes thus brought about will intensify the cardiac sensations and this will confirm the subject in his or her interpretation and anxiety, i.e. a vicious circle as described by Liebhart (1974). Tachycardia and accompanying symptoms and complaints, once established, may occur in either of two ways: continuous and chronic, or in transient but recurrent episodes.

Besides the discomfort itself, sinus tachycardia may also add considerably to the risk for later hypertension. Not all patients with borderline hypertension will develop later sustained hypertension (Julius, 1977). However there is some evidence that when borderline hypertension and tachycardia are combined, the risk for future hypertension is particularly high (Paffenbarger et al., 1968). This finding confirmed the results of a study by Levi et al. (1945). The latter study also established that tachycardia at youth even without blood pressure elevation carries an excessive risk for future hypertension. Generalizing from such epidemiological findings, Manuck and Proietti (1982) have argued from their experiments on high heart rate reactors with a parental history of hypertension, that these subjects may be among those most likely to develop essential hypertension in later life. The same inference was made by Light and Obrist (1980) when they observed that subjects with both marginally elevated casual systolic pressure and high heart rate reactivity to stress, had by far the highest incidence of parental hypertension. Steptoe et al. (1984) report evidence suggesting more directly that exaggerated cardiac responsiveness to active challenges may be characteristic of the prehypertensive profile. Lastly, an association has been found in monkeys between heart rate reactivity under stress and the development of atherosclerosis (Manuck et al., 1983).

Treatment of sinus tachycardia commonly involves beta adrenergic blocking agents. Many of these are associated with undesirable side-effects. For example, propranolol may cause or worsen heart block or cardiac failure (Winkle et al., 1975). Another effect may be irreversible reduction of glomerular filtration rate, which would limit beta blocker use for patients with pre-existing renal insufficiency (Bauer and Brooks, 1979). Other side-effects include fatigue, depression, nausea, diarrhea, hyperglycemia, and hyperosmolar coma (Winkle et al., 1975). While not all beta blocking agents require as much caution as propranolol, one general side-effect they share is the induction of bronchospasm which renders them unsuitable for patients who besides their tachycardia display asthmatic symptoms.

Thus it would seem worthwhile to explore self-control procedures such as heart rate feedback in their potential for sinus tachycardia. The present study has tried to establish evidence in support of this clinical application of heart rate feedback, so as to bring the technique from the case study level (Engel and Bleecker, 1974; Scott et al., 1973; Vaitl, 1975; Janssen, 1983) to the next higher methodological level. In a group outcome study we aimed at assessing the effectiveness of heart rate feedback for sinus tachycardia, employing several criteria such as heart rate frequency, subjective complaint, personality dimensions. As the development of self-control was considered one of the primary aims of the treatment offered, a follow-up period was scheduled to study the durability of treatment effects.

METHOD

Subjects

General practitioners were invited to refer patients for this study, when after cardiological screening, organic causes of sinus tachycardia had been excluded. Tachycardia had to be labeled by the patients as the major complaint for which they sought treatment. Other minor dysfunctions were allowed (e.g. light headpain, nervousness, irritable stomach), but not to the extent that this constituted pathology *per se*. Patients with a history of tachycardia shorter than 6 months were not included in the study. Occurrence of tachycardia was either continuous and chronic, or in transient episodes. As in the latter case occurrence of tachycardia would not always coincide with baseline recording, we also relied on documentary evidence from general practitioners and cardiologists for definition of sinus tachycardia. However a heart rate lower than 75 bpm during any baseline recording trial led to exclusion from the study. Patients were allowed to continue their medication, but it was insisted that they would not change type of medication once they had entered into the study. During baseline they also were asked to maintain a constant medication rate, but in the course of treatment they could reduce drug use, should they feel able. The final sample included 3 males and 4 females, with a mean age of 36.3 years (SD = 12.7, range = 18–55 years). The mean number of years of tachycardia complaint was 4.8 (range 0.6–20). See Table 1.

Table 1. Patient characteristics upon intake. History (Hst) refers to earliest documented tachycardia as established by medical examination and persistence of complaint and symptoms. Adapted from Janssen and Bekkering (1986).

Age	m/f	Hst	Medication	Symptoms
A 37	f	1 yr	4*isoptin 80/d 4*inderal 10/d	fear of faint; visus disturbance + tinnitus during, precordial pulsation after effort; incid. PVCs
B 51	m	7 mo	—	respiratory distress, precordial symptoms after effort
C 55	m	5 yr	—	precordial pulsations, dyspnoe, anxiety, incid. PVCs, nightmares with tachycardia
D 27	m	1 yr	—	incid. tension headache disturbed sleep, high heart rate reactor
E 40	f	6 mo*	—	papitations, disturbed sleep, feels agitated, irritated
F 18	f	4 yr	—	early fatigue, rest after effort worsens tachycardia causing panic, incid. migraine
G 23	f	2 yr	2*Lopressor 50/d	disturbed sleep, rest after effort worsens tachycardia, tingling hands + feet, headaches

*Intermittent palpitations occurred since early adulthood.

Procedure

Subjects charted their tachycardia complaint for an 18-day baseline period. Charting was done on special forms noting complaint duration and intensity (0–10) for each 4-hour interval. During the baseline period the subject's ECG-lead II was recorded in two separate sessions. Each subject was told to relax to the best of his or her ability while recordings were taken for 3 separate 3-minute trials. The second recording session was scheduled 2 or 3 days after the first session. Complaint data charted during this intersession period and physiological data from the first recording session were not considered for statistical analysis, in order to allow for a period of adaptation. After the second recording session, a personality questionnaire (Wilde, 1970) was filled out by each subject assessing neuroticism (N) and neurosomatization (NS). This questionnaire was again filled out during the follow-up session.

Treatment consisted of 12 sessions of heart rate feedback, twice weekly. These sessions comprised four feedback periods of 6 minutes, in which the subject trained to lower heart rate with the aid of both a visual and an auditory feedback signal. These signals were derived from the ear densitogram. In some subjects where this mode of pick-up proved obtrusive, the densitogram was taken from fingertip provided this allowed for reliable pulse detection. The subject was comfortably seated in a reclining chair, in front of a feedback display bar of 30 LEDs. This bar was adjustable for level of heart rate, so that five different ranges of heart rate, overlapping each other ± 30%, could be chosen. The subject was told in which range the display bar was set. Simultaneous with the visual display, the subject listened through an earphone to a tone, whose range of pitch was linked to the range of the visual feedback signal. Both signals could be switched on and off independently of each other. Between every two periods of a session (feedback and/or recording periods) there was a break of approximately 1 min to allow for discussion between subject and the therapist, and for the subject to readjust his or her position in the chair. Also it was thought to be more useful for the subject to develop skill in lowering heart rate than to learn to maintain—once achieved—a low level of heart rate.

In each heart rate feedback session the ECG was recorded during three separate intervals of 3 minutes (trials): in advance of the first feedback period (presession), during the third feedback period (insession), and after the last feedback period (postsession). Recording in all three periods in baseline sessions was done without any feedback signal. In heart rate feedback and follow-up sessions, presession and postsession recordings were likewise made in the absence of any feedback signal, but during insession recording, both feedback signals were available to the subject. Altogether the baseline covered a 2½-week period, and treatment a nominal period of 6 weeks (an incidental break of up to 10 days was allowed for holidays). The follow-up session was scheduled 3 months after termination of treatment.

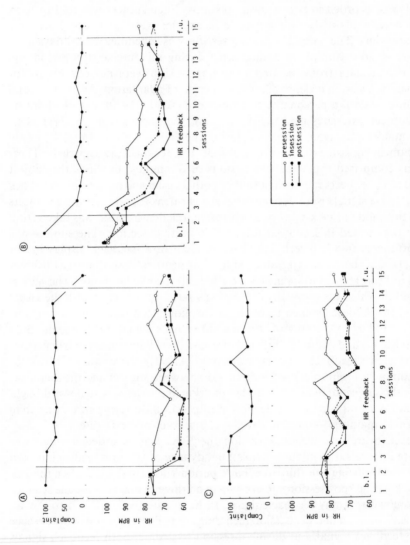

Figure 1 (see legend on p. 299).

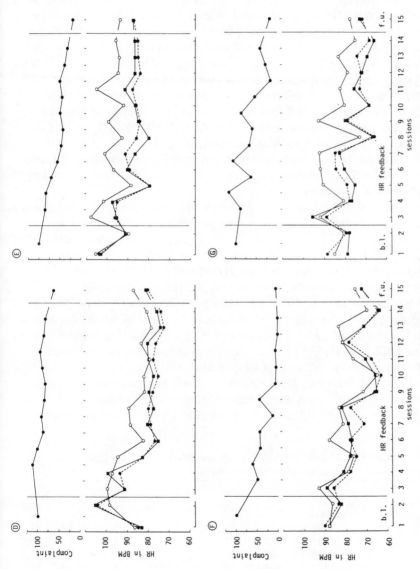

Figure 1. Treatment results per subject (plots A–G). Lower traces in each plot show average heart rate in bpm during pre-, in- and postsession recording trials. Upper trace: intersession scores of subjective complaint, expressed in percentage of baseline.

RESULTS

ECG signals of all recordings (trials) were digitized on a PDP 11/10 computer using the peak of the R wave to monitor interbeat interval. Subsequently these values were averaged over trials and expressed in bpm. These averages were plotted separately for each individual (Figure 1). This figure also shows the intersession scores of subjective complaint. Intersession scores were obtained by multiplying intensity and duration of complaints within each intersession period. In order to allow for intersubject comparisons, these product scores were expressed as percentage of baselinescores before graphical representation.

A repeated measures Subjects × Trials × Sessions ANOVA on the heart rate data from the baseline period showed no significant difference between the pre-, in- and postsession recordings ($F(2,12) = 2.5$, $p > 0.05$) and no significant difference between the two baseline sessions ($F(1,6) = 0.2$, $p > 0.20$). This indicates absence of systematic trends in heart rate fluctuations during baseline. This eliminates these fluctuations as a possible explanation for effects later in treatment or at follow-up.

Trend analysis on the heart rate data from the 12 treatment sessions showed that the linear slopes of the pre-, in- and postsession recordings did not differ significantly ($F(2,12) = 0.2$, $p > 0.20$), but that the intercepts did differ ($F(2,12) = 73.0$, $p < 0.01$). By means of Scheffé's *post hoc* procedure it could be inferred that this difference was mainly determined by the difference between the presession recordings and the in- and postsession recordings.

To further evaluate the effect of treatment on heart rate we also performed a Subjects × Trials × Sessions ANOVA on heart rate data of session 2 (baseline), 14 (end of treatment), and 15 (follow-up). This yielded a significant effect for sessions ($F(2,12) = 17.4$, $p < 0.01$). Scheffé's *post hoc* procedure revealed a very significant decline of heart rate from session 2 to 14 ($p < 0.01$). Although the mean heart rate increased from session 14 to 15, this increase was found not significant ($p > 0.20$). This would indicate that effects of heart rate feedback with these patients persisted after termination of treatment, at least over a

Table 2. Heart rate in bpm per subject per trial during baseline (session 2), end of treatment (session 14), and follow-up (session 15).

Subject	Baseline			End			Follow-up		
	pre	in	post	pre	in	post	pre	in	post
A	76.4	77.8	77.6	74.7	64.2	64.3	69.9	68.6	68.1
B	94.8	91.1	89.9	81.3	73.8	78.1	82.8	75.1	75.2
C	85.3	82.7	82.4	76.1	72.2	70.3	78.0	73.5	72.3
D	98.5	104.2	105.7	80.8	74.2	75.7	87.4	80.9	81.2
E	90.1	90.5	91.2	96.0	85.3	86.6	93.9	87.7	88.0
F	86.6	83.8	82.6	69.3	64.0	63.3	75.5	72.1	72.1
G	80.3	79.6	78.3	75.3	68.2	65.8	78.1	72.0	73.4

3-month period. For Trials a significant effect was found ($F(2,12) = 56.3$, $p < 0.01$). A significant interaction Trials × Sessions was also found ($F(4,24) = 7.7$, $p < 0.01$) and together with the insignificant Trials effect as observed in the ANOVA on Baseline sessions, this suggests that at end of treatment and at follow-up there is a sharp decrease in heart rate values during a session, whereas during baseline sessions this decrease is, on the average, much less pronounced.

As for effect of treatment on chartings of subjective complaint, a first impression can be obtained from Figure 1. Trend analysis was performed on intersession scores over the entire treatment period in order to explore this aspect further. The linear shape of subjective complaint over treatment was found to deviate significantly from zero ($p < 0.01$), indicating a significant decrease in subjective complaints during treatment. This effect of treatment was also analyzed with a repeated measures ANOVA on the product scores, as shown in Table 2.

A significant effect was observed for Sessions ($F(2,12) = 13.3$, $p < 0.01$) and Scheffé's *post hoc* analysis demonstrated that as with heart rate data, this mainly related to the contrast between baseline versus end of treatment and follow-up together. Again no difference was found between end of treatment and follow-up ($p > 0.20$).

In addition to these statistical analyses, inferential evidence can also be obtained from inspection of the individual subject results in Figure 1 and Tables 1 and 2. A gradual decline in presession heart rate from baseline towards end of treatment and follow-up phase was observed in 4 subjects. Subjects A, C, and E however did not show any apparent decrease in presession heart rate. Still subject E was able to lower heart rate within treatment sessions appreciably, as did subject A by the end of treatment. This ability had disappeared by follow-up for subject A. In subject C it was present to a minor degree, although with considerable consistency as evidenced over treatment sessions and at follow-up.

Another way to evaluate the outcome of this treatment is to consider its effect on personality variables (Table 3).

Table 3. Subjective complaint (intensity × duration scores) during baseline, end of treatment, and follow-up. Each value refers to average of a 2-week period.

Subject	Baseline	End	Follow-up
A	6.6	5.2	0.0
B	4.9	0.1	0.0
C	11.4	5.9	7.9
D	9.0	7.8	6.0
E	19.5	7.0	5.4
F	8.9	0.0	0.2
G	4.9	1.6	0.9

Table 4. Scores in percentiles for neuroticism (N) and neurosomatization (NS), sampled at baseline and at follow-up.

Subject	Baseline		Follow-up	
	N	NS	N	NS
A	37	86	08	12
B	81	58	62	29
C	89	91	96	81
D	68	76	61	57
E	57	42	18	19
F	95	86	80	76
G	85	98	55	57

N- and NS-scores were sampled at baseline and at follow-up, and we performed a Subjects × Sessions ANOVA to assess any shifts over treatment in these scores. Significant effects were found for N-scores ($F(1,6) = 10.3$, $p < 0.05$) as well as for NS-scores ($F(1,6) = 12.0$, $p < 0.05$). This indicates that treatment effect is not limited to symptom related parameters, but does spread into the domain of personality variables as well.

Finally we explored the association of effects of treatment on heart rate, subjective complaint, and personality variables. To do this, we computed correlations between level values of parameters from these three domains before treatment and after treatment. Correlation coefficients between heart rate levels and subjective complaints were low (< 0.39). Negative correlations were found between heart rate levels and both neuroticism and neurosomatization scores (largest individual $r = -0.71$, $F(1,5) = 5.1$, $p = 0.07$). Although this correlation is rather large, it was not found to differ significantly from zero due to the small sample size.

DISCUSSION

Together these findings are encouraging for the clinical application of heart rate feedback for sinus tachycardia. Gradually over treatment most of our subjects developed skill in self-control of heart rate, and were able after treatment to maintain their skill as demonstrated at the follow up session. Concomitantly there was a statistically significant decrease in the charting of subjective complaint, and this mirrored the general improvement in symptoms and well-being as reported by most of the patients at end of treatment and at follow up. They felt less tense, anxious or depressed, more self-confident, less rigid in daily activities and slept better. These findings are consistent with those from earlier case studies (Engel and Bleecker, 1974; Scott et al., 1973; Vaitl, 1975; Janssen, 1983) and thus add to the evidence for the clinical application of heart rate feedback for this form of tachycardia.

Inspection of individual subject results suggests that basically there are two different ways in which heart rate feedback therapy may have produced its effects in this group of patients. One is by inducing lower levels of tonic heart rate, as evidenced in four of our subjects by a gradual decline in their presession recordings. Another way for this therapy to come into effect is exemplified by subjects A, C, and E. Presession values remained almost stable in these subjects, while 2 of them still definitely improved with therapy. These subjects did attain however considerable insession control of their heart rate. It is likely therefore that treatment was effective here not by lowering tonic level of heart rate, but by the learning of heart rate decrease as a phasic response, one that could be invoked over several minutes. This may have helped patients to reduce their heart rate reactivity, thus limiting their episodes of sinus tachycardia.

It is an intriguing question which processes were at work in this application of heart rate feedback. Several alternative explanations can be raised for the results obtained. One is that non-specific factors were involved. Placebo effects may have been induced by the novelty of the treatment situation, and this may well have influenced the patients in the charting of their complaint. Also habituation may have made a contribution, as two baseline sessions may not have been sufficient to become at ease in the artificial situation of a recording baseline session. Besides non-specific factors there is evidence in the results obtained that would encourage the belief in specific factors in this treatment. Specificity is suggested by the finding for heart rate of a significant interaction between Sessions and Trials, indicating that at the end of treatment with aid of feedback signals patients were able to attain considerably lower levels of heart rate than without signals. It is noteworthy here to look at earlier reports on clinical heart rate feedback, where considerably longer training periods were required: Engel and Bleecker (1974) 21 sessions, Scott et al. (1973) 19 sessions. It is important that binary feedback signals were employed in these studies, since these do not allow subjects to learn how variations in heart rate occur in association with somatic and respiratory activity. Following the experimental tradition of establishing operant conditioning of heart rate without any mediation (e.g. Miller, 1969), early studies on heart rate feedback with humans merely considered somatic and respiratory activity as nuisance variables. In order to eliminate these, not only were the feedback signals employed binary, but also the subject was instructed that the response being monitored was not related to respiration nor to muscle tension. This attitude of methodological rigor, although laudable in itself, seriously hampered the development of heart rate feedback towards clinical maturity. Only later did it become clear that with analogue signals heart rate feedback yields better results than with binary signals (Blanchard and Epstein, 1978; Colgan, 1977). It is not mere speculation to suggest that the decisive factor in this effect is whether the signal allows the subject to monitor the coherence of changes in heart rate with every respiratory cycle (respiratory sinus arrhythmia: RSA). All our patients in the beginning of treatment asked for hints and instructions about how to influence their heart rate. We told them that often pacing of respiration had proven a useful tool in acquiring self-control of heart rate, without however specifying in what way this might be done most profitably. They were encouraged to try several strategies for themselves, and to monitor the effects on heart rate by means of the analogue feedback signals.

The assumption of a significant role of respiratory influences in heart rate feedback therapy has several implications for our understanding of the neurophysiological mechanisms in sinus tachycardia, as well as for its treatment with heart rate feedback. Katona and Jih (1975) established the existence of a linear and powerful relationship between variations in heart rate caused by spontaneous respiration, and degree of parasympathetic heart rate control. With spectral analysis of heart rate, RSA amplitude can be measured accurately by the integration of the heart rate power spectre in the respiration frequency band (Porges, 1986). This measure has indeed been found to reliably follow induced changes in cardiovagal tone (McCabe et al., 1979; Youngue et al., 1980). When we performed this analysis (details in Janssen and Bekkering, 1986) we found, at baseline, a virtual absence of energy in the respiratory band (0.15 – 0.50 Hz) in four of our subjects. This would suggest a deficient control of heart rate by cardiovagal tone, and that variations in heart rate occur more or less randomly as there was little energy below 0.15 Hz in these spectra either. Furthermore, there was in most subjects an increase in respiratory energy over treatment, especially during insession recordings. Such results lend support to the view that the treatment effects observed were vagally mediated, and that heart rate feedback was helpful in restoring cardiovagal tone in these subjects.

All in all these results are promising enough to warrant further clinical trials of heart rate feedback with sinus tachycardia. Heart rate and experimental heart rate feedback are among the best researched areas in psychophysiology. Although there is a great potential here, there has been little impact on clinical practice. Only further trials of heart rate feedback with clinical populations can tell whether it is possible to bridge this gap or not.

REFERENCES

Bauer, J. H. and Brooks, C. S. (1979). The long term effect of propranolol therapy on renal function. *American Journal of Medicine*, **66**, 504–510.

Blanchard, E. B. and Epstein, L. H. (1978). *A Biofeedback Primer*. Reading Ma: Addison-Wesley.

Blanchard, E. B. and Young, L. D. (1973). Self-control of cardiac functioning: A promise as yet unfulfilled. *Psychology Bulletin*, **79**, 145–163.

Cheatle, M. D. and Weiss, T. (1982). Biofeedback in heart rate control and in the treatment of cardiac arrhythmias. In White, L. and Turskey, B. (Eds), *Clinical Biofeedback: Efficacy and Mechanisms*, Guilford Press, New York, pp. 198–211.

Clemens, W. J. and Shattock, R. J. (1979). Voluntary heart rate control during static muscular effort. *Psychophysiology*, **16**, 327–332.

Colgan, M. (1977). Effects of binary and proportional feedback on bidirectional control of heart rate. *Psychophysiology*, **14**, 187–191.

Engel, B. T., Bleecker, E. R. (1974). Application of operant conditioning techniques to the control of cardiac arrhythmias. In Obrist, P. A., Black, A. H., Brener, J. and DiCara, L. V. (Eds), *Cardiovascular Psychophysiology*. Aldine, Chicago, 456–476.

Garnier, B. (1981). How to distinguish between 'health' and 'illness' in the psychosomatic cardiovascular field. In Kielholz, P., Siegenthaler, W., Taggart, P. and Zanchetti, A. (Eds), *Psychosomatic Cardiovascular Disorders*. Huber, Bern, pp. 21–27.

Guyton, A. C. (1981). *Medical Physiology*. Saunders, Philadelphia.

Janssen, K. (1983). Treatment of sinus tachycardia with heart-rate feedback. *Journal of Behavioural Medicine*, **6**, 109–114.

Janssen, K. and Bekkering, R. (1986). Spectral analysis of biofeedback-induced changes of heart-rate in sinus tachycardia. In Grossman, P., Janssen, K., Vaitl, D. (Eds) *Cardiorespiratory and Cardiosomatic Psychophysiology*. Plenum, New York, 263–277.

Julius, S. (1977). Borderline hypertension: Epidemiological and clinical implications. In Genest, A. *et al.* (Eds), *Hypertension*. McGraw-Hill, New York, pp. 630–640.

Katona, P. G. and Jih, F. (1975). Respiratory sinus arrhythmia: Noninvasive measure of parasympathetic cardiac control. *Journal of Applied Physiology*, **39**, 801–805.

Levi, R. L., White, P. D., Stroud, W. D., Hillman, C. C. (1945). Transient tachycardia: Prognostic significance alone and in association with transient hypertension. *Journal of the American Medical Association*, **129**, 585–588.

Liebhart, E. H. (1974). Attributionstherapie. Beeinflussung herzneurotischer Beschwerden durch Externalisierung kausaler Zuschreibungen. *Zeitschrift für Klinische Psychologie*, **3**, 71–94.

Light, K. C., Obrist, P. A. (1980). Cardiovascular reactivity to behavioral stress in young males with and without marginally elevated casual systolic pressures: A comparison of clinic, home and laboratory measures. *Hypertension*, **2**, 802–808.

Manuck, S. B., Proietti, J. M. (1982). Parental hypertension and cardiovascular response to cognitive and isometric challenge. *Psychophysiology*, **19**, 481–489.

Manuck, S. B., Kaplan, J. R., Clarkson, T. B. (1983). Behaviorally induced heart rate reactivity and atherosclerosis in cynomolgus monkeys. *Psychosomatic Medicine*, **45**, 95–107.

McCabe, P. M., Porges, S. W., Youngue, B. G. (1979). Spectral analysis of heart rate during depressor nerve stimulation: The validation of a non-invasive estimate of vagal tone. *Society for Neuroscience Abstract*, **5**, 156.

Miller, N. E. (1969). Learning of visceral and glandular responses. *Science*, **163**, 434–445.

Mulder, G., Mulder, L. J. M. (1981). Information processing and cardiovascular control. *Psychophysiology*, **18**, 392–402.

Paffenbarger, R. S., Thorne, M. C. and Wing, A. L. (1968). Chronic disease in former college students. VIII Characteristics in youth predisposing to hypertension in later years. *American Journal of Epidemiology*, **88**, 25–32.

Porges, S. W. (1986). Respiratory sinus arrhythmia: Physiological basis, quantitative methods, and clinical implications. In Grossman, P., Janssen, K. and Vaitl, D. (Eds), *Cardiorespiratory and Cardiosomatic Psychophysiology*. Plenum, New York, pp. 101–115.

Robles de Medina, E. O., Zimmerman, A. N. E., Meijler, F. L. (1980). *Electrocardiografie voor de hartbewaking*. Wolters-Noordhoff, Groningen.

Scott, R. W., Blanchard, E. B., Edmundson, E. D., Young, L. D. (1973). A shaping procedure for heart-rate control in chronic tachycardia. *Perception and Motor Skills*, **37**, 327–338.

Steptoe, A., Melville, D., Ross, A. (1984). Behavioral response demands, cardiovascular reactivity, and essential hypertension. *Psychosomatic Medicine*, **46**, 33–48.

Stoney, C. M., Langer, A. W., Sutterer, J. R., Gelling, P. D. (1986). Biofeedback-assisted heart rate deceleration: Specificity of cardiovascular and metabolic effects in normal and high risk subjects. In Grossman, P., Janssen, K. and Vaitl, D. (Eds), *Cardiorespiratory and Cardiosomatic Psychophysiology*. Plenum, New York, pp. 233–249.

Vaitl, D. (1975). Biofeedback-Einsatz in der Behandlung einer Patientin mit Sinustachykardie. In Legewie, H. and Nusselt, L. (Eds), *Biofeedback Therapie*. Urban & Schwarzenberg, Munich, pp. 205–217.

Wilde, G. J. S. (1970). *Neurotische labiliteit gemeten volgens de vragenlijstmethode*. Van Rossen, Amsterdam.

Williamson, D. A. and Blanchard, E. B. (1979). Heart rate and blood pressure feedback: A review of the recent experimental literature. *Biofeedback and Selfregulation*, **4**, 1–34.

Winkle, R. A., Glant, S. A., Harrison, D. C. (1975). Pharmacologic therapy of ventricular arrhythmias. *American Journal of Cardiology*, **36**, 629–635.

Youngue, B. G., McCabe, P. M., Kelley, S., Rivera, P. and Porges, S. W. (1980). Changes in a respiratorily modulated component of heart period variability as a result of pharmacological manipulations of vagal tone in rats. Paper presented at the *Society for Psychophysiological Research*, Vancouver, BC.

Behavioural Medicine in Cardiovascular Disorders
Edited by T. Elbert, W. Langosch, A. Steptoe and D. Vaitl
©1988 John Wiley & Sons Ltd

19

Cardiac Feedback Training in Patients with Cardiophobia

D. Vaitl, B. Ebert-Hampel and W. Kuhmann

University of Giessen, FRG

INTRODUCTION

Patients with heart-related behavioral and emotional disorders are very often seen in general practitioners' and cardiologists' offices. Every physician who has to deal with them would agree that it is very difficult to find an adequate treatment for them. This is mainly due to three different problems involved in this clinical disorder:

1. The cardiodiagnostic procedures as routinely applied, very scarcely reveal any clear sign indicating organic dysfunctions which might be responsible for the wide range of complaints which comprise cardiac, somatic, as well as behavioral and emotional disturbances (for details, see Nutzinger, 1987).
2. It is nearly impossible to relate the behavioral problems reported to any specific somatic dysfunction.
3. The group of patients is in itself very heterogenous. There are patients who are primarily suffering from manifest somatic and circulatory disorders. On the other hand, there are patients whose complaints are predominantly emotional and behavioral in nature.

Because of the similarities of symptoms, patients with cardiophobic and heart-related disorders have been classified by DSM-III as patients with panic disorders (for discussion see also Ehlers *et al.*, Chapter 17). Very recently, Nutzinger (1987) has suggested that cardiophobic disorders should be classified as a subcategory of panic disorders. According to his stepwise diagnostic procedure, they are characterized by lack of organic causes, duration of at least 2 months, initial panic attack (with at least four out of twelve clinical signs associated with panic attacks; see DSM-III), agoraphobia indicated by strong avoidance behaviors, and severe restrictions of everyday life activities. As stated by Nutzinger and Zapotoczky (1985), the patients' history plays an important role with respect to the prognosis of this disorder. A long history of cardiophobia before the beginning of treatment appears to reduce the chance of remedy. The majority of patients, however, permanently seeks appropriate medical and/or psychological help which is frequently ineffective for alleviating their various complaints. Therefore, the attempt was made in this study to improve and stabilize the self-control activities — which are still in existence in such groups — by providing a cardiac feedback which is directly focused at the target organ, that is the beating heart.

There are only a few studies which have examined the clinical usefulness of cardiac feedback for the management of cardiovascular disorders, including cardiophobia* (for review see Cheatle and Weiss, 1982). In single case studies, it could be shown that heart rate (HR) slowing and stabilization feedback training has been clinically effective for reducing HR levels as well as for improving sinus tachycardia attacks (e.g. Scott et al., 1973; Engel and Bleecker, 1974; Vaitl, 1975; Janssen, 1983). For other types of cardiac arrhythmia HR feedback appeared to be less effective compared to the reasonable cost-benefit ratio of pharmacological treatment available (for details see Cheatle and Weiss, 1982). This is not surprising as our present knowledge about the basic physiological mechanisms involved in cardiac feedback is very weak. Cardiac feedback, however, has been regarded as a helpful adjunct within a multimodal framework of medical and psychotherapeutic interventions in cardiophobics (Kuhmann, 1984).

Because of the relevance of excess heart period variability (HPV) for clinical issues (Skinner and Reed, 1981; Porges et al., 1982), a cardiac feedback for HP stabilization was chosen. A bidirectional HR feedback training (HR speeding and/or slowing), as previously reported in literature, would be contra-indicated, given the patients' previous experiences and heart-related complaints (e.g. tachycardia, irregular heart beats, fear of cardiac arrest). A training for HP stabilization was, therefore, more likely to be accepted by them as an aid to gain cardiac self-control.

With the HPV feedback approach, the following basic and clinical questions should be answered:

1. Are patients able to reduce (= stabilize) their instantaneous HP fluctuations by the aid of various kinds of feedback? If so, does this learned performance persist over time?
2. Are there any different effects of feedback contingency (contingent vs noncontingent) and continuity (continuous vs delayed, or cumulative on HPV?
3. Which individual control strategies for stabilizing HP are induced by different kinds of feedback?
4. Is feedback training for HP stabilization effective at all in reducing somatic, behavioral and emotional problems?

*Synonyms: cardiac neurosis (Caughey in 1939); irritable heart (Da Costa in 1871); functional cardiovascular disease (Friedman in 1947).

METHODS

Patients

Thirty-one patients (males $n = 16$, females $n = 15$) were selected out of a total of 242 patients who were referred from private practices and medical centers to the Department of Clinical Psychology at the University of Muenster. Their age ranged from 21 to 55 years (average age: 34.2 years in males, 32.8 years in females). The criteria for selection were: (a) reports of frequent and intense heart-related disturbances, (b) heart-related problems triggered by behaviorally defined situations, (c) no organic cardiovascular disorder, and (d) no psychiatric disorder.

Behavioral analyses and questionnaires (administered during two separate entry sessions; for details see Ebert-Hampel, 1982) revealed a long history of symptoms, both in males (5.4 years; range 0.8–20.0 years) and females (5.9 years; range 0.3–28.0 years). In 98% of the patients the symptoms occurred once a week up to every day. The attacks endured 2 or more hours in 53% of patients, and less than 1 hour in 47% of patients.

Table 1. Percentage of patients who believed that the specific circumstances under which the first attack occurred might be the causes of their disorder.

Circumstances	Percentage of cases
Chronic stress	
A. At work	42
B. At home	45
Physical stress	
A. Alcohol, nicotine abuse	19
B. Physical overstrain	16
C. Illness	3
Confrontation with death	
A. In general	16
B. Myocardial infarction	22
Loss of object	16

Table 1 illustrates the circumstances which have led to the onset of symptoms. They represent the beliefs of patients about the causes of the first attack they have experienced in their life.

Treatment program

The treatment program comprised ten feedback training sessions of approximately 45 minutes duration each. They consisted of a 5-minute baseline

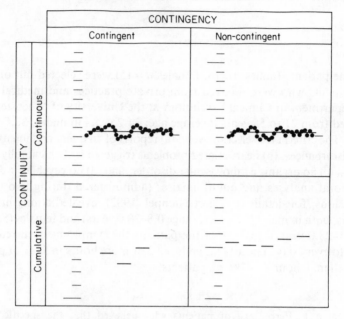

Figure 1. Visual displays of the four feedback conditions. For explanation see text. (With permission of Lawrence Erlbaum Ass., Publishers.)

period and six feedback trials (2 minutes each), each followed by transfer trials (2 minutes each) during which the patients were required to perform HPV control without the aid of feedback. Two follow-up sessions were carried out 7 weeks and 6 months after the feedback training had been terminated (for final behavioral analyses and questionnaires).

Feedback procedures

ECG (II lead) and respiration (thermistor at patient's nostril) were recorded on a physiopolygraph (Siemens Minograf) and processed by a computer (IBM 1130). Data were stored on magnetic disks. Acquisition of data, timing, and the generation of feedback signals by computer were automatically controlled by a special device.

The feedback was given on an oscilloscope (see Figure 1). Two factors of feedback characteristics were systematically crossed: contingency (yes/no) and continuity (yes/no). These four experimental conditions were designed as follows: The continuous feedback (contingent, non-contingent) was given during each training trial, whereas the non-continuous feedback (contingent, non-contingent) was delayed and given cumulatively after each trial.

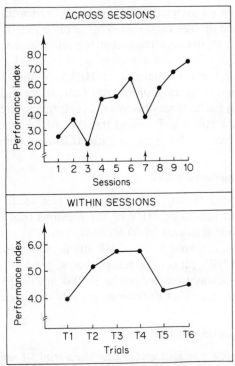

Figure 2. Manipulated learning progress across (upper panel) and within (lower panel) sessions in the noncontingent feedback conditions. Y-axis: Mean performance index (low values = high HPV; high values = low HPV). T1–T6: Feedback training trials (1–6) within sessions. Note: Relatively low performance indices within session 3 and 7 (= 'failure' feedback).

Continuous, contingent feedback

Patients received beat-to-beat information and could observe the cardiotachogram curve of the previous 50 heartbeats. The curve of the cardiotachogram moved to the rhythm of the individuals' heartbeats across the oscilloscope from right to left. The cardiotachogram curve was drawn around a target line which was determined by a moving average of 50 heartbeats. Patients were asked to reduce the instantaneous fluctuations of the cardiotachogram towards the target line which in turn should result in flattening the amplitudes of HPV. The mean HR level was indicated by the position of the target line with respect to the HR scale at the left side of the oscilloscope.

Continuous, non-contingent feedback

This kind of feedback was displayed on the oscilloscope exactly in the same form as contingent feedback. However, the variability of the cardiotachogram curve was manipulated systematically by computer routines according to a predetermined schedule (see Figure 2). This implied that HPV was gradually reduced within and across sessions except for session three and seven. Here, to stimulate subjects' effort, the non-contingent feedback displayed poor HP stabilization performance (= increase in HPV). Within session, the mean performance trend rose initially up to trial four, decreased in trial five, and rose again slightly in the last trial (this average performance trend has been found in previous feedback studies). By using this type of feedback, it was possible to manipulate the success fed back to patients in a systematic fashion.

Cumulative, contingent feedback

Instead of a cardiotachogram curve patients received feedback in the form of five horizontal lines indicating HPV of the previous trial (2.5 min duration) divided into five time segments of 30 seconds each. The scale on the left side represented nine performance levels of HP stabilization indicating low (lower segments) and high HPV (upper segments), that is, good or poor performance. This kind of feedback was presented on the oscilloscope for 30 seconds after each training trial. Onset and offset of training periods were signalled acoustically.

Cumulative, non-contingent feedback

This type of feedback was also given after each trial. It was displayed in the same manner as in cumulative, contingent feedback. However, the same predetermined schedule as in continuous, non-contingent feedback has been used to manipulate the position of the five horizontal lines with respect to the nine performance levels represented by the scale on the left side. Here again, during sessions three and seven, a 'failure' feedback was given, whereas the general trend of performance exhibited a gradual improvement of HP stabilization.

By using these four forms of feedback, it became possible to differentiate between the effects of feedback continuity and the amount of success in HP control provided by non-contingent feedback.

Patients were assigned to one of these four feedback forms. Due to technical and clinical problems (cf. Ebert-Hampel, 1982) the sample size of each group could not be kept identical ($n = 10$). The continuous, non-contingent group comprised $n = 8$ patients, the cumulative contingent feedback group $n = 6$ patients, and the cumulative, non-contingent feedback group $n = 7$ patients, respectively. The latter group was additionally instructed to relax and to breath regularly.

RESULTS

The main results of this study concern:

1. The feedback-induced cardiac control (i.e. changes in HR and HPV);

2. the control strategies used;
3. the changes in heart-related clinical symptoms.

Interestingly enough, no significant changes in mean HR level could be observed, neither within sessions nor across sessions. All patients showed HR within normal ranges (between 69 and 75 bpm during baselines). Mean changes in HR during feedback and transfer trials did not exceed 2–3 bpm. This implies that the cardiac adaptation indicated by HR deceleration regularly observed in bidirectional feedback trainings appears to be reduced in feedback trials for HP stabilization.

Feedback-induced changes in HPV, however, can be interpreted in rather different ways depending upon the variability measures employed. Increases in HR stabilization did occur when standard deviations of interbeat intervals were used as HPV measures.

Here, the mean changes in HPV across ten feedback training sessions showed very clearly that HR stabilization was mainly achieved by continuous feedback (see Figure 3). In this regard, the contingency of feedback was of minor relevance. This main effect of stabilization training, however, disappeared immediately when another variability measure was employed. Fouad *et al.* (1984) suggested that HP fluctuations should be determined simply by a peak-to-trough measure (i.e. amplitude of minimum-maximum HP during instantaneous HP fluctuations (for discussion see Grossman and Wientjes, 1986; Vaitl *et al.*, 1986).

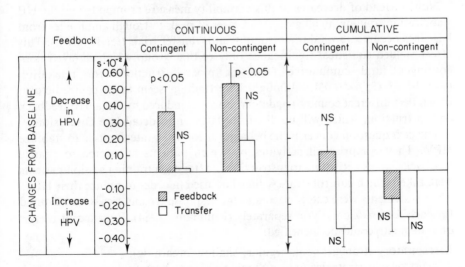

Figure 3. Mean of changes form baseline in standard deviation measures ($s \times 10^{-2}$) for HPV during training and transfer trials across 10 sessions with continuous (contingent or non-contingent) and cumulative (contingent or non-contingent) feedback ($p < 0.05$ indicates statistical significance of overall changes in HPV from baseline to training/transfer trials across 10 sessions.

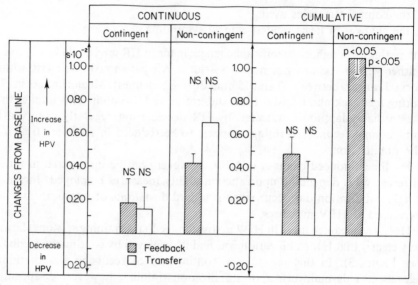

Figure 4. Mean changes from baseline in peak-to-trough measures ($s \times 10^{-2}$) for HPV during training and transfer trials across 10 sessions with continuous (contingent or non-contingent) and cumulative (contingent or non-contingent) feedback ($p < 0.05$ indicates statistical significance of overall changes in HPV from baseline to training/transfer trials across 10 sessions.) (With permission of Plenum Press.)

Now, instead of decreases of this variability measure as intended by the HP stabilization training, in all groups increases of peak-to-trough amplitudes from baselines occurred both during training and transfer trials (see Figure 4). This effect yielded statistical significance only in that group which received non-contingent and cumulative feedback plus instructions for relaxation ($F(1/10 = 7.45; p < 0.05$). Although these findings seem to be contradictory, they reflect different counter-regulatory processes induced by visual HP feedback and instruction, which will be discussed later on in detail (see Discussion).

The next question concerns the behavioral control strategies used to stabilize HPV. They comprise all activities by which patients attempted to change feedback signals according to instructions. After each training session patients were asked which control strategy they had used in order to reduce their HPV. Their statements were categorized and the response frequencies were clustered for each feedback condition separately (Kuhmann, 1984). Four major classes of statements could be identified:

1. respiratory strategies (e.g. regular, shallow breathing);
2. heart-related strategies (e.g. attending to heart beats);
3. relaxation and/or cognitive strategies (e.g. reduction of muscle tension, thought-stopping, breath-counting);
4. remainder, comprising all those strategies not included in three previous ones.

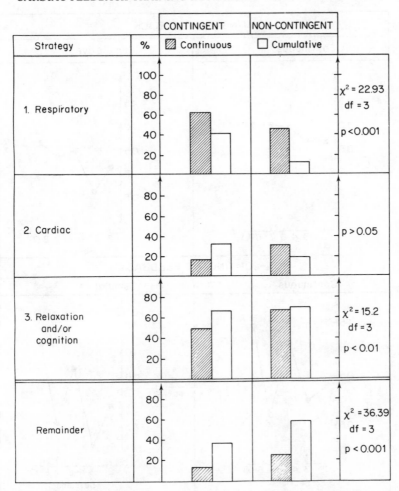

Figure 5. Percentage of strategies reported used by patients to control HPV throughout the course of ten training sessions under contingent (continuous or cumulative) and non-contingent (continuous or cumulative) feedback conditions. Chi-square statistics indicate statistical significance of the distribution of patients' statements with regard to the categories of respiratory and cardiac control strategies, bodily relaxation and/or cognitive strategies (e.g. imagery, thought stopping, breath counting), and other strategies not included in the previous ones (remainder). (With permission of Plenum Press.)

It is quite obvious that respiratory maneuvers were mainly provoked by continuous feedback both under contingent and non-contingent conditions (see Figure 5); similarly, relaxation and/or cognitive strategies were very frequently reported by those two groups which received cumulative feedback as well as by the non-contingent feedback group. Here it becomes clear that the type of feedback given does determine what behavioral control strategies are favored.

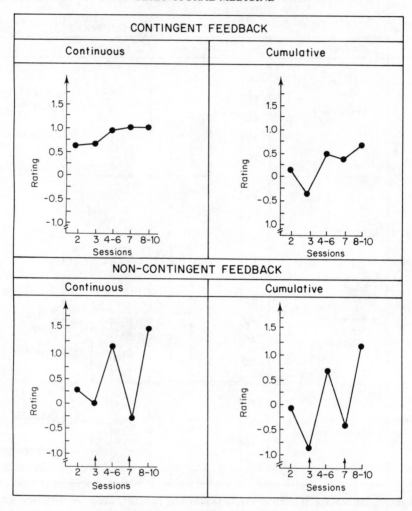

Figure 6. Mean changes in effectiveness ratings from session 1 (= reference session) for strategies used to stabilize HP during consecutive blocks of sessions with continuous (contingent or non-contingent) and cumulative (contingent or non-contingent) feedback (↑indicates 'failure' feedback in session 3 and 7).

In contrast to this finding, no significant differences between feedback groups could be obtained with respect to heart-related strategies. Furthermore, it is interesting to note that the differential feedback effects upon patients' verbal reports were mainly influenced by those feedback forms that are shown to be less effective for actual HPV control (Vaitl *et al.*, 1986), that is non-contingent and cumulative feedback. When non-contingent feedback is given, patients reported more frequently cognition-oriented and global control strategies (e.g. bodily relaxation, imagery, regular breathing) than specific ones which are more physiology-oriented (e.g. short-term respiratory maneuvers). The same is true for cumulative feedback. No differences, however, could be found between such specific and global strategies under contingent and continuous feedback conditions.

The finding that the different types of feedback information affect primarily verbal behavior (i.e. patients verbal reports after sessions) is additionally supported by the fact that no relationship could be found between strategies reported and actual performance of HPV control (i.e. HP stabilization). Nor did breathing patterns correspond to verbal reports. More specifically, a close relationship between feedback parameters and verbal reports could be obtained when patients' effectiveness ratings (completed after each training session) were analysed in order to determine how effective the control strategies used have been (see Figure 6). All groups showed an increase in rated effectiveness of their control strategies (for details see Ebert-Hampel, 1982).

Interestingly enough, this increase is exactly parallel to the improvement of HP stabilization in the group which received continuous and contingent feedback. A similar trend towards increased effectiveness could also be observed in the other three groups throughout the course of all sessions except for session three and seven, where a remarkable decrease in effectiveness ratings occurred which precisely coincided with the deliberate manipulation feedback of 'failure' during those sessions.

Thus, one may conclude that patients' verbal reports about the effectiveness of the individual strategies they have been using for HPV control were primarily influenced by the information about success given by contingent as well as by noncontingent feedback procedures, that is, by true or completely false information.

The question of whether and to what extent these feedback manipulations are effective at all in reducing clinical symptoms which are very frequently reported by patients with cardiophobic and heart-related disorders remains to be answered. Here, cardiac complaints are of central importance. They were determined by a standardized questionnaire (Zenz, 1971) and subsequently cluster-analysed (for details see Ebert-Hampel, 1982; Kuhmann, 1984).

The symptoms of cardiac disorders comprised reports of very heterogeneous heart-related problems such as irregular heart-beats, tachycardia, heart palpitations, acute chest pain or burning sensation in the heart region. Changes in those complaints were determined between pre-treatment level (data collected during two entry sessions of behavioral analysis and questionnaire completion) and three subsequent sessions: post-treatment session after the training has been terminated (session ten) and two follow-up sessions (7 weeks and 6 months after the tenth session). Here, it is obvious that all groups did profit from feedback training to some extent. Statistically significant changes were found only in those groups which received continuous feedback, either contingent or non-contingent.

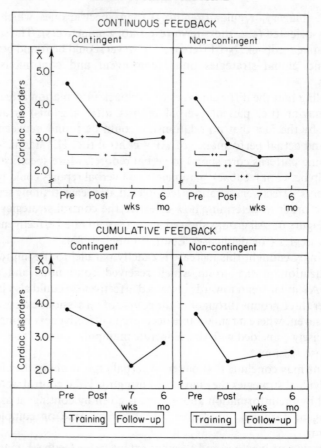

Figure 7. Mean changes in test-scores (Zenz, 1971, Liste körperlicher Symptome) for cardiac disorders under different feedback conditions (contingent–continuous, non-contingent–continuous, contingent–cumulative, non-contingent–cumulative) at pre-treatment, after 10 training sessions, 7 weeks and 6 months after training has been terminated (i.e. follow-ups): $+ = p < 0.05$. $++ = p < 0.01$. (With permission of Plenum Press.)

However, no differences between groups could be found. It is interesting to note that in all groups the most pronounced changes occurred immediately after the last training session. This is probably due to a strong attention-placebo effect emanating from the biofeedback-setting itself. Influences from the patient–therapist relationship, instructions given and/or information provided about normal and pathological cardiac functioning may be responsible for this overall positive effect.

In order to determine the overall effects of this kind of feedback training, regardless of the individual feedback form employed, the amount of clinically

Table 2. Changes (positive, negative, no changes) in clinically relevant behaviors which were brought about by feedback therapy in all groups.

Changes in behavior	Positive (%)	No (%)	Negative (%)
Claustrophobic reactions	86	14	—
Cardiac problems	77	19	4
Social avoidance behavior	72	28	—
Heart-related anxiety	71	29	—
Frequent search for medical help	68	25	7
Physicial activity	68	32	—
Excessive monitoring of bodily functions	64	29	7

relevant change was determined for the whole sample. As illustrated in Table 2, considerable improvement could be achieved.

Positive changes (improvement) were reported by the majority of patients. They concern claustrophobic reactions (86% of cases), cardiac disorders (77% of cases), and social avoidance behavior (72% of cases). An approximate ratio of 3:1 of positive to no changes could be obtained for other clinically relevant classes of behavior; that is, heart-related anxiety, search for medical aid, physical exercise, and excessive monitoring of bodily functions.

DISCUSSION

The present clinical outcome–study was conducted to explore the multimodal effects of visual feedback for HP stabilization in patients with cardiophobic disorders. This particular task was chosen because HP stabilization presumably prevents patients from developing irritations and anxiety associated with HR speeding (e.g. tachycardia) or HR slowing (e.g. fear of cardiac arrest) tasks. In addition to this clinical aspect, patients were permanently forced to act as counter-regulatory agents in order to reduce the instantaneous fluctuations of their heartbeat intervals. The possible multimodal effects of such a feedback training consisted in changes in heart period variability (HPV), in behavioral or cognitive strategies used to cope with the task requirements, as well as in heart-related symptoms.

As previous feedback studies have shown, subjects can be taught by feedback information to act in a counter-regulatory fashion in order to improve their performance of HP stabilization (Vaitl and Kenkmann, 1972; Vaitl, 1975; Vaitl et al., 1986). These effects, however, were short-term rather than long-term in nature. When contingent beat-to-beat feedback was withdrawn, as in transfer phases, cardiac control previously gained through feedback was blunted or completely abolished. Thus, there is little evidence that subjects are able to transfer the learned performance from feedback to no feedback trials (Kuhmann, 1984). During feedback trials, however, feedback-dependent changes in HPV may occur. This has been demonstrated in single-session studies (Vaitl and Kenkmann, 1972) as well as in long-term studies (Kuhmann, 1984). The type and the amount of those changes depend upon the measure employed to determine HPV. As demonstrated in the results section, contingent and continuous feedback led to HP stabilization when standard deviations were used as HPV measure, whereas an increase of HPV occurred when peak-to-trough measures were employed. Although these findings appear to be contradictory at first glance, they represent only two sides of the same coin. While standard deviations of HP are mainly influenced by long-term trends in HPV, such as inevitable non-stationarities, peak-to-trough amplitude measures are likely to be associated with respiratory sinus arrhythmias (RSA), which are short-term in nature. Throughout the course of feedback training the RSA increased slightly in all groups and yielded statistical significance only in that group which received a non-contingent and cumulative feedback and was additionally instructed to relax and to breath regularly. The result, however, that standard deviations were reduced when continuous feedback, both contingent and non-contingent, was given, needs further explanation. When subjects are required to perform a visual tracking task like in continuous beat-to-beat feedback, the non-stationarity of HR is reduced by applying involuntary respiratory maneuvers which result in flattening of the cardiotachogram curve. When the cardiotachogram curve displayed on the oscilloscope goes up (= increase in HR), subjects may try to compensate by exhaling or interrupting their inspiration cycle. The reverse may be seen when HR tends to slow down. By using weighted coherence measures and applying different forms of visual feedback (contingent, non-contingent, high vs. low information feedback, no feedback) it could be demonstrated that in normals there are possibly counter-regulatory processes which affect HPV measures in a very specific and subtle way (Vaitl et al., 1986). Spectral power analysis of the present HP data set reported elsewhere (Vaitl et al., 1986) revealed that two classes of frequency components prevailed: low frequency (LF) from 0.03 up to 0.15 Hz (band around 0.10 Hz) and high frequency (HF) from 0.15 up to 0.35 Hz. The LV band (10-second rhythm) has been interpreted as spectral component of HPV reflecting changes in baroreceptor activity (Akselrod et al., 1981), baroreceptor resonance (Wesseling and Settels, 1985) or in diastolic blood pressure (De Boor, 1985), whereas the spectrum of HF is predominantly associated with respiratory cycles. The most pronounced increases in the 10-second rhythm occurred when non-contingent cumulative feedback was given and patients were additionally instructed to relax and to breath regularly. In contrast, when high information density had to be processed continually, like in contingent beat-to-beat feedback, this rhythmic component of HPV was inhibited from developing to as full an extent as under cumulative feedback conditions. Since the 10-second rhythm is likely to be related to a central rhythm which is basically a product of common brain stem activities, as has been demonstrated by Langhorst and his colleagues (Langhorst et al., 1986), this 'noise' variability in HPV is presumably reduced when patients are required to process visual information.

The extent to which this reduction takes place appears to depend upon the density of feedback signals which are to be processed rather than upon their contingency. While reducing slow, non-stationary HPV the HF band was facilitated and enhanced. This implies that throughout the HP stabilization training the respiratory HPV component was not suppressed by feedback as one might have expected, but gradually increased due to greater respiratory regularity which is in turn facilitated by a general adaptation to the experimental setting (Vaitl et al., 1986).

At this point, one may raise the question on whether these specific feedback-induced cardiac-respiratory interaction effects corresponded to any changes in behavioral strategies used for HPV control or in symptoms reported. As to the verbal reports on strategies employed, such a relationship seems to exist. For instance, the delayed feedback which was given after each trial made patients report more frequently global control strategies including non-specific, cognitive strategies, whereas continuous feedback evoked more specific and physiology-oriented reports about respiratory maneuvers. In addition, verbal reports about the effectiveness of the strategies used were closely related to the HP stabilization fed back by the visual display.

It is tempting to speculate by which experimental manipulation or component of the therapeutic setting the long-term changes in symptom alleviation might have been brought about. Since no between group effects could be accomplished by feedback conditions, general factors must be assumed to be responsible for the relatively stable long-term effects of feedback training; one element might be the fact that patients are provided with information about their ability to influence a delicate organ such as the heart and its beating rate. To play with one's own heart-rate, and to see on the oscilloscope that a wide range of voluntarily provoked heart-rate changes occur, may create a feeling of mastery over this autonomic bodily process. It is not sufficient to reassure or to persuade patients that their heart is functioning very well. Beyond that, it is essential that they perceive themselves as active participants in the treatment and not merely as passive recipients of information and advice. The credibility of information and advice will certainly drop down to zero the next time an uncomfortable and uncontrollable alteration of cardiac functioning is experienced. In this context, feedback training is nothing but a tool for cognitive restructuring by persuading people not only verbally but by providing objective and credible information.

Acknowledgements

Research was supported by the Deutsch Forschungsgemeinschaft by a grant to D. Vaitl (Va 37/1, 37/14-1).

REFERENCES

Akselrod, S., Gordon, D., Ubel, F. A., Shannon, D. C., Barger, A. C. and Cohen, R. J. (1981). Power spectrum analysis of heart rate fluctuation: A quantitative probe of beat-to-beat cardiovascular control. *Science*, **213**, 220–222.

Cheatle, M. D. and Weiss, T. (1982). Biofeedback in heart rate control and the treatment of cardiac arrhythmias. In *Clinical Biofeedback: Efficacy and Mechanisms*. Guilford Press, New York.

DeBoer, R. W. (1985). *Beat-to-Beat Blood Pressure Fluctuations and Heart-Rate Variability in Man: Physiological Relationships, Analysis Techniques and Simple Model*. Drukkerji Elinkwijk B. V., Utrecht.

Ebert-Hampel, B. (1982). *Biofeedback und funktionelle Herzbeschwerden*. Peter Lang Verlag, Frankfurt/M.

Engel, B. T. and Bleecker, E. R. (1974). Application of operant conditioning techniques to the control of cardiac arrhythmias. In Obrist, P. A., Black, A. H., Brener, J. and DiCara, L. V. (Eds), *Cardiovascular Psychophysiology*. Aldine, Chicago.

Fouad, F. M., Tarazi, R. C., Ferrario, C. M., Fighaly, S. and Alicandri, C. (1984). Assessment of parasympathetic control of heart rate by a noninvasive method. *American Journal of Physiology*, p. 246 (*Heart, Circulation Physiology*), **15**, H838–H842.

Grossman, P. and Wientjes, K. (1986). Respiratory sinus arrhythmia and parasympathetic cardiac control: some basic issues concerning quantification, applications and implications. In Grossman, P., Janssen, K. H. L. and Vaitl, D. (Eds), *Cardiorespiratory and Cardiosomatic Psychophysiology*. Plenum Press, New York.

Janssen, K. H. L. (1983). Treatment of sinus tachycardia with heart rate feedback. *Journal of Behavioural Medicine*, **6**, 109–114.

Kuhmann, W. (1984). *Effekte und Mechanismen eines Langzeit-Biofeedback-Trainings zur Kontrolle der Variabilität der Herztätigkeit*. Dreieich: Weiss.

Langhorst, P., Schulz, G. and Lambertz, M. (1986). Integrative control mechanisms for cardiorespiratory and somatomotor functions of the lower brain stem. In Grossman, P., Janssen, K. H. L. and Vaitl, D. (Eds), *Cardiorespiratory and Cardiosomatic Psychophysiology*. Plenum Press, New York.

Nutzinger, D. O. (1987). Klassifikation und Verlauf der Herzphobie. In Nutzinger, D. O., Pfersmann, D., Welan, T. and Zapotoczky, H.-G. (Eds), *Herzphobie. Klassifikation, Diagnostik und Therapie*. Enke Verlag, Stuttgart.

Nutzinger, D. O. and Zapotoczky, H.-G. (1985). The influence of depression on the outcome of cardiac phobia (panic disorder). *Psychopathology*, **18**, 155–162.

Porges, S. W., McCabe, P. M. and Yongue, B. G. (1982). Respiratory-heart-rate interactions: Psychophysiological implications for pathophysiology and behavior. In Cacioppo, J. and Petty, R. (Eds), *Perspective in Cardiovascular Psychophysiology*. Guilford Press, New York.

Scott, R. W., Blanchard, E. B., Edmundson, E. D. and Young, L. D. (1973). A shaping procedure for heart rate control in chronic tachycardia. *Perceptual and Motor Skills*, **37**, 327–338.

Skinner, J. E. and Reed, J. C. (1981). Blockade of the frontocortical brainstem pathway prevents ventricular fibrillation of the ischemic heart in pigs. *American Journal of Physiology*, **240**, H156–H163.

Vaitl, D. (1975). Biofeedback-Einsatz in der Behandlung einer Patientin mit Sinus-Tachykardie. In Legewie, H. and Nusselt, L. (Eds), *Biofeedback-Therapie. Lernmethoden in der Psychosomatik, Neurologie und Rehabilitation*. Urban and Schwarzenberg, München.

Vaitl, D. and Kenkmann, H.-J. (1972). Stabilisation der Pulsfrequenz durch visuelle Rückmeldung. *Zeitschrift für Klinische Psychologie*, 1, 251–271.

Vaitl, D., Kuhmann, W. and Ebert-Hampel, B. (1986). Biofeedback-assisted control of heart period variability. In Grossman, P., Janssen, K. H. L. and Vaitl, D. (Eds), *Cardiorespiratory and Cardiosomatic Psychophysiology*. Plenum Press, New York.

Wesseling, K. H. and Settels, J. J. (1985). Baromodulation explains short-term blood pressure variability. In Orlebeke, J. F., Mulder, G. and van Doornen, L. J. P. (Eds), *Psychophysiology of Cardiovascular Control*. Plenum Press, New York.

Zenz, H. (1971). Empirische Befunde über die Giessener Fassung einer Beschwerdeliste. *Zeitschrift für Psychotherapie und Medizinische Psychologie*, 21, 7–13.

Index

325